Mycotoxins Study: Toxicology, Identification and Control

Mycotoxins Study: Toxicology, Identification and Control

Editor

Cristina Juan García

MDPI • Basel • Beijing • Wuhan • Barcelona • Belgrade • Manchester • Tokyo • Cluj • Tianjin

Editor
Cristina Juan García
Preventive Medicine and Public
Health, Food Sciencs, Toxicology
and Forensic Medicine
University of Valencia
Valencia
Spain

Editorial Office
MDPI
St. Alban-Anlage 66
4052 Basel, Switzerland

This is a reprint of articles from the Special Issue published online in the open access journal *Toxins* (ISSN 2072-6651) (available at: www.mdpi.com/journal/toxins/special_issues/Mycotoxins_Control).

For citation purposes, cite each article independently as indicated on the article page online and as indicated below:

LastName, A.A.; LastName, B.B.; LastName, C.C. Article Title. *Journal Name* **Year**, *Volume Number*, Page Range.

ISBN 978-3-0365-1416-1 (Hbk)
ISBN 978-3-0365-1415-4 (PDF)

Contents

About the Editor . . . vii

Preface to "Mycotoxins Study: Toxicology, Identification and Control" . . . ix

Cristina Juan García
Mycotoxins: Toxicology, Identification and Control
Reprinted from: *Toxins* **2021**, *13*, 242, doi:10.3390/toxins13040242 . . . 1

Aicha El Jai, Abdellah Zinedine, Ana Juan-García, Jordi Mañes, Samira Etahiri and Cristina Juan
Occurrence of Free and Conjugated Mycotoxins in Aromatic and Medicinal Plants and Dietary Exposure Assessment in the Moroccan Population
Reprinted from: *Toxins* **2021**, *13*, 125, doi:10.3390/toxins13020125 . . . 5

Shabbir Hussain, Muhammad Rafique Asi, Mazhar Iqbal, Nisha Khalid, Syed Wajih-ul-Hassan and Agustín Ariño
Patulin Mycotoxin in Mango and Orange Fruits, Juices, Pulps, and Jams Marketed in Pakistan
Reprinted from: *Toxins* **2020**, *12*, 52, doi:10.3390/toxins12010052 . . . 21

Liliana J. G. Silva, Ana C. Teixeira, André M. P. T. Pereira, Angelina Pena and Celeste M. Lino
Ochratoxin A in Beers Marketed in Portugal: Occurrence and Human Risk Assessment
Reprinted from: *Toxins* **2020**, *12*, 249, doi:10.3390/toxins12040249 . . . 31

Elena Efremenko, Olga Maslova, Nikolay Stepanov and Anvar Ismailov
Using Cholinesterases and Immobilized Luminescent Photobacteria for the Express-Analysis of Mycotoxins and Estimating the Efficiency of Their Enzymatic Hydrolysis
Reprinted from: *Toxins* **2021**, *13*, 34, doi:10.3390/toxins13010034 . . . 41

Yelko Rodríguez-Carrasco, Alfonso Narváez, Luana Izzo, Anna Gaspari, Giulia Graziani and Alberto Ritieni
Biomonitoring of Enniatin B1 and Its Phase I Metabolites in Human Urine: First Large-Scale Study
Reprinted from: *Toxins* **2020**, *12*, 415, doi:10.3390/toxins12060415 . . . 53

Fojan Agahi, Guillermina Font, Cristina Juan and Ana Juan-García
Individual and Combined Effect of Zearalenone Derivates and Beauvericin Mycotoxins on SH-SY5Y Cells
Reprinted from: *Toxins* **2020**, *12*, 212, doi:10.3390/toxins12040212 . . . 65

Paloma Oliveira da Cruz, Clarisse Jales de Matos, Yuri Mangueira Nascimento, Josean Fechine Tavares, Evandro Leite de Souza and Hemerson Iury Ferreira Magalhães
Efficacy of Potentially Probiotic Fruit-Derived *Lactobacillus fermentum*, *L. paracasei* and *L. plantarum* to Remove Aflatoxin M_1 In Vitro
Reprinted from: *Toxins* **2020**, *13*, 4, doi:10.3390/toxins13010004 . . . 81

Atena Abbasi Pirouz, Jinap Selamat, Shahzad Zafar Iqbal and Nik Iskandar Putra Samsudin
Efficient and Simultaneous Chitosan-Mediated Removal of 11 Mycotoxins from Palm Kernel Cake
Reprinted from: *Toxins* **2020**, *12*, 115, doi:10.3390/toxins12020115 . . . 91

Kai Yang, Ke Li, Lihong Pan, Xiaohu Luo, Jiali Xing, Jing Wang, Li Wang, Ren Wang, Yuheng Zhai and Zhengxing Chen
Effect of Ozone and Electron Beam Irradiation on Degradation of Zearalenone and Ochratoxin A
Reprinted from: *Toxins* **2020**, *12*, 138, doi:10.3390/toxins12020138 . . . . **105**

Monika Nowak, Przemysław Bernat, Julia Mrozińska and Sylwia Różalska
Acetamiprid Affects Destruxins Production but Its Accumulation in *Metarhizium* sp. Spores Increases Infection Ability of Fungi
Reprinted from: *Toxins* **2020**, *12*, 587, doi:10.3390/toxins12090587 . . . . **115**

Jingjing Wang, Qunfang Weng, Fei Yin and Qiongbo Hu
Interactions of Destruxin A with Silkworms' Arginine tRNA Synthetase and Lamin-C Proteins
Reprinted from: *Toxins* **2020**, *12*, 137, doi:10.3390/toxins12020137 . . . . **129**

Muzi Zhu, Youfei Cen, Wei Ye, Saini Li and Weimin Zhang
Recent Advances on Macrocyclic Trichothecenes, Their Bioactivities and Biosynthetic Pathway
Reprinted from: *Toxins* **2020**, *12*, 417, doi:10.3390/toxins12060417 . . . . **139**

About the Editor

Cristina Juan García

Cristina Juan García PhD is Associate Professor of Food Science at the University of Valencia (2008). Her active research concerns to develop analytical methods to identify mycotoxins in different matrices (food, feed, biological matrices, and culture cells) using mass spectrometry equipment (QqQ, Qtrap, and QTOF). She is author of more than 60 international publications (ORCID: 0000-0002-8923-3219). She has collaborated with research groups of food safety of Prof. Celeste Lino research group from University of Coimbra in Portugal; Prof. Alberto Ritieni from "Università degli Studi di Napoli "Federico II" in Italy; and Prof. Felicia Loghin research groups from University of Medicine and Pharmacy "Iuliu Haţieganu"of Cluj-Napoca in Rumania. She has been involved in several research projects supported by the Spanish Ministry of Education and participated as a member in the European MycoKey project H2020-EU.3.2. –SOCIETAL

Preface to "Mycotoxins Study: Toxicology, Identification and Control"

The evaluation of the presence of mycotoxins in different matrices is achieved through different analytical tools (including quantitative or qualitative determinations). Studies of mycotoxin isolation, using chromatographyc equipment coupled to spectrometry detectors (QTrap-MS/MS, MS/MS tandem, QTOF-MS/MS), are the most useful tools to control their presence. All these studies represent key steps in the establishment of the limits of detection, limits of quantification, points of identification, accuracy, reproducibility, and repeatability of different procedures. The maximum permitted or recommended levels for mycotoxins in different matrices are within a wide range (including the levels tolerated by infants and animals). In addition, decontaminated strategies, as well as control and evaluation of exposure, are demanded by authorities and food safety systems.

These authorities are not only concerned with the determination of mycotoxin presence but also with the toxicological effects of mycotoxins, and in vivo or in vitro assays are necessary for a complete evaluation. In fact, these assays are the basis for the control and prevention of population exposure to mycotoxins in dietary exposure studies. The most recent surveys focused on regulated mycotoxins (aflatoxins, fumonisins, trichothecenes, and zearalenones) and emerging toxins, such as enniatins and beauvericin in adult consumers, while very few studies have monitored mycotoxin levels in infant products.

This *Book of Toxins* comprises 11 original contributions and one review. New findings regarding presence of mycotoxins in aromatic and medicinal plants, mango and orange juice, juices, pulps, jams, and beer, from Morocco, Pakistan, and Portugal are reported. In these studies, innovative techniques to study their presence has been developed, including liquid chromatography coupled with time-of-flight mass spectrometry to analyse mycotoxins and conjugated mycotoxins. Novel strategies to detect mycotoxin presence and comparisons the characteristics of a rapid quantitative analysis of different mycotoxins (deoxynivalenol, ochratoxin A, patulin, sterigmatocystin, and zearalenone) are also presented using acetyl- and butyrylcholinesterases and photobacterial strains of luminescent cells. Additionally, toxicological effects of zearalenone metabolites and beauvericin on SH-SY5Y neuronal cells are presented. One important point in the control of mycotoxins is related to decontaminated strategies, and in this sense the efficacy of potentially probiotic fruit-derived Lactobacillus isolates in removing aflatoxin M1 (AFM1) is presented. Other mycotoxin decontaminated techniques included in this book are electron beam irradiation (EBI) and degradation of zearalenone and ochratoxin A using ozone. Finally, a review that summarizes the newly discovered macrocyclic trichothecenes and their bioactivities over the last decade is included.

Cristina Juan García
Editor

toxins

MDPI

Editorial

Mycotoxins: Toxicology, Identification and Control

Cristina Juan García

Laboratory of Food Chemistry and Toxicology, Faculty of Pharmacy, University of Valencia, Avda. Vicent Andrés Estellés, S/N, 46100 Burjassot-Valencia, Spain; cristina.juan@uv.es

The evaluation of the presence of mycotoxins in different matrices is achieved through different analytical tools (including quantitative or qualitative determinations). Research on optimal mycotoxins' extraction and clean-up methods, combined with chromatographic equipment coupled to mass spectrometric detectors (Triple quadrupole/linear ion trap mass spectrometry, tandem mass spectrometry, quadrupole time-of-flight mass spectrometry) is of the utmost importance for accurate measurements of mycotoxins in diverse matrices. All these techniques and methodologies imply key steps in the establishment of the limits of detection, limits of quantification, points of identification, accuracy, reproducibility, and/or repeatability of different procedures. The maximum levels or recommended levels for mycotoxins in different matrices are comprised within a wide range (including the levels tolerated by infants and animals). In addition, their control and evaluation of exposure are demanded by authorities and food safety systems.

Food and feed authorities are concerned not only with the determination of presence of mycotoxins but also with the toxicological effects of them, and in vivo or in vitro assays are necessary for a complete evaluation. In fact, these assays are the basis for the control and prevention of population exposure to mycotoxins in dietary exposure studies. Recent surveys are focused on regulated mycotoxins (aflatoxins, fumonisins, and trichothecenes) and emerging toxins such as enniatins and beauvericin in adult consumers, while very few studies have monitored mycotoxins levels in infant products.

This Special Issue of Toxins comprises 11 original contributions and one review. The issue reports new findings regarding the presence of mycotoxins in aromatic and medicinal plants, mango and orange juice, juices, pulps, jams and beer, from Morocco, Pakistan, and Portugal. In these studies, innovative techniques to study their presence have been developed. El Jai et al. [1] used liquid chromatography coupled to time-of-flight mass spectrometry to analyse mycotoxins and conjugated mycotoxins; there were a total of 14 mycotoxins in 40 samples of aromatic medicinal plants (AMPs) from Morocco. Hussain et al. [2] analyzed patulin in 274 fruit and derived products samples from Pakistan, and Silva et al. [3] evaluated the presence of ochratoxin A in 85 beer samples from Portugal. These results revealed that regular monitoring of cereals or fruits and their products (beer, juices, pulps and jams) during the harvest and processing stages is recommended to enhance the confidence in final consumers.

The Special Issue also presents novel strategies to detect the presence of mycotoxins as reported by Efremenco et al. [4]. They compared the characteristics of a rapid quantitative analysis of different mycotoxins (deoxynivalenol, ochratoxin A, patulin, sterigmatocystin, and zearalenone) using acetyl-, butyrylcholinesterases and photobacterial strains of luminescent cells. The best bioindicators in terms of sensitivity and working range (μg/mL) were as follows: *Photobacterium* sp. 17 cells for analysis of deoxynivalenol (0.8–89) and patulin (0.2–32); *Photobacterium* sp. 9.2 cells for analysis of ochratoxin A (0.4–72) and zearalenone (0.2–32); and acetylcholinesterase for analysis of sterigmatocystin (0.12–219).

Related with this highlighted scenario, Rodríguez-Carrasco et al. [5] have evaluated the exposure to enniatin B1 by biomonitoring metabolites in urine and identifying as major products: hydroxylated metabolites (78% samples) and carbonylated metabolites (66% samples). Also toxicological effects of zearalenone metabolites and beauvericin were

Citation: Juan García, C. Mycotoxins: Toxicology, Identification and Control. *Toxins* **2021**, *13*, 242. https://doi.org/10.3390/toxins13040242

Received: 8 March 2021
Accepted: 24 March 2021
Published: 29 March 2021

evaluated by Agahi et al. [6]. They evaluated the metabolism and toxicological effects on SH-SY5Y neuronal cells and IC_{50} values for the individual and combined treatments of the mentioned mycotoxins.

One important point in control of mycotoxins is decontamination strategies, and in this sense, Oliveria da Cruz et al. (2021) [7] evaluated the efficacy of potentially probiotic fruit-derived *Lactobacillus* isolates to remove aflatoxin M_1 (AFM_1) from a phosphate buffer solution (PBS; spiked with 0.15 μg/mL AFM_1). The authors concluded that *L. paracasei 108, L. plantarum 49,* and *L. fermentum 111* could have potential application to reduce AFM_1 to safe levels in foods and feeds.

Abbasi Pirouz et al. [8] present a simultaneous removal of 11 mycotoxins in palm kernel cake (PKC) using chitosan. PKC is used in ruminant feed; its use in poultry, swine, and fish diets is as a valuable source of protein and energy, while chitosan is a polyaminosaccharide and the second most abundant bio-polymers after cellulose. Mycotoxins studied were: aflatoxins (AFB_1, AFB_2, AFG_1 and AFG_2), ochratoxin A (OTA), zearalenone (ZEN), fumonisins (FB_1 and FB_2), trichothecenes (deoxynivalenol (DON), HT-2, and T-2 toxin) [8].

Another mycotoxin decontamination technique was tested by Yang et al. [9]. They used electron beam irradiation (EBI) and ozone on the degradation of ZEN and OTA. It was observed that 2 mL of 50 μg/mL of ZEN and OTA was completely reduced for ZEN and when 50 mg/L ozone is used, OTA is reduced at 34%. Acetamiprid was used by Nowak et al. [10] to reduce the production of destruxins produced by *Metarhizium* sp. Acetamiprid at concentrations from 5–50 mg/L did not inhibit the growth of all tested *Metarhizium* sp.; however, it reduced the level of 19 produced destruxins in direct proportion to the dosage used. Also, Wang et al. [11] studied a destruxin mycotoxin: destruxin A (DA), a cyclodepsipeptidic mycotoxin with pesticide proprieties involved in regulation of transcription and protein synthesis. It was suggested that silkworms' arginine tRNA synthetase (BmArgRS), Lamin-C Proteins (BmLamin-C), and ATP-dependent RNA helicase PRP1 (BmPRP1) were candidates of DA-binding proteins.

Finally, this Special Issue includes a review by Zhu et al. [12], which summarizes the newly discovered macrocyclic trichothecenes and their bioactivities over the last decade, as well as identifications of genes tri17 and tri18 involved in the trichothecene biosynthesis and putative biosynthetic pathway [12].

Funding: This research received no external funding.

Acknowledgments: The guest editor of this Special Issue, Cristina Juan García is grateful to the authors for their contributions and particularly to the referees for their invaluable work. Without their effort this special issue would have not been possible. The valuable contributions, organization, and editorial support of the MDPI management team and staff are greatly appreciated.

References

1. El Jai, A.; Zinedine, A.; Juan-García, A.; Mañes, J.; Etahiri, S.; Juan, C. Occurrence of Free and Conjugated Mycotoxins in Aromatic and Medicinal Plants and Dietary Exposure Assessment in the Moroccan Population. *Toxins* **2021**, *13*, 125. [CrossRef]
2. Hussain, S.; Rafique Asi, M.; Iqbal, M.; Khalid, N.; Wajih-ul-Hassan, S.; Ariño, A. Patulin Mycotoxin in Mango and Orange Fruits, Juices, Pulps, and Jams Marketed in Pakistan. *Toxins* **2020**, *12*, 52. [CrossRef] [PubMed]
3. Silva, J.G.L.; Teixeira, A.C.; Pereira, A.M.P.T.; Pena, A.; Lino, C.M. Ochratoxin A in Beers Marketed in Portugal: Occurrence and Human Risk Assessment. *Toxins* **2020**, *12*, 249. [CrossRef]
4. Efremenko, E.; Maslova, O.; Stepanov, N.; Ismailov, A. Using Cholinesterases and Immobilized Luminescent Photobacteria for the Express-Analysis of Mycotoxins and Estimating the Efficiency of Their Enzymatic Hydrolysis. *Toxins* **2021**, *13*, 34. [CrossRef]
5. Rodríguez-Carrasco, Y.; Narváez, A.; Izzo, L.; Gaspari, A.; Graziani, G.; Ritieni, A. Biomonitoring of Enniatin B1 and Its Phase I Metabolites in Human Urine: First Large-Scale Study. *Toxins* **2020**, *12*, 415. [CrossRef]
6. Agahi, F.; Font, G.; Juan, C.; Juan-García, A. Individual and Combined Effect of Zearalenone Derivates and Beauvericin Mycotoxins on SH-SY5Y Cells. *Toxins* **2020**, *12*, 212. [CrossRef]
7. Oliveira da Cruz, P.; Jales de Matos, C.; Mangueira Nascimento, Y.; Fechine Tavares, J.; Leite de Souza, E.; Iury Ferreira Magalhães, H. Efficacy of Potentially Probiotic Fruit-Derived *Lactobacillus fermentum*, *L. paracasei* and *L. plantarum* to Remove Aflatoxin M1 *In Vitro*. *Toxins* **2021**, *13*, 4. [CrossRef]
8. Abbasi Pirouz, A.; Selamat, J.; Iqbal, S.Z.; Putra Samsudin, N.I. Efficient and Simultaneous Chitosan-Mediated Removal of 11 Mycotoxins from Palm Kernel Cake. *Toxins* **2020**, *12*, 115. [CrossRef]

9. Yang, K.; Li, K.; Pan, L.; Luo, X.; Xing, J.; Wang, J.; Wang, L.; Wang, R.; Zhai, Y.; Chen, Z. Effect of Ozone and Electron Beam Irradiation on Degradation of Zearalenone and Ochratoxin A. *Toxins* **2020**, *12*, 138. [CrossRef]
10. Nowak, M.; Bernat, P.; Mrozińska, J.; Różalska, S. Acetamiprid Affects Destruxins Production but Its Accumulation in Metarhizium sp. Spores Increases Infection Ability of Fungi. *Toxins* **2020**, *12*, 587. [CrossRef] [PubMed]
11. Wang, J.; Weng, Q.; Yin, F.; Hu, Q. Interactions of Destruxin A with Silkworms' Arginine tRNA Synthetase and Lamin-C Proteins. *Toxins* **2020**, *12*, 137. [CrossRef] [PubMed]
12. Zhu, M.; Cen, Y.; Ye, W.; Li, S.; Zhang, W. Recent Advances on Macrocyclic Trichothecenes, Their Bioactivities and Biosynthetic Pathway. *Toxins* **2020**, *12*, 417. [CrossRef] [PubMed]

toxins

MDPI

Article

Occurrence of Free and Conjugated Mycotoxins in Aromatic and Medicinal Plants and Dietary Exposure Assessment in the Moroccan Population

Aicha El Jai [1], Abdellah Zinedine [1,*], Ana Juan-García [2], Jordi Mañes [2], Samira Etahiri [1] and Cristina Juan [2]

1 Laboratory of Marine Biotechnologies and Environment (BIOMARE), Faculty of Sciences, Chouaib Doukkali University, P.O. Box. 20, El Jadida 24000, Morocco; aichaeljai01@gmail.com (A.E.J.); setahiri@hotmail.com (S.E.)
2 Laboratory of Food Chemistry and Toxicology, Faculty of Pharmacy, University of Valencia, E-46100 Valencia, Spain; ana.juan@uv.es (A.J.-G.); jordi.manes@uv.es (J.M.); cristina.juan@uv.es (C.J.)
* Correspondence: zinedineab@yahoo.fr

Abstract: Aromatic and medicinal plants (AMPs), as herbal material, are subjected to contamination by various mycotoxin-producing fungi, either free and conjugated. Such a problem is associated with poor storage practices, and lack of adopting good agricultural practices and good harvesting practices. Nevertheless, AMPs are poorly investigated. The purpose of this study was to investigate the co-occurrence of 15 mycotoxins (four aflatoxins (AFB1, AFB2, AFG1, and AFG2), ochratoxin A (OTA), beauvericin (BEA), four enniatins (ENA, ENA1, ENB, and ENB1), zearalenone (ZEN), alternariol (AOH), tentoxin (TENT), T-2, and HT-2 toxins) in 40 samples of AMPs frequently consumed in Morocco by using liquid chromatography tandem mass spectrometry. Evaluation of conjugated mycotoxins and their identification using liquid chromatography coupled to time-of-flight mass spectrometry with ion mass exact was also carried out. Results showed that 90% of the analyzed samples presented at least one mycotoxin, and 52% presented co-occurrence of them. Mycotoxins detected were: AOH (85%), ZEN (27.5%), β-ZEL (22%), AFG1 (17.5%), TENT (17.5%), ENB (10%), AFG2 (7.5%), α-ZEL (5%), ENA1 (2.5%), and HT-2 (2.5%), while the conjugated mycotoxins were ZEN-14-Glc (11%) and ZEN-14-Sulf (9%). The highest observed level was for AOH, with 309 ng/g. Ten samples exceeded the recommended levels set by the European Pharmacopoeia for AF mycotoxins in plant material (4 ng/g), and three samples exceeded the maximum limits for AFs (10 ng/g) in species established by the European Commission. Although the co-occurrence of several mycotoxins in AMP samples was observed, the dietary exposure assessment showed that the intake of mycotoxins through the consumption of AMP beverages does not represent a risk for the population.

Keywords: mycotoxins; co-occurrence; Q-TOF-LC/MS; exposure; Morocco

Key Contribution: Aromatic and medicinal plants (AMPs) from Morocco presented levels of mycotoxins including conjugated mycotoxins such as ZEN-14-Glc (11%) and ZEN-14-Sulf (9%).

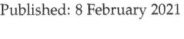

Citation: El Jai, A.; Zinedine, A.; Juan-García, A.; Mañes, J.; Etahiri, S.; Juan, C. Occurrence of Free and Conjugated Mycotoxins in Aromatic and Medicinal Plants and Dietary Exposure Assessment in the Moroccan Population. *Toxins* **2021**, *13*, 125. https://doi.org/10.3390/toxins13020125

Received: 8 January 2021
Accepted: 4 February 2021
Published: 8 February 2021

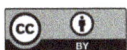

1. Introduction

Aromatic and medicinal plants (AMPs) are known to contain various compounds that can be valorized for several purposes, including preservative, therapeutic, and organoleptic proprieties, most of which are precursors for chemo-pharmaceutical semi-synthesis [1,2]. AMPs have been widely used to treat and/or prevent diseases and promote health since ancient times. However, AMPs are frequently exposed to various fungi responsible for the decrease in market quality, as their growth allows the presence of mycotoxins. Such fungi respond to contamination in soil, or during harvesting, drying, transport, manipulation, or storage [3,4].

Nowadays, several studies have reported the presence of mycotoxins in herbal plants and derivative products, considering that this contamination is a global issue, particularly in developing countries [5]. In fact, previous investigations reported that, under specific conditions, toxigenic fungal species from *Aspergillus, Penicillium, Fusarium,* and *Alternaria* genus can generate mycotoxins and contaminate herbal medicines. Indeed, these reports described mycotoxin contamination of medicinal herbs and related products, showing that mycotoxins, such as aflatoxins (AFs), ochratoxin A (OTA), zearalenone (ZEN), fumonisins, and trichothecenes are the most commonly present [6]. Another important point is related to the metabolization that can partially suffer from some mycotoxins, such as ZEN and deoxynivalenol (DON), by the fungus producer and by the infected host plant. The Phase I and II reactions in the metabolism process aim to eliminate these compounds, and this is often accomplished by the attachment of hydrophilic groups. The most indicated enzymatic system in the literature is the UDP-glucosyltransferase (UGT), which is capable of converting ZEN into ZEN-4-glucoside (ZEN-4-Glc) [7–9], or in Zearalenone-14-Glucoside (ZEN-14-Glc) and Zearalenone-16-Glucoside (ZEN-16-Glc) [10]. Furthermore, α-zearalenol (α-ZEL) and β-zearalenol (β-ZEL) suffer glycosylation as part of the host plant's metabolism, leading to α–ZEL-14-glucoside (α-ZEL-14-Glc) and β–ZEL-14-glucoside (β-ZEL-14-Glc), respectively [11]. This happens with other mycotoxins, such as DON, which is converted to DON-3-glucoside (DON-3-Glc) [12,13]. Moreover, during fungal metabolism, the sulfate form of ZEN, which is partially converted to Zearalenone-4-sulfate (ZEN-4-Sulf), has been found [14,15]. Despite their chemical alteration, there is evidence that metabolites have a similar toxic potential to those of their precursors when it is ingested, as attached functional groups like glycosylic or sulfate residues are likely to be enzymatically cleaved during digestion [14,16]. In most of the analytical approaches published, the main target of study has been the parental molecules forgetting the detection of their metabolites, resulting in an underestimation of the inherent toxicity of a contaminated sample. Altered metabolites of mycotoxins are also referred to as masked mycotoxins [16], thus, it is important to perform a non-target analysis to study the formation, determination, and significance of masked and other conjugated mycotoxins present in foodstuffs [17].

There is legislation established for mycotoxins in some spices and plants to avoid hazardous effects associated with their presence in herbal material [18]. The European Commission has established maximum limits (MLs) for mycotoxins, such as AFB1 (5 ng/g) and AFs (10 ng/g) in various spices (*Capsicum spp., Piper spp., Myristica fragrans, Zingiber officinale,* and *Curcuma longa*); however, no MLs have been established for aromatic plants [19]. In the European Pharmacopoeia (2016) [20], MLs have been set for AFs as 2 ng/g for AFB1 in herbal drugs and 4 ng/g for the sum of AFs [21]; while in the US Pharmacopeia (USP), ML of 5 ng/g for AFB1 and 20 ng/g for AFs have been implemented for certain types of raw medicinal herb materials, as well as their by-products (in powder and/or dry extract) [6].

In Morocco, several reports have evaluated the presence of mycotoxins in spices and herbal materials [22–24]. Recent Moroccan regulations have set MLs for certain mycotoxins in food products. For example, the ML is set at 5 ng/g for AFB1, 10 ng/g for the sum of AFs, and 15 ng/g for OTA in selected spices, such as *Capsicum spp., Piper spp., Myristica fragrans, Zingiber officinale,* and *Curcuma longa* [25]. However, no information is available regarding the possible co-occurrence of mycotoxins in AMP samples consumed in the country. Thus, the aims of the present study were: (i) to develop a liquid chromatography tandem mass spectrometry (LC-MS/MS) method to determinate 15 mycotoxins in AMPs from Morocco; (ii) to develop a liquid chromatography coupled with a time-of-flight mass spectrometry (LC-QTOF-MS) method as the screening tool to obtain not only confirmation, but also the detection of possible co-occurrence non-target mycotoxins, including masked mycotoxins; and (iii) to apply the developed method in the most consumed Moroccan AMP varieties supplied from the Moroccan market to investigating their co-occurrence. Data obtained from contamination levels will permit the assessment of the risk of dietary exposure for the Moroccan population to these mycotoxins through AMP intake.

2. Results and Discussion

2.1. Validation

Mycotoxin analysis in food and plant ingredients is always based on several factors, including the composition and nature of the matrix or ingredients to control, and the mycotoxin to investigate. In this study, the used modified dispersive liquid−liquid microextraction (DLLME) and LC-MS/MS methods were checked, and validation of the parameters of recoveries, linearity, LOD, and LOQ were carried out (Table 1 and Supplementary Table S1).

Table 1. Values of repeatability (mean recoveries of the triplicate and matrix effect ME) and sensitivity with a mix of blank AMP samples spiked at 10 times LOD.

Mycotoxin	Repeatability		Sensitivity	
	R ± SD (%)	ME ± SD [a] (%)	LOD (ng/g)	LOQ (ng/g)
AFB1	102 ± 1.4	9 ± 1.9	4.05	13.52
AFB2	112 ± 5.1	9.9 ± 3.8	3.30	11.00
AFG1	86 ± 0.5	13.5 ± 4.8	1.22	4.06
AFG2	97 ± 0.02	8.1 ± 2.4	2.07	6.90
OTA	92 ± 13	4.5 ± 0.96	0.93	3.11
BEA	85 ± 16	7.2 ± 0.3	0.37	1.22
ENA	100 ± 0.1	4.5 ± 0.7	0.29	0.95
ENA1	125 ± 14	3.6 ± 0.5	0.29	0.95
ENB	103 ± 4.5	4.5 ± 0.6	0.09	1.02
ENB1	112 ± 13	5.4 ± 1.2	0.52	1.74
ZEN	100 ± 2.5	3.6 ± 0.9	12.90	43.00
AOH	109 ± 0.8	4.5 ± 0.7	0.20	6.67
TENT	87 ± 6	5.4 ± 0.8	0.28	0.92
T-2	99 ± 0.01	7.2 ± 1.2	4.75	15.84
HT-2	81 ± 4.3	10.3 ± 1.3	1.59	5.30

[a] SD: Standard deviation.

Linearity was evaluated with calibration curves, which were constructed for each mycotoxin with methanol and a blank sample at concentration levels ranging from the LOQ to 1 µg/mL. All studied mycotoxins presented good linearity, with correlation coefficients (r^2) higher than 0.9995. Substances present in the matrix that modified the instrumental response of the analyte were evaluated by matrix effects (MEs), resulting in enhancement or suppression of the signal, so that signal suppression/enhancement was evaluated comparing the slopes of calibration curves obtained with methanol and in the blank sample. ME values higher than 100% indicated enhancement of the signal, ME values lower than 100% indicated suppression of the signal, and ME values near 100% indicated no significant matrix effects. The accuracy has been evaluated with recoveries (R) of the analytical method, so that a mix of blank samples (negative, < LOD) were spiked at three levels (LOQ, 2 LOQ. and 10 LOQ). Recovery values ranged from 81 ± 4.26% (HT-2) to 125 ± 14.18% (EN A1) at 10 times LOQ (Table 2). In Supplementary Table S2, the R at 10 times LOQ (n = 3, intraday study) and the ME observed by each studied AMP sample (n = 3) are shown. High ion suppression in *Rosmarinus officinalis, Matricaria chamomilla,* and *Myrtus communis* samples were observed.

2.2. Natural Occurrence of Mycotoxins

Out of 40 total AMP samples, 36 samples (90%) presented at least one mycotoxin (Table 3). All analyzed samples of *Mentha spicata, Lavandula intermedia, Matricaria chamomilla,* and *Myrtus communis* were contaminated by at least one mycotoxin. The most frequent mycotoxins in AMP were AOH (85%), ZEN (27.5%), AFG1 (17.5%), TENT (17.5%), ENB (10%), AFG2 (7.5%), ENA1 (2.5%), and HT-2 (2.5%) (Table 3), while the mycotoxins AFB1, AFB2, OTA, BEA, ENA, ENB1, and T-2 were under the LOD. The highest mycotoxin value found in AMP samples was registered in a sample of *Origanum vulgare*, with 309 ng/g of AOH (Table 3). Below, the occurrence in the analyzed samples by group of mycotoxins is detailed.

Table 2. MS/MS parameters for mycotoxin detection by multiple reaction monitoring (MRM).

Analyte	Rt [a] (min)	Parent Ion Q1 (*m/z*)	Product Ions Q3						DP [c]	CEP [c]
			Q (*m/z*) [b]	CE [c]	CXP [c]	q (*m/z*) [b]	CE[c]	CXP [c]		
AFB_1	7.8	313.1 $[M+H]^+$	241	41	4	285	39	4	46	18
AFB_2	7.7	315.1 $[M+H]^+$	259	39	6	287	33	6	81	18
AFG_1	7.6	329.1 $[M+H]^+$	311	29	6	243	39	6	76	18
AFG_2	7.5	331.1 $[M+H]^+$	245	39	6	313	27	6	61	18
OTA	8.7	404.1 $[M+H]^+$	102	97	6	239	27	6	55	21
ENA	10.3	699.4 $[M+NH_4]^+$	228	59	16	210	35	14	66	30
ENA_1	10.1	685.4 $[M+NH_4]^+$	214	59	10	210	37	8	66	30
ENB	9.7	657.3 $[M+NH_4]^+$	214	59	10	196	39	8	51	29
ENB1	9.9	671.2 $[M+NH_4]^+$	228	57	12	214	61	10	66	29
AOH	8.5	259.0 $[M+H]^+$	184	42	3	128	65	3	39	16
TENT	7.8	415.0 $[M+H]^+$	256	39	2	312	29	2	55	21
BEA	10	801.2 $[M+NH_4]^+$	244	39	6	784	27	10	116	33
HT-2	8.2	442.1 $[M+NH_4]^+$	215	19	8	263	19	4	21	22
T-2	8.4	484.1 $[M+NH_4]^+$	215	29	4	185	22	4	21	23
ZEN	8.9	319.1 $[M+H]^+$	282	19	4	301	15	10	26	18

[a] Rt: Retention time; [b] Q: quantification transition; q: qualification transition; [c] de-clustering potential (DP), collision energy (CE), collision cell entrance potential (CEP), and collision cell exit potential (CXP) are all expressed in voltage.

Table 3. Mycotoxin incidence, mean of positive (Mp) samples, and range levels distributed according to the eight studied species of AMP varieties.

AMP	Detected Mycotoxins	Incidence (%)	Mp ± SD (ng/g)	Range (ng/g)
Origanum vulgare (*n* = 12)	AOH	9 (75)	174 ± 96	8.6–309
	ZEN	3 (25)	72 ± 29	86.6–91
Rosmarinus officinalis (*n* = 7)	AFG2	3(43)	27.7 ± 2.1	26.2–41
	ZEN	6 (86)	45 ± 21	33.7–88
	AOH	6(86)	38 ± 16	10.9–53
Myrtus communis (*n* = 5)	AFG1	5 (100)	6.4 ± 1.3	4.9–9
	AOH	4 (80)	40.7 ± 16	34.5–72
	TENT	5 (100)	1.7 ± 2	0.7–4.5
Verveine officinale (*n* = 4)	ENA1	1 (25)	0.3	LOD–0.3
	ENB	1 (25)	0.1	LOD–0.1
	HT-2	1 (25)	2.9	LOD-2.0
	AOH	4 (100)	199.3 ± 70	124.6–293
Mentha spicata (*n* = 2)	ZEN	2 (100)	95.7 ± 27	76.7–115
	AOH	2 (100)	138.9 ± 1.2	138.1–140
Lavandula intermedia (*n* = 3)	AFG1	2 (67)	7.1 ± 1.5	6–8
	ENB	3 (100)	0.2 ± 0.1	LOD–0.4
	AOH	3 (100)	53.3 ± 21	29.8–69
	TENT	2 (67)	1.6 ± 0.1	1.5–1.6
Artemisia absinthium (*n* = 2)	AOH	1 (50)	2.3	LOD–2.3
Matricaria chamomilla (*n* = 5)	AOH	5 (100)	204.6 ± 102	30.9–279

Raw tea and herbal infusion materials were reported to contain up to 76 μg/kg of fumonisin B1, but no mycotoxins were detected in infusions [25]. In China, the presence of ZEN and its metabolite α-zearalenol (α-ZEL) in 100 widely-consumed foods and medicinal plants was investigated. Authors reported that 12% of these tested samples were contaminated with ZEN at levels ranging from 5.3 to 295.8 μg/kg [26]. Another study from Spain reported the occurrence of T-2 and HT-2 in seeds of milk thistle (*Silybum marianum*) at levels ranging from 363 to 453.9 μg/kg and from 826.9 to 943.7 μg/kg, respectively [27]. A study from India reported that dried market samples of stem portions of *Tinospora cordifolia*, an important medicinal plant, were contaminated with AFB1, AFB2, OTA, patulin, and citrinine; however, fusarial species and their toxins were not detected in those samples [28]. In Latvia, the occurrence of 12 mycotoxins has been recently investigated in 60 herbal teas. Among the dry tea samples, 90% were positive from one to eight mycotoxins. ENB, DON, AFB1, and OTA were the most frequently detected mycotoxins in 55%, 45%, 20%, and 10% of samples, respectively. The authors reported that 32% and 100% of DON and ZEN, respectively, present in dry teas were extracted into the infusions ready for its consumption [29]. A study from Spain showed the presence of AFB2 (19.1–134.7 μg/L) and AFG2 (2.2 to 13.5 μg/L) in botanical dietary supplement infusion beverages, and ENB in two samples, although at low levels [30]. More recently, AFs were detected in green tea samples obtained from retail shops and supermarkets in three Moroccan areas; however, the rate transfer of AFs from herbal green tea to infusion was unavailable, as it was not investigated [31].

2.2.1. Aflatoxins (AFG1 and AFG2)

AFG1 was detected in seven samples (17.5%), including two samples of *Lavandula intermedia* (5%) and five samples of *Myrtus communis* (12.5%) (Tables 3 and 4). Levels of AFG1 ranged from 4.9 to 8.6 ng/g, and the mean level of AFG1 in positive samples was 4.6 ± 1.4 ng/g (Table 4). Concerning the presence of AFG2, it was detected in three samples of *Rosmarinus officinalis* (7.5%). Levels of the AFG2 in this plant ranged from 26.2 to 41.1 ng/g, with a mean value of 27.7 ± 2.1 ng/g (Tables 3 and 4). It should be highlighted that three positive AMP samples (*Lavandula intermedia, Myrtus communis,* and *Rosmarinus officinalis*) exceeded the ML (10 ng/g) of Moroccan regulation set for the sum of AFs [32].

Table 4. Occurrence, mean levels, probable daily intake (PDI), and risk of dietary exposure of studied mycotoxins through analyzed Moroccan AMPs.

Mycotoxin	Incidence (%)	Range Levels (ng/g)	Mp ± SD [a] (ng/g)	Mt ± SD (ng/g)		PDI (ng/kg b.w./day) [%TDI]		TDI (ng/kg b.w./day)
				LB [b]	UB [c]	LB	UB	
AFG1	7 (17.5)	4.9–8.6	4.6 ± 1.4	1.16 ± 4.7	3.97 ± 1.35	-	-	-
AFG2	3 (7.5)	26.2–41.1	27.7 ± 2.1	2.42 ± 8.8	7.27 ± 8.8	-	-	-
AFs	-	-	-	-	-	-	-	-
ENA1	1 (2.5)	0.35	0.16 ± 0.3	0.019 ± 0.05	1.3 ± 0.32	-	-	-
ENB	1 (10)	LOD (0.1) [d]	0.05 ± 0.1	0.02 ± 0.063	1.01 ± 0.06	-	-	-
ENs	-	-	-	-	-	-	-	-
ZEN	11 (27.5)	33.7–114.7	55.5 ± 26	18.2 ± 32.7	37.8 ± 32.7	0.67 [0.56]	1.39 [0.82]	250
AOH	34 (85)	2.3–309.5	126.2 ± 40.4	99.7 ± 97.8	116.2 ± 97	-	-	-
TENT	7 (17.5)	0.7–4.5	1.47 ± 0.8	0.29 ± 1.2	0.88 ± 0.3	-	-	-
HT-2	1 (2.5)	LOD–LOQ (2.9) [e]	1.47 ± 2.6	0.072 ± 2.05	5.49 ± 0.5	0.003	0.203	-
T2+HT2	-	-	-	-	-	0.003	0.203	100

[a] Mp: mean of positive samples; Mt: mean of total analyzed samples; SD: Standard deviation; [b] LB: Lower bound; [c] UB: Upper bound; [d] Values close to LOD; [e] Value between LOD and LOQ.

2.2.2. *Fusarium* Toxins (ZEN and HT-2)

Determination of ZEN in AMP samples showed that 27.5% of samples were positive for this mycotoxin (Table 4) specifically: two samples of *Mentha spicata*, six samples of *Rosmarinus officinalis*, and three samples of *Origanum vulgare*. Levels of ZEN varied between 33.7 and 114.7 ng/g, and the mean ZEN level was 55.7 ± 26 ng/g. Recent studies have also detected ZEN in AMP as Duarte et al., who detected them in 19 herb samples with smaller ranged values (1.82–19.02 ng/g) than those detected in our analyzed samples [33]. Concerning the presence of HT-2, one AMP sample of *Verveine officinale* (2.5%) contained this mycotoxin, with levels up to 2.9 ng/g, and a mean level of 1.47 ± 2.6 ng/g.

2.2.3. Emerging Mycotoxins (ENA1 and ENB)

In this survey, only ENA1 and ENB were detected among emerging mycotoxins in AMP samples. Regarding the occurrence of ENA1 in AMP samples, this toxin was detected only in one sample (2.5%) of *Verveine officinale*, with a contamination level up to 0.3 ng/g and a mean level of 0.16 ± 0.3 ng/g. For the presence of ENB in AMP samples, four samples (10%) were contaminated: one sample of *Verveine officinale* and three samples of *Lavandula intermedia* (Table 3). Levels of the ENB were detected in a range of 0.04–0.1 ng/g, and the mean level was 0.05 ± 0.1 ng/g.

2.2.4. *Alternaria* Toxins (AOH and TENT)

Alternaria mycotoxins gain more and more interest due to their frequent contamination of food commodities. Indeed, these toxins are often detected in fruits, vegetables, and wines [34]. Besides the estrogenic activity demonstrated in vitro for certain *Alternaria* toxins, AOH causes DNA damage and cell cycle arrest [35]. In the present survey, 34 samples (85%) presented levels of AOH. Nine of them were *Origanum vulgare*. Levels of AOH ranged from 2.3 to 309 ng/g, and the mean level was 126.2 ± 40.4 ng/g. TENT was detected in seven samples (17.5%) as follows: five samples of *Myrtus communis* and two samples of *Lavandula intermedia*. Levels of TENT varied from 0.7 to 4.5 ng/g, and the mean level was 1.47 ± 0.85 ng/g.

2.3. *Co-Occurrence of Mycotoxins in AMP*

The co-presence of mycotoxins in a single sample could be a health concern due to the exposure of consumers to multiple fungal metabolites, which might exert greater toxicity than the exposure to a single one. The multi-mycotoxin occurrence in food and feed could be associated with health and reproductive disorders, lower performance in animals, and higher medical costs [36]. Concerning the mycotoxins' co-occurrence in AMP samples, this happened in 52% of samples. Figure 1 summarizes the data obtained on the multi-contamination of AMP samples, revealing that the ZEN + AOH combination was the most commonly present (20%).

Analytical results showed that four mycotoxins co-occurred in samples of *Verveine officinale* (AOH + HT-2 + ENA1 + ENB) and *Lavandula intermedia* (AFG1 + ENB + AOH + TENT), three mycotoxins were present in samples of *Rosmarinus officinalis* (AFG2 + AOH + ZEN), and *Myrtus communis* (AFG1 + AOH + TENT), while two mycotoxins (AOH + ZEN) co-occurred in *Origanum vulgare* and *Mentha spicata* samples (Figure 1). Finally, positive samples of *Artemisia absinthium* and *Matricaria chamomilla* were contaminated individually by AOH.

To the best of our knowledge, limited data have been published on the multi-presence of mycotoxin in aromatic and medicinal herbs available worldwide. Indeed, a recent investigation from Spain was performed to screen the multi-contamination by mycotoxins (AFs, OTA, ZEN, T-2, DON, citrinin, and fumonisins) in 84 samples of aromatic and/or medicinal herbs, showing that 99% of the samples were contaminated with T-2 (99%), ZEN (98%), AFs (96%), OTA (63%), DON (62%), citrinin (61%), and fumonisins (13%) [37].

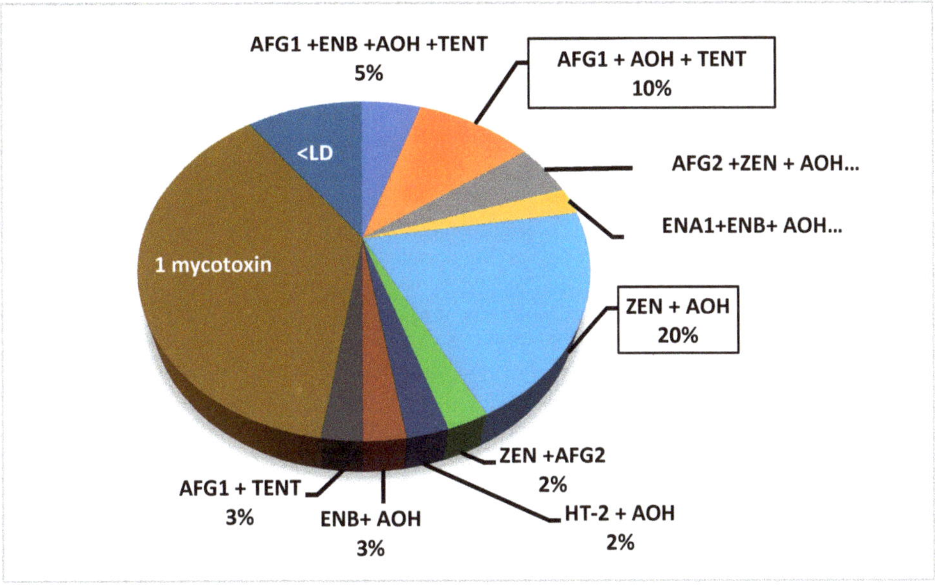

Figure 1. Co-occurrence mycotoxin distribution.

2.4. *Conjugated Mycotoxins in AMP*

Samples with contamination levels of target mycotoxins were injected into the LC–QTOF–MS system to confirm their presence and to study the possible co-occurrence of lesser known non-target mycotoxin metabolites formed during detoxification and glycosylated and sulfated conjugates, since the probability of identifying these compounds was reasonably greater when more mycotoxins were present.

In the present work, the exact mass and isotope pattern calculated from the molecular formula and plus/minus the expected adduct(s) of the suspected substance and experimental information (retention time behavior and presence of related substances) were used to screen that substance in the samples. Afterwards, non-target components of modified and conjugated compounds were studied to gain confidence through library match and/or diagnostic fragments.

All target mycotoxins previously quantified by LC–MS/MS were confirmed by LC–QTOF–MS (Table 4). However, the results of the study of non-target components derived from metabolism were only presented for ZEN. Although AOH was the most detected mycotoxin, ZEN was the second mycotoxin highly present in Moroccan AMP samples, and more susceptible to suffering from glycosylation, sulphuration, and hydroxylation reactions than AOH, as reported in the literature in the last decade [7,11,38]. After automatic acquisition mode MS/MS, α-ZEN, β-ZEL, ZEN-4-Glc, ZEN-14-Glc, ZEN-16-Glc, α-ZEL-14-Glc, β-ZEL-14-Glc, and ZEL-4-Sulf were selected to be identified by MassHunter Qualitative Analysis B.10.0. Mycotoxins or metabolites that have an available commercial standard (α-ZEL, β-ZEL, ZEN) were confirmed and quantified with the same program, and a "Find by Formula" data-mining algorithm with a mass error below $\pm$ 5 ppm with score values ≥ 70 (including isotope abundance and isotope spacing) was also used. A retention time window of $\pm$ 1 min was specified for peak detection to compensate for retention time shifts due to system-to-system variability. All relevant compound species including adducts: $[M+H]^+$, $[M+Na]^+$, $[M-H]^-$, $[M+HCOO]^-$, $[M-OH]^-$, and $[M+HCOOH-H]^-$ were used as target masses. Mycotoxin metabolites' annotation was also supported by comparing the obtained MS/MS fragmentation spectra with the experimental spectra proposed in the databases of mycotoxins and related metabolites, Personal Compound Database and

Library (PCDL) Manager MassHunter. Metlin Metabolites PCDL MassHunter contains an accurate mass compound database, a collision cross section database, and an MS/MS accurate mass spectral library for mycotoxins.

In the present study, the ZEN conjugates and metabolites selected were α-ZEL, β-ZEL, ZEN-14-Glc, β-ZEL-14-Glc, and ZEN-4-Sulf. All were selected based on purity score values ≥ 70 and a mass error < ± 5 ppm. Tentative identification is listed in Table 5. β-ZEL was the most abundant metabolite found (22%). The glycosylated ZEN (ZEN-14-Glc) compound was detected in five samples (11%), with low intensity. Regarding ZEN sulfate conjugate (ZEN-4-Sulf), it was detected in four samples (9%). Previous studies have indicated the presence of ZEN-4-Sulf in fungal cell cultures in molar ratios from 1:12 to 1:1, compared with ZEN [14], and in wheat flour samples at levels of 9.7% ZEN-4-Sulf [38]. Here, in AMP samples, ZEN-4-Sulf was present at levels ranging from 5 to 2% of the ZEN level. As far as we know, this is the first time that these non-target metabolites have been reported in AMP samples, and the first time they have been identified by LC–QTOF–MS in AMP. QTOF-MS data cannot support quantification of compounds without the use of a reference compound so that the conjugated mycotoxins detected were not quantified, although their presence was positive. Supplementary Figure S1 shows a total ion current (TIC) chromatogram from a positive sample and its extracted ion chromatogram (EIC) of β-ZEL and ZEN-14-Glc detected. Their corresponding scan and product ion spectrum are included in Supplementary Figure S1.

Table 5. Identification of conjugated mycotoxins and ZEA's metabolites detected in AMP analyzed samples.

Samples Code	Mycotoxins Conjugate and Metabolites	Molecular Formula	Precursor Ion Mass (*m*/*z*)	Exact Molecular Mass (Da)	Mass Error (ppm)	Purity Score	Area	Retention Time (min)
PAM 2.d	β-ZEL	C18 H24 O5	365.1616	320.1633	1.2	82.27	273957	9.1
PAM 3.d		C18 H24 O5	379.1771	320.1623	2.3	82.95	317981	9.1
PAM 4.d		C18 H24 O5	379.1773	320.1623	1.3	98.15	312003	9.3
PAM 5.d		C18 H24 O5	319.1553	320.1615	1.62	84.71	387715	9.3
PAM 6.d		C18 H24 O5	379.1769	320.1630	0.9	98.23	326655	9.3
PAM 9.d		C18 H24 O5	379.1769	320.1630	1.5	83.70	439643	9.3
PAM 27.d		C18 H24 O5	379.1763	320.1627	2.4	98.06	599853	9.3
PAM 28.d		C18 H24 O5	365.1614	320.1631	−1.3	94.51	274979	9.2
PAM 32.d		C18 H24 O5	365.1614	320.1633	1.04	80.27	14188	9.1
PAM 8.d	α-ZEL	C18 H24 O5	319.1553	320.1629	1.3	96.50	450446	10.4
PAM 27.d		C18 H24 O5	319.1560	320.1636	1.4	97.38	185920	10.2
PAM 2.d	ZEN-14-Glc *	C24 H32 O10	525.2144	480.1992	2.5	71.67	24470	6.8
PAM 3.d		C24 H32 O10	539.2156	480.2017	2.6	69.62	20691	6.5
PAM 6.d		C24 H32 O10	525.1971	480.2028	−2.3	73.19	9149	6.6
PAM 8.d		C24 H34 O10	537.2128	481.2165	2.4	69.49	29254	6.3
PAM 8.d	β-ZEL-14-Glc *	C24 H34 O10	481.2058	482.2139	2.05	67.21	9817	15.9
PAM 8.d	ZEN-4-Sulf *	C18 H22 O8 S	399.2550	400.2624	1.1	71.02	32229	11.1
PAM 27.d		C18 H22 O8 S	399.2555	400.2625	−1.03	75.04	10390	11.1
PAM 28.d		C18 H22 O8 S	399.2539	400.2608	−2.2	92.11	11117	11.1
PAM 32.d		C18 H20 O8 S	397.0968	398.1031	−1.29	93.36	22950	13.5

* Tentative identification by Metlin Metabolites PCDL MassHunter (PCDL contains an accurate mass compound database, a collision cross section database, and an MS/MS accurate mass spectral library).

2.5. Dietary Exposure

Several studies have reported the presence of mycotoxins in food and feed, while few data are still available of mycotoxins present in medicinal plants. The effect of mycotoxins found in some herbal plants on biochemical parameters of blood from mice were reported by Alwakeel (2009) [39]. The authors showed that analytical parameters, such as mean creatinine, urea, alanine aminotransferase, aspartate aminotransferase, and gamma-glutamyl transpeptidase, were higher in the mice group fed or treated with herbal and fungal extracts than the control group, and the study confirms the implication of the AFs with induction of nephrotoxicity and hepatoxicity in animals.

No data is currently available on the annual consumption of AMPs in Morocco, and as for estimation, it is assumed that the annual AMP consumption is half of the annual raw tea consumption. According to FAO, the annual consumption per capita of green tea in Morocco averages 1.89 kg/year, so the annual consumption per capita of AMPs in Morocco is supposed to be 0.94 kg/year [40]. The risk of mycotoxins was assessed herein following both lower bound (LB) and upper bound (UB) approaches. For the LB approach, mean values were obtained by assigning a level of zero to free mycotoxin samples (where no mycotoxins were detected), or at levels below the LOQ (where mycotoxins were detected), whereas, in the UB approach, values equal to the LOD were assigned to samples where no mycotoxins were detected, and values equal to the LOQ were assigned to samples in which mycotoxin levels were below the LOQ.

In this study, mycotoxins AFG1, AFG2, ZEN, HT-2, AOH, TENT, ENA1, and ENB were detected in positive samples. For the AFs, these substances are confirmed as carcinogenic and classified by IARC in Group 1 (do not have an established TDI), so it is not possible to determine the threshold levels at which AFs have no effect [41]. It is recommended by JECFA, with regard to the safe level of AFs in foods, that AF levels must be reduced according to the "As Low As Reasonably Achievable" (ALARA) principle [42]. Furthermore, no TDI values have been established for emerging mycotoxins (BEA and ENs) and *Alternaria* toxins (AOH and TENT), so a risk assessment is not possible to calculate for these mycotoxins. For ZEN, the PDIs calculated were 0.67 ± 1.21 ng.kg^{-1}.bw.day^{-1} (LB approach) and 1.39 ± 1.20 ng.kg^{-1}.bw.day^{-1} (UB approach), and the TDIs (ZEN 250 ng.kg^{-1}.bw.day^{-1}) were 0.56% and 0.82% by the LB and UB approaches, respectively (Table 4).

Risk assessment shows that the intake of mycotoxins through the consumption of AMP beverages does not represent a risk for the population, except for AFs that are classified as carcinogenic compounds. Nevertheless, the presence of mycotoxins in AMPs could increase the exposure in large consumers. A focus on plants is relevant to gather more knowledge on larger spectra of mycotoxin contamination related with AMP handling conditions, their presence in extracted essential oils, the apparition of any toxic effect, or the effect on human health.

Another important point is that the conjugated metabolites, as well as their reductive forms, are not a part of ZEN´s regulations. In vitro analyses of the gastrointestinal digestive process showed no cleavage of ZEN´s conjugates, but in human microbiota fermentation, the conjugates were cleaved by the microbial enzymes [43,44]. Thus, ZEN uptake might be underestimated, due to the release of absorbable ZEN.

Recently, the EU-CONTAM Panel found it appropriate to set a group TDI for ZEN and its modified forms [45]. It must be considered that the estrogenic potency of ZEN derivatives differs. Potency factors assigned to these derivatives by the EFSA CONTAM Panel are 0.2 for β-ZEL and 60 for α-ZEL relative to ZEN. Moreover, for sulfate and glucoside conjugates, the same factors as the free forms are proposed. However, to obtain more data on the occurrence of ZEN metabolites in food and feed, standard compounds are needed.

3. Conclusions

Mycotoxin analysis showed that 90% of Moroccan AMP samples were positive and 52% presented co-occurrence. Besides the high incidence in samples, the concentration ranged from 0.35 ng/g (ENA1) to 309 ng/g (AOH). The most detected were AOH (85%) and ZEN (27.5 %), while ZEN + AOH was the most frequent co-occurrent mycotoxins (20% of positive samples). AFs were present in 25% of samples (*Lavandula intermedia, Myrtus communis,* and *Rosmarinus officinalis),* seven of which exceeded the European and Moroccan recommended levels [19,20,32].

In the present study, a sensitive, rapid, robust, and reliable LC–MS/MS method was validated for the simultaneous determination of 15 target mycotoxins in five different species of AMP: *Origanum vulgare, Rosmarinus officinalis, Matricaria chamomilla, Myrtus communis,* and *Verveine officinale.* A new LC–QTOF–MS method was applied for the simultaneous screening of non-target mycotoxins and conjugated mycotoxins in positive AMP samples. ZEN-14-Glc (11%) and ZEN-14-Sulf (9%) conjugated mycotoxins were detected in AMP samples. The strategy of combining QTOF–MS and MS/MS detectors with LC is a powerful approach for the routine monitoring of mycotoxin and conjugated mycotoxins in contaminated AMPs and other foodstuffs, providing quality and safety to the food industry and consumers.

4. Material and Methods

4.1. Chemicals and Reagents

Standards of mycotoxins (four aflatoxins (AFB1, AFB2, AFG1 and AFG2), ochratoxin A (OTA), beauvericin (BEA), four enniatins (ENA, ENA1, ENB, and ENB1), zearalenone (ZEN), α-zearalenol (α-ZEL), β-zearalenol (β-ZEL), alternariol (AOH), tentoxin (TENT), T-2, and HT-2 toxins) were purchased from Sigma Aldrich (St. Louis, MO, USA). Individual stock solutions containing a concentration of 1000 µg/mL were prepared in methanol. Working solutions were prepared starting from the appropriate individual stock solutions. All solutions were prepared and stored in the dark at −20 °C. Methanol and acetonitrile ($\geq$ 99.9% purity) liquid chromatography tandem mass spectrometry grades (LC-MS/MS) were supplied by VWR international Eurolab (Barcelona, Spain). Formic acid ($\geq$ 98%) was obtained from Sigma Aldrich (St. Louis, MO, USA). Ammonium formate ($\geq$ 99.995%) and chloroform ($CHCl_3$) (99%) were obtained from Merck KGaA (Darmstadt, Germany). Ethyl acetate (EtOAc) (HPLC-grade, > 99.5%) was purchased from Alfa Aesar (Karlsruhe, Germany). The water used was purified ($\leq$ 10 MΩ cm^{-1} resistivity) in the laboratory using a Milli-Q SP® Reagent water system (Millipore, Bedford, MA, USA).

4.2. Plant Sampling

A total of forty AMP samples were randomly collected in 2019 from local markets (retailers and supermarkets) in three different areas of Rabat (Morocco): Témara, Bitat, and Kamra. All samples belonged to eight varieties of AMP plants (*Origanum vulgare* (n = 12), *Rosmarinus officinalis* (n = 7), *Myrtus communis* (n = 5), *Matricaria chamomilla* (n = 5), *Verveine officinale* (n = 4), *Mentha spicata* (n = 2), *Lavandula Intermedia* (n = 3), and *Artemisia absinthium* (n = 2)). The selection of these plants was based on the criteria that they are among the most traditionally used plants and consumed by the Moroccan population for their aromatic and/or therapeutic properties [46]. The amount of each AMP sample was at least 50 g, packed in bags and stored in a dark and dry place until analysis.

4.3. Mycotoxin Extraction Procedure

The sensitive and accurate analysis of mycotoxins in complicated matrices (e.g., herbs) typically involves challenging sample pretreatment procedures and an efficient detection instrument. A modified DLLME method [47] was applied to extract the studied mycotoxins. Firstly, 2 g of AMP samples were boiled with 200 mL of water for 5 min in a glass container. Next, 10 mL of the aqueous solution tea filtrated with Whatman filter paper was placed in a conical polytetrafluoroethyl (PTFE) centrifuge tube (15 mL), and 2 g of NaCl was added. Then, 1.9 mL of acetonitrile (dispersion solvent) and 1.24 mL of ethyl acetate (extraction solvent) was added and vortexed for 1 min. It was centrifuged for 5 min at 4000 rev/min at 5 °C, using Eppendorf centrifuge 5810R (Eppendorf, Hamburg, Germany), and a cloudy solution of the three phases was formed. The organic phase at the top (Tube 1) was recovered and placed in a second PTFE centrifuge tube (15 mL, Tube 2), while the remaining residue (Tube 1) was saved for a second extraction with 3.2 mL of a mixture of methanol and chloroform (60:40, *v*/*v*). Then, Tube 1 was vortexed for 1 min, and, with a centrifugation at 4000 rev/min for 5 min at 5 °C, the separated organic phase was recovered and added to the collected organic phase in Tube 2.

Both separated organic phases in PTFE centrifuge Tube 2 were evaporated to dryness under a nitrogen stream using a TurboVap LV evaporator (Zymark, Hopkinton, MA). The dried residue was reconstituted with 1 mL of methanol and water (70:30, *v*/*v*), and filtered through a 13 mm/0.22 µm nylon filter (Membrane Solutions, Plano, TX, USA). Next, 20 µL of the filtrate was injected into the LC-MS/MS analysis.

4.4. Analysis of Mycotoxins by LC-MS/MS

Analysis of the mycotoxins was performed using an LC Agilent 1200 with a binary pump and an automatic injector, and coupled to a 3200 QTRAP®ABSCIEX (Applied Biosystems, Foster City, CA, USA) equipped with a Turbo-V™ source (ESI) interface. The chromatographic separation of the analytes was conducted at 25 °C with a reverse phase analytical column Gemini® NX-C18 (3 µm, 150 × 2 mm ID) and a guard column C18 (4 × 2 mm, ID; 3 µm). The mobile phase was a time programmed gradient using water (0.1% formic acid and 5 mM of ammonium formate) as phase A, and methanol (0.1% formic acid and 5 mM of ammonium formate) as phase B [48]. The following gradient was used: equilibration for 2 min at 90% A, 80–20% A in 3 min, 20% A for 1 min, 20–10% A in 2 min, 10% A for 6 min, 10–0% A in 3 min, 100% B for 1 min, 100–50% B in 3 min, return to initial conditions in 2 min and maintain during 2 min. The flow rate was 0.25 mL/min in all steps. The total run time was 21 min.

Regarding mycotoxin analysis, the QTRAP System was used as the triple quadrupole mass spectrometry detector (MS/MS). The Turbo-V™ source was used in a positive mode to analyze the 15 mycotoxins with the following settings for source/gas parameters: Vacuum Gauge (10×10^{-5} Torr) 3.1, curtain gas (CUR) 20, ion spray voltage (IS) 5500, source temperature (TEM) 450 °C, and ion source gas 1 (GS1) and ion source gas 2 (GS2) 50. The fragments monitored (retention time, quantification, ion, and confirmation ion) and spectrometric parameters (de-clustering potential, collision energy, and cell exit potential) used were those performed previously (Juan et al. 2019), and are shown in Table 1.

4.5. Method Validation

Validation of the LC-MS/MS method was performed for linearity, repeatability (intraday and inter-day precision), and sensitivity, following the EU Commission Decision 2002/657/EC (EC, 2002). Matrix-matched calibration curves were constructed at concentration levels between the LOQ to 1 µg/mL. The matrix effect (ME) was assessed for each analyte by comparing the slope of the standard calibration curve (standard) with that of the matrix-matched calibration curve (matrix) for the same concentration levels. The limit of detection (LOD) and limit of quantification (LOQ) were estimated for a signal-to-noise ratio (S/N) ≥ 3 and ≥ 10, respectively, from chromatograms of samples spiked at the lowest level validated. LOD and LOQ values were established as a mean of the LOD and LOQ for each matrix and a mix with all studied matrixes, in this way taking into account the possible heterogeneity of the samples. Accuracy of the studied mycotoxin extraction from AMP samples was determined by a mix blank samples fortification procedure. The mix blank was prepared using each AMP sample studied (*Origanum vulgare, Rosmarinus officinalis, Matricaria chamomilla Myrtus communis, Verveine officinale, Mentha spicata, Lavandula Intermedia,* and *Artemisia absinthium*), which initially tested negative, and was fortified before the extraction procedure with three different mycotoxin levels. The concentrations of studied mycotoxins for reproducibility and repeatability studies in AMP samples were at LOQ, 2 LOQ, and 10 LOQ. Three replicates were prepared for each spiking level. Intra-day precision (repeatability) and inter-day precision (reproducibility) of the method were carried out by spiking the mix blank at the three levels previously indicated. Method precision was estimated by calculating the relative standard deviation (RSD_R) using the results obtained during intra-day and inter-day replicate analysis ($n = 9$).

4.6. Analysis of Mycotoxin Metabolites by LC-QTOF-MS

The QTOF LC/MS analysis was carried out using an Agilent Technologies 1200 Infinity Series LC coupled with an Agilent Technologies 6540 UHD Accurate-Mass Q-TOF-LC/MS (Agilent Technologies, Santa Clara, CA, USA), equipped with an electrospray ionization Agilent Technologies Dual Jet Stream ion source (Dual AJS ESI). Chromatographic separation was achieved on a Gemini® NX-C18 (3 µm, 150 × 2 mm ID) and a guard column C18 (4 × 2 mm, ID; 3µm). The mobile phase consisted of 0.1% formic acid in water milli-Q (solvent A) and methanol (solvent B) with a 25 min gradient. The mobile phase gradient (10–95% B) steps were applied as follows: 0–2 min, 10% B; 2–5 min, 70% B; 5–7 min, 80% B; 7–8 min, 90% B; maintained 4 min at 90% B; 12–16 min, 95% B; 16–18 min, 50% B; 18–22 min, and 10% B. The injection volume was 10 µL.

A mass spectrometry analysis was used with the following QTOF-MS conditions: drying gas flow (N_2), 8.0 L min−1; nebulizer pressure, 45 psi; gas drying temperature, 370 °C; capillary voltage, 3500 V; fragmentor voltage, 130 V; skimmer voltage, 65 V; and octopole RF peak, 750 V. The Agilent Dual Jet Stream electrospray ionization (Dual AJS ESI) interface was used in the positive and negative ionization modes, and ions were acquired in the range of 100–1000 *m*/*z* for MS scans, and 50–1000 *m*/*z* for auto MS/MS scans, at a scan rate of five spectra/s for MS and three spectra/s for MS/MS, respectively. Automatic acquisition mode MS/MS was carried out using the following collision energy values: *m*/*z*, 20 eV; *m*/*z*, 30 eV and 40 eV. Internal mass correction was enabled by using two reference masses at 121.0509 and 922.0098 *m*/*z*. Instrument control and data acquisition were performed using Agilent MassHunter Workstation software B.08.00. All of the MS and MS/MS data of the validation standards were integrated by MassHunter Qualitative Analysis B.10.0 and MassHunter Quantitative Analysis B.10.0 (Agilent Technologies).

4.7. Risk of Dietary Exposure

Risk of dietary exposure calculation/evaluation, in the present study, consisted of measuring the presence of mycotoxins in analyzed samples. It also consisted of characterizing the distribution of one or more mycotoxin for estimating population exposure upon the consumption of average or extremely high amounts [49]. The probable daily intake (PDI, ng.kg^{-1}.bw.day^{-1}) of each mycotoxin through AMP consumption was estimated based on the concentration of each mycotoxin detected in the samples, the daily consumption rate of AMPs, and the average body weight of an individual consumer (70 kg). It is important to highlight that this is for genotoxic substances and substances classified as carcinogenic by the International Agency for Research on Cancer (IARC) [41] (such as AFs or OTA). EFSA, through a CONTAM Panel, considered the possibility of applying a margin of exposure (MOE) approach, with a benchmark dose lower confidence limit, for a benchmark response of 10% (BMDL10) [50]. Nonetheless, recent studies from Portugal [26] have conducted this calculation for AFs by using the TDI of 0.2 ng/kg b.w./day already proposed [51]. To characterize the risk for each mycotoxin, the PDIs were compared with the TDIs of mycotoxins established by JECFA (2001) [52] and SCF (2002) [53]. The percentage of tolerable daily intake (%TDI) from the consumption of green tea was calculated as follows: %TDI = PDI/TDI × 100.

Supplementary Materials: The following are available online at https://www.mdpi.com/2072-6651/13/2/125/s1, Figure S1: Total ion current (TIC) chromatogram from a positive sample and its extracted ion chromatogram (EIC) of β-ZEL and ZEN-14-Glc (a), scan and product ion spectrum of β-ZEL (b), and scan and product ion spectrum of ZEN-14-Glc (**c**)., Table S1: Recoveries of intraday (*n* = 3) study of spiked AMP samples and matrix.

Author Contributions: Data curation, A.E.J.; Formal analysis, C.J.; Funding acquisition, A.Z.; Investigation, A.J.-G. and C.J.; Methodology, C.J.; Project administration, A.Z. and J.M.; Resources, A.E.J. and A.Z.; Supervision, A.Z., A.J.-G., J.M., S.E., and C.J.; Visualization, C.J.; Writing—original draft, A.E.J. and C.J.; Writing—review & editing, A.E.J., A.J.-G., and C.J. All authors have read and agreed to the published version of the manuscript.

Funding: This research was funded by Spanish Ministry of Science and Innovation PID2019-108070RB-I00ALI and the Generalitat Valenciana GVPROMETEO2018-126, Generalitat Valenciana GV 2020/020 and PHC Maghreb project (09MAG20). A. Zinedine would like to thank the CNRST of Morocco and the Moroccan Ministry of Higher Education and Scientific Research (MENESRSFC) for their support.

Institutional Review Board Statement: Not applicable.

Informed Consent Statement: Not applicable.

Conflicts of Interest: The authors declare that there are no conflicts of interest regarding the publication of this paper.

Abbreviations

AFB1	aflatoxin B1
AFB2	aflatoxin B2
AFG1	aflatoxin G1
AFG2	aflatoxin G2
AFs	aflatoxins
AMP	aromatic and medicinal plants
AOH	alternariol
BEA	beauvericin
DON-3-G	DON-3-glucoside
DON	deoxynivalenol
PDI	probable daily intake
ENA	enniatin A
ENA1	enniatin A1
ENB	enniatin B
ENB1	enniatin B1
ENs	enniatins
OTA	ochratoxin A
TENT	tentoxin
TDI	tolerable daily intake
ZEN	zearalenone
α-ZEL	α-zearalenol
β-ZEL	β-zearalenol
ZEN-4-Glc	zearalenone-4-glucoside
ZEN-4-Sulf	zearalenone-4-sulfate
α-ZEL-14-Glc	α–ZEL-14-glucoside
β-ZEL-14-Glc	β–ZEL-14-glucoside
ZEN-16-Glc	zearalenone-16-glucoside

References

1. Tripathy, V.; Basak, B.; Varghese, T.S.; Saha, A. Residues and contaminants in medicinal herbs—A review. *Phytochem. Lett.* **2015**, *14*, 67–78. [CrossRef]
2. WHO. *Promotion and Development of Training and Research in Traditional Medicine*; World Health Organization: Geneva, Switzerland, 1977; pp. 30–49.
3. Calixto, J.B. Efficacy, safety, quality control, marketing and regulatory guidelines for herbal medicines (phytotherapeutic agents). *Braz. J. Med Biol. Res.* **2000**, *33*, 179–189. [CrossRef] [PubMed]
4. Rizzo, I.; Vedoya, G.; Maurutto, S.; Haidukowski, M.; Varsavsky, E. Assessment of toxigenic fungi on Argentinean medicinal herbs. *Microbiol. Res.* **2004**, *159*, 113–120. [CrossRef] [PubMed]
5. Ałtyn, I.; Twarużek, M. Mycotoxin Contamination Concerns of Herbs and Medicinal Plants. *Toxins* **2020**, *12*, 182. [CrossRef] [PubMed]
6. Zhang, L.; Dou, X.-W.; Zhang, C.; Logrieco, A.F.; Yang, M. A Review of Current Methods for Analysis of Mycotoxins in Herbal Medicines. *Toxins* **2018**, *10*, 65. [CrossRef] [PubMed]
7. Borzekowski, A.; Drewitz, T.; Keller, J.; Pfeifer, D.; Kunte, H.J.; Koch, M.; Rohn, S.; Maul, R. Biosynthesis and Characterization of Zearalenone-14-Sulfate, Zearalenone-14-Glucoside and Zearalenone-16-Glucoside Using Common Fungal Strains. *Toxins* **2018**, *10*, 104. [CrossRef]
8. Engelhardt, G.; Ruhland, M.; Wallnofer, P.R. Metabolism of mycotoxins in plants. *Adv. Food Sci.* **1999**, *21*, 71–78.

9. Karlovsky, P. Biological detoxification of fungal toxins and its use in plant breeding, feed and food production. *Nat. Toxins* **1999**, *7*, 1–23. [CrossRef]
10. Engelhardt, G.; Zill, G.; Wohner, B.; Wallnfer, P.R. Transformation of the Fusarium mycotoxin zearalenone in maize cell suspension cultures. *Naturwissenschaften* **1988**, *75*, 309–310. [CrossRef]
11. Berthiller, F.; Werner, U.; Sulyok, M.; Krska, R.; Hauser, M.-T.; Schuhmacher, R. Liquid chromatography coupled to tandem mass spectrometry (LC-MS/MS) determination of phase II metabolites of the mycotoxin zearalenone in the model plant Arabidopsis thaliana. *Food Addit. Contam.* **2006**, *23*, 1194–1200. [CrossRef] [PubMed]
12. Sewald, N.; Von Gleissenthall, J.L.; Schuster, M.; Müller, G.; Aplin, R.T. Structure elucidation of a plant metabolite of 4-desoxynivalenol. *Tetrahedron Asymmetry* **1992**, *3*, 953–960. [CrossRef]
13. Berthiller, F.; Dall'Asta, C.; Schuhmacher, R.; Lemmens, M.; Adam, G.; Krska, R. Masked mycotoxins: Determination of a deoxynivalenol glucoside in artificially and naturally contaminated wheat by liquid chromatography-tandem mass spectrometry. *J. Agric. Food Chem.* **2005**, *53*, 3421–3425. [CrossRef]
14. Plasencia, J.; Mirocha, C.J. Isolation and characterization of zearalenone sulfate produced by *Fusarium* spp. *Appl. Environ. Microbiol.* **1991**, *57*, 146–150. [CrossRef] [PubMed]
15. Böswald, C.; Engelhardt, G.; Vogel, H.; Wallnöfer, P.R. Metabolism of the Fusarium mycotoxins zearalenone and deoxynivalenol by yeast strains of technological relevance. *Nat. Toxins* **1995**, *3*, 138–144. [CrossRef]
16. Gareis, M.; Bauer, J.; Thiem, J.; Plank, G.; Grabley, S.; Gedek, B. Cleavage of Zearalenone-Glycoside, a "Masked" Mycotoxin, during Digestion in Swine. *J. Vet. Med. Ser. B* **1990**, *37*, 236–240. [CrossRef]
17. Berthiller, F.; Hametner, C.; Krenn, P.; Schweiger, W.; Ludwig, R.; Adam, G.; Krska, R.; Schuhmacher, R. Preparation and characterization of the conjugated Fusarium mycotoxins zearalenone-4-O-β-D-glucopyranoside, α-zearalenol-4-O-β-D-glucopyranoside and β-zearalenol-4-O-β-D-glucopyranoside by MS/MS and two-dimensional NMR. *Food Addit. Contam.* **2009**, *26*, 207–213. [CrossRef] [PubMed]
18. Steinhoff, B. Review: Quality of herbal medicinal products: State of the art of purity assessment. *Phytomedicine* **2019**, *60*, 153003. [CrossRef] [PubMed]
19. European Commission. Commission Directive 2006/1881/EC of 19 December 2006, setting maximum levels for certain contaminants in food stuffs. *Off. J. Eur. Union* **2006**, *L364*, 5–24.
20. European Pharmacopoeia. Determination of Aflatoxin B1 in Herbal drugs. In *European Pharmacopoeia 9th Edition 2.8.18*; Council of Europe: Strasbourg, France, 2016; Volume 1, p. 289.
21. European Pharmacopoeia. *Council of Europe European Directorate for the Quality of Medicines (EDQM)*, 7th ed.; European Pharmacopoeia: Strasbourg, France, 2011.
22. Zinedine, A.; Brera, C.; Elakhdari, S.; Catano, C.; Debegnach, F.; Angelini, S.; De Santis, B.; Faid, M.; Benlemlih, M.; Minardi, V.; et al. Natural occurrence of mycotoxins in cereals and spices commercialized in Morocco. *Food Control* **2006**, *17*, 868–874. [CrossRef]
23. Zinedine, A.; Mañes, J. Occurrence and legislation of mycotoxins in food and feed from Morocco. *Food Control* **2009**, *20*, 334–344. [CrossRef]
24. Zinedine, A. Ochratoxin A in Moroccan Foods: Occurrence and Legislation. *Toxins* **2010**, *2*, 1121–1133. [CrossRef]
25. Monbaliu, S.; Wu, A.; Zhang, D.; Van Peteghem, C.; De Saeger, S. Multimycotoxin UPLC−MS/MS for Tea, Herbal Infusions and the Derived Drinkable Products. *J. Agric. Food Chem.* **2010**, *58*, 12664–12671. [CrossRef] [PubMed]
26. Kong, W.-J.; Shen, H.-H.; Zhang, X.-F.; Yang, X.-L.; Qiu, F.; Ou-Yang, Z.; Yang, M.-H. Analysis of zearalenone and α -zearalenol in 100 foods and medicinal plants determined by HPLC-FLD and positive confirmation by LC-MS-MS. *J. Sci. Food Agric.* **2013**, *93*, 1584–1590. [CrossRef] [PubMed]
27. Arroyo-Manzanares, N.; García-Campaña, A.M.; Gámiz-Gracia, L. Multiclass mycotoxin analysis in Silybum marianum by ultra high performance liquid chromatography–tandem mass spectrometry using a procedure based on QuEChERS and dispersive liquid–liquid microextraction. *J. Chromatogr. A* **2013**, *1282*, 11–19. [CrossRef] [PubMed]
28. Sharma, S.K.; Sumbali, G.; Sharma, V. Mycobial contamination and mycotoxinogenesis of Tinospora cordifolia: An important medicinal plant of India. *Int. J. Agric. Res. Innov. Technol.* **2014**, *3*, 16–21. [CrossRef]
29. Reinholds, I.; Bogdanova, E.; Pugajeva, I.; Bartkevics, V. Mycotoxins in herbal teas marketed in Latvia and dietary exposure assessment. *Food Addit. Contam. Part B* **2019**, *12*, 199–208. [CrossRef]
30. Pallarés, N.; Tolosa, J.; Mañes, J.; Ferrer, E. Occurrence of Mycotoxins in Botanical Dietary Supplement Infusion Beverages. *J. Nat. Prod.* **2019**, *82*, 403–406. [CrossRef]
31. Mannani, N.; Tabarani, A.; Abdennebi, E.H.; Zinedine, A. Assessment of aflatoxin levels in herbal green tea available on the Moroccan market. *Food Control* **2020**, *108*, 106882. [CrossRef]
32. *Bulletin Officiel 6514/2016. Arrêté Conjoint du Ministre de l'Agriculture et de la Pêche Maritime et du Ministre de la Santé n°1643-16 du 30 Mai 2016 Fixant les Limites Maximales de Contaminants Autorisées dans ou sur les Produits Primaires et les Produits Alimentaires*; Ministre de l'Agriculture et de la Pêche Maritime: Paris, France, 2016; p. 1681.
33. Duarte, S.; Salvador, N.; Machado, F.; Costa, E.; Almeida, A.; Silva, L.J.; Pereira, A.M.; Lino, C.; Pena, A. Mycotoxins in teas and medicinal plants destined to prepare infusions in Portugal. *Food Control* **2020**, *115*, 107290. [CrossRef]
34. Fraeyman, S.; Croubels, S.; Devreese, M.; Antonissen, G. Emerging Fusarium and Alternaria Mycotoxins: Occurrence, Toxicity and Toxicokinetics. *Toxins* **2017**, *9*, 228. [CrossRef] [PubMed]

35. Schoevers, E.J.; Santos, R.R.; Roelen, B.A.J. Alternariol disturbs oocyte maturation and preimplantation development. *Mycotoxin Res.* **2019**, *36*, 93–101. [CrossRef]
36. Abbas, M. Co-Occurrence of Mycotoxins and Its Detoxification Strategies. In *Mycotoxins—Impact and Management Strategies*; Njobeh, P.B., Stepman, F., Eds.; IntechOpen: London, UK, 2019. [CrossRef]
37. Santos, L.; Marín, S.; Sanchis, V.; Ramos, A.J. Screening of mycotoxin multicontamination in medicinal and aromatic herbs sampled in Spain. *J. Sci. Food Agric.* **2009**, *89*, 1802–1807. [CrossRef]
38. Vendl, O.; Crews, C.; MacDonald, S.; Krska, R.; Berthiller, F. Occurrence of free and conjugated Fusarium mycotoxins in cereal-based food. *Food Addit. Contam.* **2010**, *27*, 1148–1152. [CrossRef]
39. Alwakeel, S.S. The Effect of Mycotoxins found in some Herbal Plants on Biochemical Parameters in Blood of Female Albino Mice. *Pak. J. Biol. Sci.* **2009**, *12*, 637–642. [CrossRef] [PubMed]
40. FAO; Committee on Commodity Problems; Intergovernmental Group on Tea. *Twenty-Third Session*; CCP:TE 18/CRS1; FAO: Hangzhou, China, 2018.
41. IARC (International Agency for Research on Cancer). *IARC Monograph on the Evaluation of Carcinogenic Risk to Humans. Some Naturally Occurring Substances: Food Items and Constituent Heterocyclic Aromatic Amines and Mycotoxins*; IARC: Lyon, France, 1993.
42. JECFA (Joint FAO/WHO Expert Committee on Food Additives). *Safety Evaluation of Certain Mycotoxins in Food*; Series N°47; JECFA: Geneva, Switzerland, 2011.
43. Kovalsky Paris, M.P.; Schweiger, W.; Hametner, C.; Stückler, R.; Muehlbauer, G.J.; Varga, E.; Krska, R.; Berthiller, F.; Adam, G. Zearalenone-16-O-glucoside: A New Masked Mycotoxin. *J. Agric. Food Chem.* **2014**, *62*, 1181–1189. [CrossRef] [PubMed]
44. Dall'Erta, A.; Cirlini, M.; Dall'Asta, M.; Del Rio, D.; Galaverna, G.; Dall'Asta, C. Masked mycotoxins are efficiently hydrolyzed by human colonic microbiota releasing their aglycones. *Chem. Res. Toxicol.* **2013**, *26*, 305–312. [CrossRef]
45. EFSA. Appropriateness to set a group health-based guidance value for zearalenone and its modified forms. *EFSA J.* **2016**, *14*, 4425.
46. Tahraoui, A.; El-Hilaly, J.; Israili, Z.H.; Lyoussi, B. Ethnopharmacological survey of plants used in the traditional treatment of hypertension and diabetes in south-eastern Morocco (Errachidia province). *J. Ethnopharm.* **2007**, *110*, 105–117. [CrossRef]
47. Pallarés, N.; Font, G.; Mañes, J.; Ferrer, E. Multimycotoxin LC–MS/MS Analysis in Tea Beverages after Dispersive Liquid–Liquid Microextraction (DLLME). *J. Agric. Food Chem.* **2017**, *65*, 10282–10289. [CrossRef] [PubMed]
48. Juan, C.; Covarelli, L.; Beccari, G.; Colasante, V.; Mañes, J. Simultaneous analysis of twenty-six mycotoxins in durum wheat grain from Italy. *Food Control* **2016**, *62*, 322–329. [CrossRef]
49. European Food Safety Authority. Management of left-censored data in dietary exposure assessment of chemical substances. *EFSA J.* **2010**, *8*, 1557.
50. Schrenk, D.; Bignami, M.; Bodin, L.; Chipman, J.K.; del Mazo, J.; Grasl-Kraupp, B.; Wallace, H. European Food Safety Authority CONTAM Panel (EFSA Panel on Contaminants in the Food Chain). Scientific opinion—Risk assessment of aflatoxins in food. *EFSA J.* **2020**, *18*, 112.
51. Kuiper-Goodman, T. Uncertainties in the risk assessment of three mycotoxins: Aflatoxin, ochratoxin, and zearalenone. *Can. J. Physiol. Pharmacol.* **1990**, *68*, 1017–1024. [CrossRef] [PubMed]
52. JECFA—Joint FAO/WHO Expert Committee on Food Additives. *Safety Evaluation of Certain Mycotoxins in Food Prepared by the Fifty Sixth Meeting of the Joint FAO/WHO Expert Committee on Food Additives (Vol. 47)*; WHO Food Additives Series; FAO Food and Nutrition Paper 74; World Health Organization: Geneva, Switzerland, 2001; ISBN1 (FAO) 92 5104664 6. ISBN2 (WH0) 92 4166047 3. Available online: www.fao.org/3/a-bc528e.pdf (accessed on 8 February 2021).
53. SCF—Scientific Committee on Food. *Part. 6: Group Evaluation of T-2 Toxin, HT2 Toxin, Nivalenol and Deoxynivalenol*; Opinion of the Scientific Committee on Food on Fusarium Toxins; SCF: Brussels, Belgium, 2002; Available online: https://ec.europa.eu/food/sites/food/files/safety/docs/cs_contaminants_catalogue_fusarium_out123_en.pdf (accessed on 27 February 2002).

toxins

MDPI

Article

Patulin Mycotoxin in Mango and Orange Fruits, Juices, Pulps, and Jams Marketed in Pakistan

Shabbir Hussain [1,2], Muhammad Rafique Asi [1,*], Mazhar Iqbal [3,*], Nisha Khalid [1], Syed Wajih-ul-Hassan [1] and Agustín Ariño [4]

1 Food Toxicology Laboratory, Nuclear Institute for Agriculture and Biology College (NIAB-C), Pakistan Institute of Engineering and Applied Sciences (PIEAS), Jhang Road, Faisalabad 38000, Pakistan; shabbir.ne@gmail.com (S.H.); nishakhalid22@gmail.com (N.K.); wajih599@yahoo.com (S.W.-u.-H.)

2 Central Analytical Facility Division, Pakistan Institute of Nuclear Science and Technology (PINSTECH), P. O. Nilore, Islamabad 45650, Pakistan

3 Health Biotechnology Division, National Institute for Biotechnology and Genetic Engineering College (NIBGE-C), Pakistan Institute of Engineering and Applied Sciences (PIEAS), Jhang Road, Faisalabad 38000, Pakistan

4 Instituto Agroalimentario de Aragón—IA2 (Universidad de Zaragoza-CITA), Facultad de Veterinaria, 50013 Zaragoza, Spain; aarino@unizar.es

* Correspondence: asimuhammad@yahoo.co.uk (M.R.A.); hamzamgondal@gmail.com (M.I.)

Received: 19 November 2019; Accepted: 13 January 2020; Published: 16 January 2020

Abstract: The objective of the study was to explore the incidence of patulin (PAT) mycotoxin in mango and orange fruits and derived products marketed in Pakistan. A total of 274 samples, including 70 mango fruits, 63 mango-based products (juices, pulp, and jam), 77 orange fruits, and 64 orange-based products, were collected. PAT was determined by reverse-phase high-performance liquid chromatography (HPLC) with UV-Vis detector (276 nm). Linear detector response was observed ($R^2 > 0.99$), the limit of detection (LOD) was 5 μg/kg and recovery percentage was 97.4%. The incidence of PAT in mango samples was 61.7%, and the concentration ranged from <LOD to 6415 μg/kg with a mean of 110.9 μg/kg. Our results showed the high susceptibility of mango fruits to patulin, and it was observed that decayed mango fruits were most contaminated with PAT. Among the mango samples, PAT concentration was higher in fruits than in processed products such as mango juice, pulp, and jam. Toxin incidence in orange samples was 52.5% with concentrations from <LOD to 61 μg/kg and a mean of 6.3 μg/kg. As much as 29 samples of mango (21.8%) contained PAT concentration above the regulatory limit (50 μg/kg), whereas there was only one exceeding orange sample (0.7%). Our results show that PAT seems to be a problem in fruits, juices, and derived solid products, especially from mango, and needs surveillance on regular basis.

Keywords: patulin; mango; orange; fruit-derived products; food safety; regulatory limits

Key Contribution: Patulin mycotoxin was present in more than 50% samples of mango, orange, and fruit-derived products, with a significant number of exceeding samples. Results showed for the first time the high susceptibility of mango to patulin.

1. Introduction

Mycotoxins are compounds produced by naturally occurring fungi having toxic nature for animals and humans [1–3]. It has been considered that approximately 25% of total world food crops annually are contaminated with mycotoxins [4]. Patulin mycotoxin (a polyketide lactone 4-hydroxy-4H-furo (3,2c) pyran-2 (6H)-one; Figure 1) [5,6] belongs to a class of toxic compound with low molecular weight (154.121 g/mol) [7,8]. The molecular formula of patulin (PAT) is $C_7H_6O_4$; it is stable in aqueous media at 105–125 °C with melting point of 110 °C. It is a colorless and crystalline compound [9,10]. PAT is often associated with fruits, juices, and derived products, including foods intended for young children, because of the contamination with fungal species such as *Penicillium expansum*, *Aspergillus clavatus*, and *Byssochlamys nivea* [11]. These patulin-producing fungi attack susceptible products during growth, harvest, storage, or food processing. Among different fungi species, *Penicillium expansum*, which is commonly present in many varieties of fruits, is the major producer of PAT [12–14]. Patulin has been primarily associated with apple and apple-based products. However, the toxin may also contaminate other fruits, moldy feed, rotten vegetables, and wheat straw residue. It has been suggested that cold regions may become liable to temperate problems concerning patulin in foodstuffs due to climate change [15].

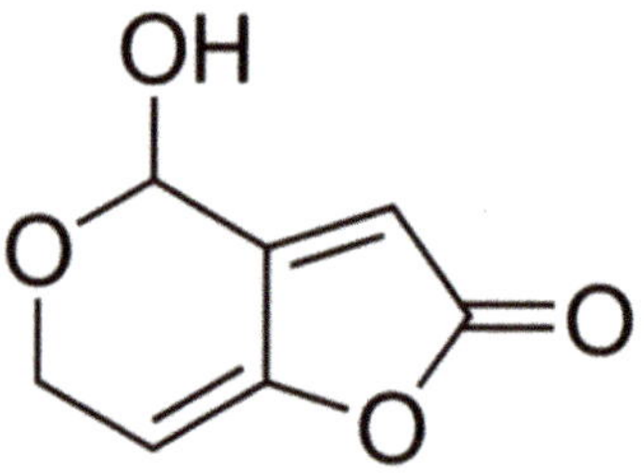

Figure 1. Molecular structure of patulin.

Due to contamination of food and feed at all phases of processing, storage, transportation, and sale, PAT has a critical effect in agriculture zone and food industry. PAT mycotoxin causes health hazards after ingestion of contaminated fruits and derived products. PAT toxicity relates to deleterious formation of adducts with sulfhydryl groups, producing acute and chronic toxicity problems in animals and humans [16]. Exposure to this mycotoxin is associated with immunological, neurological, and gastrointestinal outcomes such as distension, ulceration, and hemorrhage [17,18]. Body organs affected by PAT include kidney, liver, intestine, spleen, and stomach. PAT toxicity in mammalian cells and animals includes genotoxicity, teratogenicity, embryotoxicity, and immunotoxicity [19,20]. According to the International Agency for Research on Cancer (IARC), PAT is classified in the group 3 as "not classifiable as to its carcinogenicity to humans" [20].

The adverse health effects of PAT have led to the establishment of safe levels of PAT in foodstuffs. The Codex Alimentarius established the maximum level of PAT in fruits and juices at 50 μg/kg [21]. According to Commission Regulation (EC) No. 1881/2006, the European Union (EU) fixed maximum levels of PAT in fruit juices (50 μg/kg), solid apple products (25 μg/kg), and foods intended for infants and young children (10 μg/kg) [22]. Countries such as China, USA, and Canada have also established maximum levels for PAT in foods, primarily in apple-based products, in the range between 25 and 50 μg/kg [23–25]. Furthermore, the Joint Expert Committee for Food Additives has established a provisional maximum tolerable daily intake of 0.4 μg/kg body weight [26].

It is well established that the main sources of PAT in human diet are apples and apple-derived products, so the majority of reported studies concern patulin determination in apple-based foodstuffs [27,28]. However, monitoring of PAT in other fruits and fruit-derived products should not be neglected. A previous study carried out in Pakistan on various fruits, juices and smoothies showed the presence of PAT in more than 50% of samples with a mean concentration of 182 μg/kg (Iqbal et al., 2018) [29]. However, mango and orange fruits, and their derived products were not included in the survey.

In view of the above details, the present research has focused on exploring the current occurrence of PAT in mango and orange fruits, fruit juices and derived products, and to compare the levels of PAT with maximum regulatory levels.

2. Results

2.1. Method Validation

The patulin contamination in fruits and fruit-based products is a worldwide problem, and effective control of PAT strongly depends on reliable analytical methods. The validation of the analytical method for PAT included determination of linearity, recovery, precision (repeatability and reproducibility), and sensitivity (limit of detection, LOD, and limit of quantification, LOQ). Linearity was checked by injection into HPLC-UV of PAT standards in the range from 5 to 100 μg/L (Table 1), the correlation coefficient obtained was 0.9916. The average retention time of PAT was 6.383 ± 0.05 min with good coefficient of variation (0.75%). Recovery experiments were done by spiking negative samples of mango and orange at PAT concentrations of 10, 50, and 100 μg/kg. After 1 h, the spiked samples were processed and analyzed by HPLC. The average recovery was 97.4%, with good values for repeatability (relative standard deviation, RSD_r less than 5%) and reproducibility (RSD_R less than 15%). The limit of detection (LOD) and quantification (LOQ) were determined by signal-to-noise ratio and were 5 μg/kg and 15 μg/kg, respectively. In conclusion, the analytical method used allowed for accurate quantitative determination of patulin in mango and orange samples and fulfilled performance requirements of Commission Regulation (EC) No. 401/2006 [30].

Table 1. Linearity of standard working solutions of patulin (PAT). Values are mean of triplicate analysis.

Retention Time (min)	Concentration PAT μg/L	Average Peak Area (mV)	Standard Deviation	Coefficient of Variation (%)
6.383	5	327	16	4.89
6.430	10	533	21	3.94
6.381	30	1473	51	3.46
6.338	50	3451	129	3.74
6.444	70	4714	218	4.62
6.323	100	7181	283	3.94

The analytical method used is based on AOAC method 995.10, which was successfully validated through collaborative studies for patulin determination in apple products [31]. In detail, the method consists of four steps, including liquid–liquid extraction with ethyl acetate, sodium carbonate clean-up, sodium sulfate drying, and LC-UV determination. Na_2CO_3 neutralization is used to lower interference from the phenolic compounds in fruit matrices, such as the 5-hydroxymethylfurfural (5-HMF) [32]. The main shortcoming of the method is the presence of interfering matrix components that might affect chromatographic separation. To better remove interferences for patulin determination, a series of representative random samples were additionally subjected to a second purification step using multifunctional clean-up columns MFC 228. The chromatographic separation was improved, though no significant differences were observed in recovery percentage and patulin concentration. Figure 2 represents HPLC chromatograms of natural occurrence of patulin in mango and orange samples.

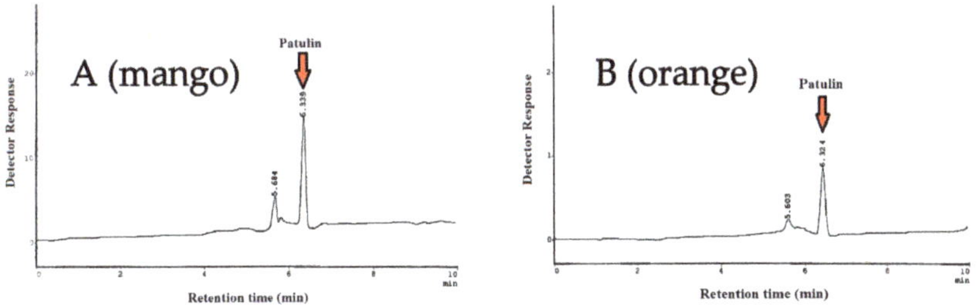

Figure 2. HPLC chromatograms of natural occurrence of patulin in mango sample (**A**) and orange sample (**B**).

2.2. Occurrence of Patulin in Fruits and Derived Products

Results of PAT occurrence in 133 samples of mango fruits and derived products are shown in Table 2. A total of 70 samples of mango fruits along with 63 samples of mango-based products (juices, pulp, and jam) were randomly collected from different sites of Punjab, Pakistan. From the data, it is evident that 82 samples were found PAT-contaminated with an incidence level (61.7%) and a total mean concentration of 110.9 μg/kg. The percentage of positive samples of Faisalabad, Sheikhupura, Multan, Shorkot, and Rawalpindi was 50%, 33.3%, 53.3%, 71.4%, and 40%, respectively, whereas the percentage of contamination in mango juice, pulp, and jam was 75%, 87.5%, and 60%, respectively. The average PAT levels in mango fruits were 348 μg/kg, 42.6 μg/kg, 87.5 μg/kg, 254.2 μg/kg, and 14.7 μg/kg in samples collected from Faisalabad, Sheikhupura, Multan, Shorkot, and Rawalpindi, respectively. The average PAT levels in mango juices, pulp, and jam of different brands were 24.3 μg/kg, 82.3 μg/kg, and 5.0 μg/kg, respectively. Although the incidence of patulin was very similar between samples of mango fruit and derived products, the concentration was higher in the first (186.6 μg/kg) compared with the second (26.9 μg/kg). Among the mango fruit samples, it is noteworthy a sample from a Faisalabad's local market with an extremely high PAT content (6415 μg/kg), as well as another sample from Shorkot with a very high PAT content of 2030 μg/kg. In the present study, healthy mango fruits were less contaminated with PAT in comparison with decayed ones.

Table 2. Incidence of patulin (μg/kg) in mango fruits and derived products.

Sample	Sampling Site	n Total (Positive)	Incidence %	Mean ± SD μg/kg	Maximum Value μg/kg	n (%) > 50 μg/kg
Mango fruit	Faisalabad	22 (11)	50%	348.0 ± 1360.2	6415	7 (31.8%)
Mango fruit	Sheikhupura	9 (3)	33.3%	42.6 ± 106.1	313	2 (22.2%)
Mango fruit	Multan	15 (8)	53.3%	87.5 ± 166.6	611	5 (33.3%)
Mango fruit	Shorkot	14 (10)	71.4%	254.2 ± 536.9	2030	8 (57.1%)
Mango fruit	Rawalpindi	10 (4)	40%	14.7 ± 34.2	113	1 (10%)
Mango juice	Local markets	40 (30)	75%	24.3 ± 38.1	226	4 (10%)
Mango pulp	Super markets	8 (7)	87.5%	82.3 ± 115.0	301	2 (25%)
Mango jam	General stores	15 (9)	60%	5.0 ± 4.3	13	0 (0%)
TOTAL	–	133 (82)	61.7%	110.9 ± 586.4	6415	29 (21.8%)

Table 3 reports the PAT incidence and concentration in 141 samples of orange fruits and derived products, comprising 77 samples of orange fruits along with 64 samples of orange-based products (juices, pulp, and jam), which were randomly collected from different sites of Punjab, Pakistan. A total of 74 samples were found positive for PAT (52.5%) with a total mean concentration of 6.3 μg/kg, much lower than that of 110.9 μg/kg found in mango. The incidences in orange fruits were 60%, 88.9%, 28.6%, 53.9%, and 18.2% in samples taken from Faisalabad, Sargodha, Layyah, Toba Tek Singh, and Sahiwal, respectively, while 71.4%, 60%, and 21% was assessed in orange juices, pulp, and jams, respectively. The average concentration of PAT in orange fruits was 7.6 μg/kg, 8.1 μg/kg, 8.7 μg/kg, 5.1 μg/kg, and 1.6 μg/kg in samples from Faisalabad, Sargodha, Layyah, Toba Tek Singh, and Sahiwal, respectively. Additionally, orange juices, pulp, and jams contained 8.3 μg/kg, 6.5 μg/kg, and 1.1 μg/kg, respectively. Both incidence and levels of PAT were similar in orange fruits and derived products.

Table 3. Incidence of patulin (μg/kg) in orange fruits and derived products.

Sample	Sampling Site	n Total (Positive)	Incidence %	Mean ± SD μg/kg	Maximum Value μg/kg	n (%) > 50 μg/kg
Orange fruit	Faisalabad	30 (18)	60%	7.6 ± 7.4	25	0 (0%)
Orange fruit	Sargodha	9 (8)	88.9%	8.1 ± 4.6	15	0 (0%)
Orange fruit	Layyah	14 (4)	28.6%	8.7 ± 19.9	61	1 (7.2%)
Orange fruit	Toba Tek Singh	13 (7)	53.9%	5.1 ± 5.4	15	0 (0%)
Orange fruit	Sahiwal	11 (2)	18.2%	1.6 ± 3.9	12	0 (0%)
Orange juice	Local markets	35 (25)	71.4%	8.3 ± 7.7	31	0 (0%)
Orange pulp	Super markets	10 (6)	60%	6.5 ± 10.9	37	0 (0%)
Orange jam	General stores	19 (4)	21%	1.1 ± 2.2	6	0 (0%)
TOTAL	–	141 (74)	52.5%	6.3 ± 9.1	61	1 (0.7%)

The percentage of mango samples that exceeded the maximum level of PAT (50 μg/kg) was 29 out of 133 (21.8%) (Table 2), while only 1 out 141 (0.7%) orange samples surpassed the maximum level (Table 3). The maximum percentage of violative mango samples came from Shorkot (57.1%), a city situated southwest of Faisalabad, while northern Rawalpindi, whose elevation above sea level is 508 m, showed the least noncompliant samples (10%). Similarly, exceeding orange samples only came from Layyah, a city located southwest of Faisalabad.

3. Discussion

The contamination with PAT in analyzed fruits and derived products showed higher incidence and concentration values in mango as compared with orange samples. Some mango samples exhibited PAT levels well above the regulatory limit (50 μg/kg), with a maximum of 6415 μg/kg in a sample from Faisalabad. Patulin-producing molds are responsible for the rotting of some fruits and vegetables, especially pomaceous fruits such as apples and pears [1]. Regarding mango samples, fruits that were decayed showed higher PAT levels as compared with apparently healthy fruits. In Pakistan, management by Good Agriculture Practices (GAPs) is not generally applied to mango production, and fungicides are not applied during the growth stage of mango fruits. In general, external wounds and ripening make fruits more sensitive to contamination by molds, so wounded and ripened fruits have a higher risk of contamination in the absence of fungicide use. Not in vain, extraordinarily high patulin levels up to 113343 μg/kg have been reported in the rotten area of an apple [33]. Therefore, wounded and ripened mangoes can be very exposed to postharvest diseases. To the best of our knowledge, there is no previous publication reporting the high susceptibility of mango to patulin-producing molds and the subsequent patulin contamination.

The extremely high level of patulin found in a mango sample (6415 μg/kg) is only comparable to those of 7339, 13808, and 19662 μg/kg reported in samples of fruit juices from Argentina [34]. Present results are also in agreement with a previous study carried out in Pakistan on patulin in different fruits, juices, and smoothies [29], with a maximum of 1100 μg/kg in a sample of red globe grapes. Other samples type such as seedless grapes, apples, pears, and tomato exceeded 500 μg/kg. Similarly, other authors have reported high patulin concentrations in apple juice from the USA (2700 μg/kg) [35] and concentrated juices from Tunisia (889 μg/kg) [2]. In Turkey, the maximum concentration of patulin in apple sour reached 1416 μg/kg [36]. In addition, fifty samples of apple juices were investigated for patulin levels in India [37], with an incidence of 24% positives and a maximum of 845 μg/kg. Beretta et al. analyzed 82 samples of apple-based foods for PAT, with maximum concentrations in juice made with apple pulp and in fruits. In rotten apples, not only was the amount of patulin very high in the rotten area (1150 μg/kg), but the mycotoxin had also spread to areas unaffected by fungus [38]. Finally, Yurdun et al. [39] reported a sample of apple juice with a patulin level of 733 μg/kg. In turn, PAT was not detected in mango juice from two studies carried out in Malaysia [40,41].

In other studies, patulin concentrations attained levels in the range of 5–50 μg/kg, such as Al-Hazmi et al. in samples of apple juice from Saudi Arabia [42]. In Greece, a study revealed the presence of PAT in 100% of the fruit juice samples examined [43]. The mean values of PAT in concentrated fruit juices and in commercial fruit juices were 10.54 μg/kg and 5.57 μg/kg, respectively. The most contaminated samples were four concentrated juices, ranging from 18.10 to 36.8 μg/kg. The mean concentration of patulin in orange juices was 6.80 μg/kg. In South Korea, a study on 72 samples of fruit juices reported nine positive for patulin (three apple, two orange, and four grape juices), with a maximum concentration of 30.9 μg/kg in an orange juice sample [44].

In the undertaken study, results on occurrence of PAT in mango and orange fruits and their derived products, which are consumed in Punjab, Pakistan, depicted higher contamination levels, especially from mango. PAT contamination in fruits and derived products is a burning issue for the health implications, so their surveillance is a basic and urgent need. In Pakistan, a variety of fruits with good flavor and taste are grown in tropical and subtropical climate and are available throughout the year. The various varieties of fruits are grown on an area of about 800,000 hectares with worth production of 7.05 million tones. During crop season 2017–2018, 10% of the total fruit production was exported [45]. Good agriculture practices (GAP) and postharvest control strategies must be adopted to inhibit PAT formation in fruits and derived products for the prevention and reduction of exposure to this mycotoxin. Proper picking, handling, and packaging operations, as well as storage and transportation of fruits can limit fungal growth and patulin production.

4. Conclusions

Patulin contamination in fruits and derived products is a worldwide problem due to its risky toxicity. An HPLC method with UV detection for the determination of PAT, which is fast, reliable, and sensitive, was successfully validated and could be applied for routine analysis and monitoring of fruits, pulps, juices, and derived products. PAT concentrations were higher in mango than in orange samples, and greater in whole fruits than in derived products such as juice, pulp, and jam. A significant percentage of mango samples exceeded the maximum levels established for patulin. Further studies are needed to develop strategies that are helpful to reduce the presence of patulin-producing fungi in these commodities. Therefore, a better understanding of the underlying mechanisms of patulin toxigenesis in mango is needed. Regular monitoring of fruits and their products during the harvest and processing stages is recommended to enhance the confidence of end users. The results of the present study would be highly beneficial for the horticulturists, processors, traders, and consumers.

5. Materials and Methods

5.1. Sampling

A total of 274 samples including 70 mango fruits, 40 mango juice, 8 mango pulp, 15 mango jam, 77 orange fruits, 35 orange juice, 10 orange pulp, and 19 orange jam were purchased in different areas of Central Punjab (Pakistan) from January to December 2018. The mango (*Mangifera indica*) and orange (*Citrus sinensis*) fruits were collected in supermarkets and local markets from Faisalabad, and from cities north (Rawalpindi, Sargodha, and Sheikhupura) or south (Multan, Shorkot, Layyah, Toba Tek Singh, and Sahiwal) Faisalabad. The mango- and orange-based products (juice, pulp, and jam) were from commercial brands of nationwide distribution purchased from supermarkets, local markets, and general stores in Faisalabad district. All samples were stored in their original packages at 4 °C until they were analyzed. The samples were opened and thoroughly homogenized.

5.2. Chemicals and Reagents

Acetonitrile (HPLC grade), glacial acetic acid, sodium chloride, and sodium carbonate were purchased from Merck. Ethyl acetate, methanol, sodium sulfate anhydrous (analytical grade), 5-hydroximethyl furfural (5-HMF), and patulin (5 mg of solid crystalline) were purchased from

Sigma-Aldrich (Saint-Louis, MO, USA). Stock solution of patulin 1 mg /mL was prepared in acetonitrile and stored at −4 °C. Necessary volumes of stock solution were taken for working solutions (5, 10, 30, 50, 70, 100 μg/L) in 0.1% acetic acid. PriboFast multifunctional cleanup columns MFC 228 (Pribolab Pte. Ltd., Singapore) were applied for the optimization of the purification process.

5.3. Sample Preparation and Extraction

The purchased fruit samples were chosen free from debris, washed with water, shade-dried, and cut into small pieces with sharp knife. A sample of about 500 g was homogenized using high-speed blender (Braun Blender Mix 2000, Marktheidenfel, Germany). Samples of products (juice, pulp, and jam) were taken directly from the original packages. Analytical method for PAT was based on AOAC method 995.10 with little modifications [31]. Homogenized samples (25 g or 25 mL in triplicate) were extracted twice with 50 mL ethyl acetate along with 2 g sodium chloride in 250 mL Erlenmeyer flask (Pyrex, Germany) by shaking at high speed in horizontal shaker (Gunther and Co, Bremen, Germany) for one hour. The upper organic layers were combined and cleaned up with sodium carbonate solution (1.5% Na_2CO_3). Cleaned extract was rapidly dehydrated with 10 g anhydrous sodium sulfate (Na_2SO_4) and filtered with Whatman No. 1 filter paper. For alternative second-time clean-up, 9 mL cleaned extract was passed through a multifunctional column MFC 228, and 4 mL purified extract was collected. The extracts were evaporated to dryness under a stream of nitrogen. The dry residue was immediately dissolved in 1000 μL of 0.1% acetic acid and passed through syringe filter (0.22 μm, Millipore, Darmstadt, Germany). The samples were analyzed for PAT by reverse-phase HPLC equipped with UV-Vis detector (SPD-10AS, Shimadzu, Japan) in isocratic mode. The injection volume was 20 μL, and total run time was 10 min for PAT analysis.

5.4. Apparatus and HPLC Conditions

HPLC comprised a delivery pump (LS-10AS), system controller (SCL-10A), column oven (CTO-10A), UV-Vis detector (SPD-10AS), and Communication Bus Module (CBM-101), Shimadzu, Japan. Separations were performed in a Discovery HS C18 silica-based column (250 × 4.6 mm, 5 μm particle size; Supelco, Bellefonte, PA, USA), maintained at 30 °C with a flow rate of 1.5 mL/min in isocratic mode. Mobile phase was a mixture of acetonitrile:water (10:90, *v/v*) filtrated with 0.45μm filter (Nylon 66 membranes filter, Supelco, Bellefonte, PA, USA). Cleaned sample extracts and standards were injected using a Rheodyne injector (20 μL loop) in reverse-phase system, and wavelength of detection was 276 nm. Chromatograms were received with CLASS LC-10 Acquisition software. Qualitative and quantitative determinations of PAT were made comparing the retention time and peak area of reference standards. For method validation, a test was performed to confirm the peak separation of PAT and its principal interference 5-HMF. A solution containing 2 μg/mL of 5-HMF and 2 μg/mL of PAT was prepared and injected into HPLC (Figure 3).

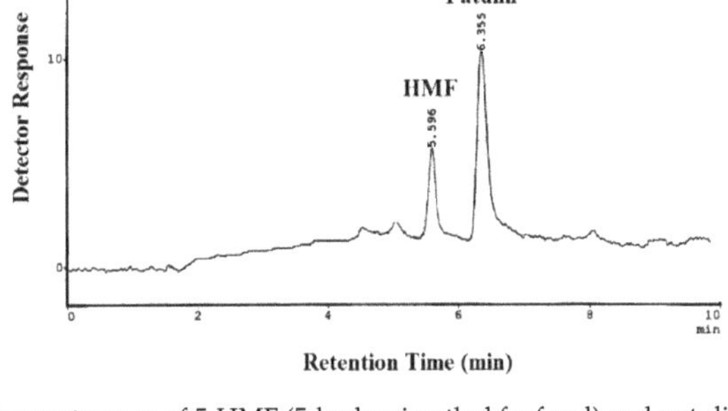

Figure 3. Chromatogram of 5-HMF (5-hydroximethyl furfural) and patulin standards.

5.5. Statistical Analysis

The compiled data were subjected to statistical analysis. Triplicate results of PAT in fruits, juices, and derived products were calculated in Excel software, and data were given as mean with standard deviation. Samples with a concentration of PAT higher than the LOD were considered positive. For samples with a concentration below the LOD, a value of zero was considered for calculating the mean. The significance differences in PAT level between the groups were analyzed by one-way ANOVA test ($p < 0.05$) using SPSS (IBM SPSS Statistics 19, Armonk, NY, USA, 2010).

Author Contributions: M.R.A. conceptualized the work and conceived the experimental design; S.H. collected samples and carried out formal analysis; M.I., N.K., and S.W.-u.-H. contributed to the methodology and helped with laboratory analyses. S.H. performed statistical analyses and helped in the interpretation of the results. M.R.A. and A.A. contributed to the analysis and interpretation of the results. S.H., M.R.A., and A.A. wrote the paper. All authors read and approved the published version of the document.

Funding: Author Ariño thanks the Government of Aragón and FEDER 2014–2020 (grant Grupo A06_17R) for support.

Acknowledgments: Authors are highly thankful to PAEC and NIAB management to provide the permission and analytical facilities to carry out PhD study and complete the research work in Food Toxicology Laboratories.

Conflicts of Interest: The authors declare no conflict of interest.

References

1. Marín, S.; Mateo, E.M.; Sanchis, V.; Valle-Algarra, F.M.; Ramos, A.J.; Jiménez, M. Patulin contamination in fruit derivatives, including baby food, from the Spanish market. *Food Chem.* **2011**, *124*, 563–568. [CrossRef]
2. Zouaoui, N.; Sbaii, N.; Bacha, H.; Abid-Essefi, S. Occurrence of patulin in various fruit juice marketed in Tunisia. *Food Control* **2015**, *51*, 356–360. [CrossRef]
3. Raiola, A.; Tenore, G.C.; Manyes, L.; Meca, G.; Ritieni, A. Risk analysis of main mycotoxins occurring in food for children: An overview. *Food Chem. Toxicol.* **2015**, *84*, 169–180. [CrossRef]
4. Negedu, A.; Atawodi, S.E.; Ameh, J.B.; Umoh, V.J.; Tanko, H.Y. Economic and health perspectives of mycotoxins: A review. *Cont. J. Biomed. Sci.* **2011**, *5*, 5–26.
5. Brase, S.; Encinas, A.; Keck, J.; Nising, C.F. Chemistry and biology of mycotoxins and related fungal metabolites. *Chem. Rev.* **2009**, *109*, 3903–3990. [CrossRef] [PubMed]
6. Guo, W.; Pi, F.; Zhang, H.; Sun, J.; Zhang, Y.; Sun, X. A novel molecularly imprinted electrochemical sensor modified with carbon dots, chitosan, gold nanoparticles for the determination of patulin. *Biosens. Bioelectron.* **2017**, *98*, 299–304. [CrossRef] [PubMed]
7. Tannous, J.; Atoui, A.; El Khoury, A.; Francis, Z.; Oswald, I.P.; Puel, O.; Lteif, R. A study on the physicochemical parameters for Penicillium expansum growth and patulin production: Effect of temperature, pH, and water activity. *Food Sci. Nutr.* **2016**, *4*, 611–622. [CrossRef] [PubMed]
8. Magan, N.; Olsen, M. *Mycotoxins in Food: Detection and Control*; Woodhead Publishing Limited: Cambridge, UK, 2004.
9. González-Osnaya, L.; Soriano, J.M.; Moltó, J.C.; Manes, J. Exposure to patulin from consumption of apple-based products. *Food Addit. Contam.* **2007**, *24*, 1268–1274. [CrossRef]
10. Cunha, S.C.; Faria, M.A.; Pereira, V.L.; Oliveira, T.M.; Lima, A.C.; Pinto, E. Patulin assessment and fungi identification in organic and conventional fruits and derived products. *Food Control* **2014**, *44*, 185–190. [CrossRef]
11. Tannous, J.; Keller, N.P.; Atoui, A.; El Khoury, A.; Lteif, R.; Oswald, I.P.; Puel, O. Secondary metabolism in Penicillium expansum: Emphasis on recent advances in patulin research. *Crit. Rev. Food Sci. Nutr.* **2018**, *58*, 2082–2098. [CrossRef]
12. Marin, S.; Ramos, A.J.; Cano-Sancho, G.; Sanchis, V. Mycotoxins: Occurrence, toxicology, and exposure assessment. *Food Chem. Toxicol.* **2013**, *60*, 218–237. [CrossRef] [PubMed]
13. Moake, M.M.; Padilla-Zakour, O.I.; Worobo, R.W. Comprehensive review of patulin control methods in foods. *Compr. Rev. Food Sci. Food Saf.* **2005**, *4*, 8–21. [CrossRef]

14. Cheraghali, A.M.; Mohammadi, H.R.; Amirahmadi, M.; Yazdanpanah, H.; Abouhossain, G.; Zamanian, F.; Khansari, M.G.; Afshar, M. Incidence of patulin contamination in apple juice produced in Iran. *Food Control* **2005**, *16*, 165–167. [CrossRef]
15. Paterson, R.R.M.; Lima, N. How will climate change affect mycotoxins in food? *Food Res. Int.* **2010**, *43*, 1902–1914. [CrossRef]
16. Boussabbeh, M.; Ben Salem, I.; Prola, A.; Guilbert, A.; Bacha, H.; Abid-Essefi, S.; Lemaire, C. Patulin induces apoptosis through ROS-mediated endoplasmic reticulum stress pathway. *Toxicol. Sci.* **2015**, *144*, 328–337. [CrossRef]
17. Pal, S.; Singh, N.; Ansari, K.M. Toxicological effects of patulin mycotoxin on the mammalian system: An overview. *Toxicol. Res.* **2017**, *6*, 764–771. [CrossRef]
18. da Rocha, M.E.B.; Freire, F.D.C.O.; Maia, F.E.F.; Guedes, M.I.F.; Rondina, D. Mycotoxins and their effects on human and animal health. *Food Control* **2014**, *36*, 159–165. [CrossRef]
19. Puel, O.; Galtier, P.; Oswald, I.P. Biosynthesis and toxicological effects of patulin. *Toxins* **2010**, *2*, 613–631. [CrossRef]
20. Donmez-Altuntas, H.; Gokalp-Yildiz, P.; Bitgen, N.; Hamurcu, Z. Evaluation of genotoxicity, cytotoxicity and cytostasis in human lymphocytes exposed to patulin by using the cytokinesis-block micronucleus cytome (CBMN cyt) assay. *Mycotoxin Res.* **2013**, *29*, 63–70. [CrossRef]
21. Codex Alimentarius Commission (CAC). Codex General Standard for Contaminants and Toxins in Food and Feed. Codex STAN 193-1995; 1995, p. 44. Available online: http://www.fao.org/fao-who-codexalimentarius/codex-texts/list-standards/en/ (accessed on 16 January 2020).
22. European Commission. European Union Commission Regulation No. 1881/2006 setting maximum levels for certain contaminants in foodstuffs. *Off. J. Eur. Union* **2006**, *364*, 5–24.
23. van Egmond, H.P.; Schothorst, R.C.; Jonker, M.A. Regulations relating to mycotoxins in food. *Anal. Bioanal. Chem.* **2007**, *389*, 147–157. [CrossRef] [PubMed]
24. Food and Drug Administration (FDA). Compliance policy guidance for FDA staff. Sec. 510.150 Apple juice, apple juice concentrates, and apple juice products, Adulteration with patulin. In *Compliance Policy Guide*; U.S. Food and Drug Administration: Silver Spring, MD, USA, 2004.
25. Health Canada. Canadian Standards for Various Chemical Contaminants in Foods. In *Food and Drug Regulations*; Health Canada, Ed.: Ottawa, ON, Canada, 2014.
26. *Joint Expert Committee on Food Additives*; 44th Report of the JECFA. Technical Report Series 589; World Health Organization: Rome, Italy, 1995.
27. Ioi, J.D.; Zhou, T.; Tsao, R.; Marcone, M.F. Mitigation of patulin in fresh and processed foods and beverages. *Toxins* **2017**, *9*, 157. [CrossRef] [PubMed]
28. Zhong, L.; Carere, J.; Lu, Z.; Lu, F.; Zhou, T. Patulin in apples and apple-based food products: The burdens and the mitigation strategies. *Toxins* **2018**, *10*, 475. [CrossRef] [PubMed]
29. Iqbal, S.Z.; Malik, S.; Asi, M.R.; Selamat, J.; Malik, N. Natural occurrence of patulin in different fruits, juices and smoothies and evaluation of dietary intake in Punjab, Pakistan. *Food Control* **2018**, *84*, 370–374. [CrossRef]
30. European Union Commission Regulation No 401/2006 laying down the methods of sampling and analysis for the official control of the levels of mycotoxins in foodstuffs. *Off. J. Eur. Union* **2006**, *70*, 12–34.
31. AOAC International. AOAC Official Method 995.10 Patulin in apple juice. In *Official Methods of Analysis of AOAC International*, 18th ed.; Horwitz, W., Ed.; AOAC International: Gaithersburg, MD, USA, 2005.
32. Li, X.; Li, H.; Li, X.; Zhang, Q. Determination of trace patulin in apple-based food matrices. *Food Chem.* **2017**, *233*, 290–301. [CrossRef]
33. Majerus, P.; Kapp, K. *Assessment of Dietary Intake of Patulin by the Population of EU Member States*; Reports on Tasks for Scientific Cooperation, Task 3.2.8; SCOOP Report: Brussels, Belgium, 2002.
34. Oteiza, J.M.; Khaneghah, A.M.; Campagnollo, F.B.; Granato, D.; Mahmoudi, M.R.; Sant'Ana, A.S.; Gianuzzi, L. Influence of production on the presence of patulin and ochratoxin A in fruit juices and wines of Argentina. *LWT Food Sci. Technol.* **2017**, *80*, 200–207. [CrossRef]
35. Harris, K.L.; Bobe, G.; Bourquin, L.D. Patulin surveillance in apple cider and juice marketed in Michigan. *J. Food Prot.* **2009**, *72*, 1255–1261. [CrossRef]
36. İçli, N. Occurrence of patulin and 5-hydroxymethylfurfural in apple sour, which is a traditional product of Kastamonu, Turkey. *Food Addit. Contam. Part A* **2019**, *36*, 952–963. [CrossRef]

37. Saxena, N.; Dwivedi, P.D.; Ansari, K.M.; Das, M. Patulin in apple juices: Incidence and likely intake in an Indian population. *Food Addit. Contam.* **2008**, *1*, 140–146. [CrossRef]
38. Beretta, B.; Gaiaschi, A.; Galli, C.L.; Restani, P. Patulin in apple-based foods: Occurrence and safety evaluation. *Food Addit. Contam.* **2000**, *17*, 399–406. [CrossRef] [PubMed]
39. Yurdun, T.; Omurtag, G.Z.; Ersoy, O. Incidence of patulin in apple juices marketed in Turkey. *J. Food Prot.* **2001**, *64*, 1851–1853. [CrossRef] [PubMed]
40. Abu-Bakar, N.B.; Makahleh, A.; Saad, B. Vortex-assisted liquid-liquid microextraction coupled with high performance liquid chromatography for the determination of furfurals and patulin in fruit juices. *Talanta* **2014**, *120*, 47–54. [CrossRef] [PubMed]
41. Lee, T.P.; Sakai, R.; Abdul Manaf, N.; Mohd Rodhi, A.; Saad, B. High performance liquid chromatography method for the determination of patulin and 5-hydroxymethylfurfural in fruit juices marketed in Malaysia. *Food Control* **2014**, *38*, 142–149. [CrossRef]
42. Al-Hazmi, N. Determination of patulin and ochratoxin A using HPLC in apple juice samples in Saudi Arabia. *Saudi J. Biol. Sci.* **2010**, *17*, 353–359. [CrossRef]
43. Moukas, A.; Panagiotopoulou, V.; Markaki, P. Determination of patulin in fruit juices using HPLCDAD and GCMSD techniques. *Food Chem.* **2008**, *109*, 860–867. [CrossRef]
44. Cho, M.S.; Kim, K.; Seo, E.; Kassim, N.; Mtenga, A.B.; Shim, W.B.; Lee, S.H.; Chung, D.H. Occurrence of patulin in various fruit juices from South Korea: An exposure assessment. *Food Sci. Biotechnol.* **2010**, *19*, 1–5. [CrossRef]
45. Government of Pakistan. *Fruit, Vegetables and Condiments Statistics of Pakistan 2017–2018*; Government of Pakistan, Ministry of National Food Security & Research, Economic Wing: Islamabad, Pakistan, 2019.

toxins

MDPI

Article

Ochratoxin A in Beers Marketed in Portugal: Occurrence and Human Risk Assessment

Liliana J. G. Silva *, Ana C. Teixeira, André M. P. T. Pereira, Angelina Pena and Celeste M. Lino

LAQV, REQUIMTE, Laboratory of Bromatology and Pharmacognosy, Faculty of Pharmacy, University of Coimbra, Polo III, Azinhaga de Stª Comba, 3000-548 Coimbra, Portugal; catarina_tex@hotmail.com (A.C.T.); andrepereira@ff.uc.pt (A.M.P.T.P.); apena@ci.uc.pt (A.P.); cmlino@ci.uc.pt (C.M.L.)

* Correspondence: ljgsilva@ff.uc.pt

Received: 24 February 2020; Accepted: 11 April 2020; Published: 12 April 2020

Abstract: Ochratoxin A (OTA) is produced by fungi present in several agricultural products with much relevance to food safety. Since this mycotoxin is widely found in cereals, beer has a potential contamination risk. Therefore, it was deemed essential to quantify, for the first time, the levels of OTA in beer, a cereal-based product that is marketed in Portugal, as well as to calculate the human estimated weekly intake (EWI) and risk assessment. A total of 85 samples were analyzed through immunoaffinity clean-up, followed by liquid chromatography-fluorescence detection (LC-FD). This analytical methodology allowed a limit of quantification (LOQ) of 0.43 μg/L. The results showed that 10.6% were contaminated at levels ranging between <LOQ and 11.25 μg/L, with an average of 3.14 ± 4.09 μg/L. Samples of industrial production presented lower incidence and contamination levels than homemade and craft beers. On what concerns human risk, the calculated EWI was significantly lower than the tolerable weekly intake (TWI). However, in the worst case scenario, based on a high concentration, the rate EWI/TWI was 138.01%.

Keywords: ochratoxin A; beer; immunoaffinity clean-up; LC-FD; human risk assessment

Key Contribution: The first immunoaffinity column (IAC)-LC–FD OTA analysis of beer marketed in Portugal showed that only 10.59% of the samples were positive with a mean of 3.14 ± 4.09 μg/L, with homemade and craft production beers presenting higher frequencies and levels. Regarding human risk assessment, the EWI was considerably lower than the TWI established.

1. Introduction

Mycotoxins, secondary metabolites produced by fungi, affect 25% of crops worldwide [1]. Mycotoxin contamination usually takes place during crop growth due to adverse environmental conditions, inappropriate harvesting, storage, or processing procedures [2].

Ochratoxin A (OTA), the major mycotoxin of the ochratoxins' group and the one presenting great toxicological concern, is produced by *Penicillium verrucosum*, *Aspergillus ochraceus*, and rarely by some strains of *Aspergillus niger* [3]. OTA has been reported as nephrotoxic, carcinogenic, teratogenic, genotoxic, and immunotoxic. This mycotoxin also disturbs blood coagulation, hinders protein synthesis, endorses cell membrane peroxidation, abolishes calcium homeostasis, and constrains mitochondrial respiration [4]. In addition, it is epidemiologically associated to the human Balkan endemic nephropathy (BEN) disease and to urinary tract tumors [5,6]. Moreover, it is described as a cumulative mycotoxin since it is easily assimilated by the digestive tract and is gradually excreted by the urinary system [4]. Since 1993, OTA has been described as a possible carcinogen to humans, group 2B, by the International Agency for Research on Cancer (IARC) [7].

OTA generally occurs in numerous food products. This includes cereals, oleaginous seeds, green coffee, wine, meat, cocoa, spices, and fruit berries, which are contaminated at levels that vary according to environmental and processing conditions [8,9]. Moreover, some studies report that the prevalence and levels of OTA in organic cereals is higher when compared to non-organic cereals [10].

Due to the fact that OTA widely occurs in cereals, beer, which is a cereal product, has a potential contamination risk [11]. OTA was first reported in beer in 1983 [12]. Since then, several analytical methodologies were developed to study the natural incidence of OTA in this beverage. Most studies employed solid phase extraction through immunoaffinity columns (IAC) [12–17]. For detection and quantification, most authors employed liquid chromatography with fluorescence detection (LC-FD) [8,13,14,18,19], with limits of detection (LODs) varying between 0.002 μg/L and 1 μg/L. Liquid chromatography with tandem mass detection (LC-MS-MS) or ultra-pressure liquid chromatography with mass detection (UPLC-MS) was also applied, with LODs varying between 0.75 and 0.0003 μg/L, respectively [12,20].

Worldwide, several studies have investigated the presence of OTA in beer. Its occurrence was reported in Brazil [14], South Africa [18], Iran [21,22], Turkey [23], China [24], Japan [25], and Europe [13,20]. Namely, European studies reported it in Germany [26], Belgium [17], Spain [2], Italy [21,27], and the Czech Republic [19,28].

According to the scientific literature, the occurrence of OTA in beer samples is usually at low levels. In these studies, the minimum levels found ranged between 0.0009 and 2.7 μg/L, in Iran and Europe, respectively [20,22]. Some studies reported higher concentrations, up to 18 μg/L in Brazil [14]. However, one of the studies showed significantly higher values, up to 2340 μg/L [18].

The incidence of OTA in beer depends on the contamination of brewing materials, such as barley and barley malt, with ochratoxigenic fungi species [12]. During the production of beer, considerable OTA losses (40–89%) have been perceived in the grist during mashing, most possibly owing to proteolytic degradation [11]. Another 16% may be eliminated with spent grains [11]. With the fermentation process, OTA decreases in the range of 2% to 69% [11]. The remaining OTA passes on to the final beer product [12].

This contaminant may eventually reach consumers, and a frequent consumption of contaminated products could suppose a risk for human health [20]. There is no maximum allowable limit established by the European Commission (EC) for OTA content in beer [12]. Although there is no defined limit for beer, a maximum of 3 μg/kg for malt has been established by the European Union [29]. However, there are guideline levels established by the Netherlands (0.5 μg/L), Finland (0.3 μg/L), and Italy (0.2 μg/L) [8]. A tolerable weekly intake (TWI) of 120 ng/kg body weight (b.w.) was set for OTA in 2006 by the European Food Safety Authority (EFSA) [30].

Our main goal was to verify, for the first time, the OTA contamination of the beer marketed and consumed in Portugal, as well as to calculate the human estimated daily intake and risk assessment.

2. Results and Discussion

2.1. Validation and Quality Control

Validation and quality control fulfilled the European guidelines [31] and the results are presented in Table 1.

Table 1. Analytical quality control data obtained for OTA in beer spiked samples.

Spiking Level (μg/L)	Recovery (%)	RSD within-day (%)	RSD between-day (%)
0.5	81.0	2.43	2.74
1	86.0	2.36	5.26
2	85.0	1.72	6.25

Linearity results, both on standard and matrix-matched assays, were suitable, with correlation coefficients (r^2) of 0.998 and 0.999, respectively. The obtained limit of detection (LOD) and limit of quantification (LOQ) were 0.14 μg/L and 0.43 μg/L, respectively. The value of matrix effect (ME) obtained was considered negligible, 109%.

Accuracy and precision were adequate. Recoveries varied from 81.0% to 86.0%. Intra-day repeatability ranged from 1.72% to 2.43% and inter-day repeatability ranged from 2.74% to 6.25%. Both accuracy and precision results were adequate according to the requirements established by the EC 401/2006 directive [31].

2.2. Frequency and Occurrence of OTA in Beer Samples

In the present study, from the 85 analyzed beers, nine samples (10.6%) were contaminated at concentrations ranging from < LOQ to 11.25 μg/L, with an average level of 3.14 ± 4.09 μg/L (median of 1.74%). One of the contaminated samples presented a concentration between the LOD and the LOQ. Therefore, for results' analysis, half of the LOQ value was considered (Table 2).

Table 2. OTA contamination levels (μg/L) found in the positive samples.

Sample	Production	Type	Color	Type of Cereal	Alcohol Content (%)	Origin	Contamination (μg/L)
17	Craft beer	Ale	Pale	Barley and wheat malt	4.7	Portugal	1.81
20	Craft beer	Lager	Pale	Barley and wheat malt	5.1	Portugal	0.5
22	Craft beer	Lager	Pale	Barley malt, maize	6	Portugal	0.54
31	Homemade	Ale	Pale	Barley malt	4.2	New Zealand	9.21
32	Homemade	Ale	Pale	Barley malt	5.6	New Zealand	11.25
6	Industrial	Lager	Pale	Barley malt, maize, barley	5	Portugal	<LOQ
18	Industrial	Lager	Pale	Barley malt	5	Portugal	1.81
19	Industrial	Ale	Pale	Barley malt	8.5	Belgium	1.74
21	Industrial	Lager	Pale	Barley malt, maize, barley	5.2	Portugal	1.22
				Total			
Frequency (%)	-	-	-	-	-	-	10.6
Range (μg/L)	-	-	-	-	-	-	<LOQ-11.25
Mean ± SD (μg/L)	-	-	-	-	-	-	3.14 ± 4.09
Median							1.74

Among the contaminated samples, three contained maize, two contained wheat, and the other four indicated only the presence of barley and/or barley malt. The concentrations found in samples containing maize were 1.22, and 0.54, μg/L. In samples containing wheat, the contamination values were similar, 1.81 μg/L and 0.50 μg/L. In samples that indicated the presence of barley alone, the values were higher, at 1.81, 1.74, 9.21, and 11.25 μg/L, with the latter two being homemade beer samples. Samples with just barley in their composition represented 44.4% of the contaminated samples (Table 3). A similar higher percentage was found in samples with mixed cereals (55.5%). The difference in the OTA levels was 6.00 μg/L (median 5.51 μg/L) versus 0.86 μg/L (median 0.54 μg/L), which was due to the high levels found in the two homemade samples that were analyzed. Regarding these homemade samples, a limited number was possible to achieve. Although these are preliminary results, we thought it was interesting to include them in the study.

Although there is evidence that organic foods often contain high concentrations of natural toxins produced by fungi [10], whereas conventional foods tend to contain more synthetic compounds such as pesticide residues, none of the contaminated samples were of organic origin. In addition, the use of fungicides or preservatives in insufficient amounts can lead to a more serious situation due to stress caused in fungi, which leads to a stimulation of mycotoxin production [32].

Regarding the type of production, homemade beers presented the highest contamination levels at 10.23 ± 1.44 μg/L. Industrial and craft beers showed higher frequencies at 44.4% and 33.3%, but lower mean levels which were measured at 1.25 ± 0.74 µg/L (median 1.48 µg/L) and 0.95 ± 0.66 µg/L (median 0.54 µg/L), respectively.

Table 3. Frequency (%), OTA mean, and median contamination levels (µg/L) in different categories of contaminated beer.

Category		**Frequency Positive (total)**	**Mean ± SD**	**Median**
Production	Industrial	44.4 (4.7)	1.25 ± 0.74	1.48
	Craft	33.3 (3.5)	0.95 ± 0.66	0.54
	Homemade	22.2 (2.4)	10.23 ± 1.44	10.23
Type of beer	Lager	55.5 (5.9)	0.86 ± 0.65	0.54
	Ale	44.4 (4.7)	6.00 ± 4.95	3
Alcohol (%)	<6%	77.8 (8.2)	3.72 ± 4.53	1.81
	≥6%	22.2 (2.4)	1.14 ± 0.85	1.14
Type of cereal	Barley	44.4 (4.7)	6.00 ± 4.95	5.51
	Mixture	55.5 (5.9)	0.86 ± 0.65	0.54
Origin	Portugal	66.7 (7.1)	1.02 ± 0.70	0.88
	Abroad	33.3 (3.5)	7.40 ± 5.00	9.21

Two homemade samples showed really high levels, with 9.21 µg/L and 11.25 µg/L. Given that the maximum level of OTA is not currently established for beer but taking into account the limit established for wine (2 µg/L) (EC No. 1881/2006), these two samples exceeded at least 4.5 times and 5.5 times, respectively, this limit. Cereals used in homemade brewing are sold in plastic packaging presenting a greater risk of inadequate storage due to the moisture content, which favors their contamination. Another reason is that these types of beers are not subject to rigorous quality control and the cereals used are not as strictly controlled as those used in craft/industrial brewed beers.

Mycotoxins are highly stable and able to resist high temperatures and pH levels. The procedures involved in beer production use maximum operation temperatures lower than those able to destroy mycotoxins. However, they may impact mycotoxin levels given the physical, chemical, and biochemical alterations that take place [33]. The presence of OTA has been associated with barley malt contamination with ochratoxigenic species, namely *Penicillium verrucosum*. The OTA produced in the grains passes on to the wort and, although fermentation decreases its levels, the toxin is not completely removed [34]. Steeping, kilning, mashing, fermentation, and clarification are the most important steps of beer production presenting a negative impact on mycotoxins' levels. During these phases, mycotoxins may be removed through the drainage water, with the spent grains or with the fermentation residue. Moreover, they can also be diluted or destroyed as a result of the thermic treatment [33].

In the present study, every contaminated sample was pale beer. Drying (kilning) conditions are unfavorable for fungi (especially the first phase with a temperature of 50 °C and grain moisture of 45%). Knowing that the intensity of kilning and roasting (if applied) is crucial in malt flavor and color formation [33], fungi are removed during this process but thermostable mycotoxins produced before kilning persist [35]. Nowadays, the largest percentage of malt in most beers is pale malt which is only mildly dried at moderate temperature and might explain our results. Lager beers presented a higher contamination frequency (55.5%) but lower mean levels 0.86 ± 0.65 µg/L (median 0.54 µg/L) when compared to ale beers, the latter of which presented a frequency of 44.4% and 6.00 ± 4.95 µg/L (median 3 µg/L) mean contamination levels. On the contrary to Mateo et al. [34], a longer fermentation process and, consequently, a higher alcohol content, did not reduced the OTA level.

The studied samples were purchased from different retail outlets located in Coimbra (Portugal) but originated from 10 different countries. It was observed that from the nine contaminated samples, six (66.7%) were produced in Portugal, which provides evidence for the necessity of a greater control. Nonetheless, the mean levels found in the Portuguese samples which were 1.02 ± 0.70 µg/L (median 0.88 µg/L), were lower than in those from abroad.

The levels found in the present study are similar to those of other studies carried out in different countries. According to the scientific reported literature, the mean OTA content varies from 0.02 μg/L to 1.47 μg/L, for the samples analyzed in Turkey [23] and Germany [26], respectively. The minimum and maximum values vary between 0.012–0.045 μg/L and 1.5–2,34 μg/L in samples from Turkey [23] and South Africa [18], respectively. More recently, in 2017 Peters et al. reported the presence of mycotoxins, including OTA, in more than 1000 beers collected from 47 countries. OTA was found in five samples from Norway and England, ranging from 0.3 to 0.6 μg/L [36]. Bertuzzi et al. found OTA in the most sold beers in Italy with a mean concentration of 0.007 μg/L, with a maximum value of 0.07 μg/L [37].

With regard to the incidence of contamination, a frequency of 100% was found in samples collected in countries such as Spain [15], Hungary [2], Italy [27], Iran [22], Germany [26], and the Czech Republic [19]. The lowest OTA frequency was found in countries such as Brazil (0–5.3%) [14], China (0%) [24], Korea [16] and Turkey (14%) [23]. Recently, OTA was found in 45.8% of the most sold beers in Italy [37].

2.3. Human Estimated Daily Intake and Risk Assessment

The consumption of wine and beer make up part of the European culture. While Southern Europe is usually associated with wine consumption, Northern Europe is associated with beer. Nonetheless, since the 1960s wine consumption in Portugal has declined and beer is now the most consumed alcoholic beverage [38]. The number of brewing companies and the number of microbreweries increased, reflecting growth in the craft beer and specialty beer segment [39].

Three different scenarios were used to perform three EDI evaluations: the OTA contamination levels of the total analyzed samples (I); the mean OTA content regarding the nine positive samples; and the worst case scenario using the highest OTA level. In the first evaluation the EDI was 0.67 ng/kg b.w./day, in the second a value of 6.35 ng/kg b.w./day was obtained, and for the worst case scenario the value was 22.74 ng/kg b.w./day. When considering the estimated weekly intake (EWI) the obtained results for the three different scenarios were 4.71, 44.48, and 159.16 ng/kg b.w./week, respectively (Table 4).

Table 4. Estimated daily intake and risk assessment.

Scenarios	EDI (ng/kg b.w./day)	EWI (ng/kg b.w./week)	EWI/TWI [d] (%)
I [a]	0.67	4.71	3.92
II [b]	6.35	44.48	37.06
III [c]	22.74	159.16	132.63

[a] n = 85 samples. [b] n = 9 samples. [c] The most contaminated sample was considered. [d] TWI of 120 ng/kg b.w./week was considered [30].

For risk assessment, the most recent tolerable weekly intake (TWI) value established by EFSA [30] was used (120 ng/kg b.w./week). In the first evaluation scenario, the percentage of estimated weekly intake (EWI) versus TWI was 3.92%. In the second, it was 37.06%, and in the third scenario it was 132.63%. In the first two situations, the ingestion of OTA through the consumption of beer presents no risk to the respective consumers. The inverse situation was observed for the worst case scenario.

This risk evaluation has its limitations since it is based on consumption and occurrence data which contained a high number of negative samples in this study. Nonetheless, it is a contribution to assess the human risk posed by the consumption of beer.

In food monitoring studies, the driving force is often enforcement of legal limits [40]. Current legislation does not include limits for the occurrence of OTA in beer, but the identified concentrations, especially in homemade beers, should be considered.

3. Conclusions

The proposed analytical methodology, sample pre-treatment with sodium bicarbonate and PBS followed by IAC clean-up and LC-FD, enabled low detection and quantification levels and good results regarding accuracy and precision.

The application of this method to 85 samples showed that 10.59% were contaminated, two of which were homemade and presented considerable concentrations (9.21 and 11.25 μg/L). The discrepancy found can be explained by the storage of cereals already prepared for homemade brewing that may not be as strictly controlled as the others.

Three risk assessments were carried out based on three different scenarios. In the first two, the ingestion of OTA through the consumption of beer presents no risk to the respective consumers. The inverse situation was observed for the worst case scenario, where the most contaminated sample was considered.

The EU established maximum limits for OTA in some products. Current legislation does not include limits for the occurrence of OTA in beer, but the identified concentrations, especially in homemade beers, should be considered. For this reason, it is important to adopt preventive measures and develop control programs, reviewing the critical points where OTA production can occur in order to minimize human exposure to OTA.

4. Materials and Methods

4.1. Chemicals and Materials

HPLC grade acetonitrile and methanol and PBS tablets were purchased from Sigma Chemicals Co. (St. Louis, MO, USA). Toluene was acquired from Carlo Erba (Milan, Italy). Acetic acid was obtained from Merck (Darmstadt, Germany) and 98% purity degree OTA was obtained from Sigma Chemicals Co. (St. Louis, MO, USA).

The OTA stock solution was prepared at 250 μg/mL in toluene-acetic acid (99:1) and stored at −20 °C. The intermediate solution was prepared at 10 μg/mL, in mobile phase, and diluted accordingly to obtain the external calibration solutions.

Bi-distilled water was obtained from a Milli-Q System (Millipore, Bedford, MA, USA). A mixture of acetonitrile–water–acetic acid (49.5:49.5:1 *v*/*v*/*v*) was used as mobile phase. All chromatographic solvents were filtered through a 0.20 μm membrane filter (Whatman GmbH, Dassel, Germany) and degassed.

Immunoaffinity columns (IACs) OchraTest^{TM} (Vicam/Waters, Milford, MA, USA) were used for clean-up. Micro-glass fiber paper (150 mm, Munktell & Filtrak GmbH, Bärenstein, Germany), cellulose nitrate (0.45 μm, Sartorius Stedim Biotech GmbH, Göttingen, Germany), and Durapore membrane filter (0.22 μm, GVPP, Millipore, Ireland) were also used.

4.2. Sampling and Sample Characterization

In 2018, 84 bottled commercial beer samples and one draft beer, representing 59 brands, were randomly acquired from different retail outlets and supermarkets located in Coimbra (Coimbra, Portugal). The samples were classified based on the type of production, type of beer, color, fermentation, alcohol content, and country of origin.

In total, 61 samples were industrial manufactured, 21 were craft beers, and 3 were homemade beers. Regarding the type of beer, 44 were ale with top-fermentation, and 41 were lager, two of which were fruit/vegetable beers with bottom-fermentation. Of all the samples, 59 were of pale color, 2 were pale-red, and 24 were dark beers. Of the 85 beer samples, 30 were strong beers, with an alcohol content ≥6% and 55 contained alcohol <6% (3 samples were non-alcoholic, with <1% alcohol).

The majority of the samples (79) were of European origin and six were from abroad. Of all the beers, 36 were produced in Portugal. The imported beers originated from Belgium (n = 15), the Czech Republic (n = 3), Germany (n = 11), Ireland (n = 1), Mexico (n = 1), the Netherlands (n = 5), New Zealand (n = 2), Poland (n = 1), Russia (n = 3), Scotland (n = 2), and Spain (n = 5).

Among these samples, seven were brewed with organically produced materials and were labelled as organic beers. None of the samples was analyzed beyond their expiration date. Until analysis, they were stored in the dark at 4 °C and all the information available on the labels was assembled.

4.3. Experimental Procedure

Based on a previously reported analytical methodology [41], degassed and consecutively filtered beer samples (10 mL) were added, of 4% sodium bicarbonate (1.25 mL) and 10 mL of PBS. After centrifugation, the extract was loaded into an IAC cartridge for clean-up. After a washing step with 5 mL of water, OTA was eluted with 4 mL of methanol. Afterwards, the solvent was evaporated at 40 °C under a gentle nitrogen stream, and the dried residue was stored at −20 °C until analysis. For liquid chromatography with fluorescence detection (LC-FD), redissolution was accomplished with 1 mL of mobile phase. Following filtration through a Durapore membrane filter, 20 µL were injected into the HPLC system that consisted of a 805 manometric module Gilson, and a fluorimetric detector from Jasco (Tokio, Japan) FP-2020 Plus. Excitation and emission wavelengths were 336 nm and 440 nm, respectively. A C18 Nucleosil 5 µm (4.6 × 250 mm i.d.) column (Hichrom, Leicestershire, UK) was used and the flow rate was set at 1 mL min $^{-1}$. The total run time was 15 min.

4.4. Validation and Quality Control Assays

Validation and quality control assays were performed as set by European guidelines [31]. Different parameters were evaluated, including linearity, limit of detection (LOD) and limit of quantification (LOQ), matrix effect (ME), accuracy and precision. Linearity was assessed using standards (2.5–25 µg/L), and matrix-matched solutions (0.25–2.5 µg/L). Sensitivity was evaluated through the matrix-matched calibration curve.

The LOD was set as |3.3Sy/x|/b and the LOQ as |10Sy/x|/b, respectively, knowing that b corresponds to the slope and Sy/x corresponds to the residual standard deviation of the linear function.

The ME (%) corresponds to the percentage of the ratio of matrix-matched calibration curve slope (B) and the slope of the standard calibration curve (A). The results were interpreted as follows: 100% signifies an absence of ME; a result higher than 100% corresponds to a signal enhancement; and a result lower than 100% corresponds to a signal suppression.

Accuracy and precision were evaluated using blanks and fortified samples at three levels (0.5, 1.0, and 2.0 µg/L). Three replicates were made (n = 3), in three different days for each fortification level. The relative standard deviation (RSD) of intra-day and inter-day repeatability were assessed to evaluate the precision of the analytical methodology.

4.5. Calculation of the Human Estimated Daily Intake and Risk Assessment

A deterministic method [42] was used to calculate the OTA estimated daily intake (EDI) through the consumption of beer through the following equation (*1*):

$$\text{EDI} = \left(\sum c\right).\left(\text{CN}^{-1}\ \text{D}^{-1}\ \text{K}^{-1}\right), \tag{1}$$

where $\sum c$ is the OTA sum in the positive samples (µg/L), C corresponds to the mean annual beer consumption estimated per inhabitant, N is the samples' number, D corresponds to the days of a year, and K is the body weight (kg). According to Statistics Portugal (INE) data, the beer consumption in 2016 was 50.9 L/inhabitant (C) [43]. The mean body weight considered for the Portuguese adult population was 69 kg (K) [44].

Three different scenarios were used to perform three EDI evaluations. In the first scenario, the OTA contamination levels were taken into consideration for the total of all analyzed samples. For the second scenario, the mean OTA content was considered. Finally, the worst case scenario was observed using the highest OTA level.

Author Contributions: Conceptualization of this study was made by C.M.L. and A.P.; methodology was optimized by A.C.T. and L.J.G.S., investigation and data collection were performed by A.C.T., A.M.P.T.P., L.J.G.S., writing—original draft preparation by A.C.T.; writing, review and editing, C.M.L. and L.J.G.S.; overall supervision by C.M.L. All authors have read and agreed to the published version of the manuscript.

Funding: Fundação para a Ciência e a Tecnologia: UIDB 50006/2020

Acknowledgments: The authors gratefully acknowledge the Portuguese governmental Fundação para a Ciência e a Tecnologia—FCT for funding support through the project UIDB 50006/2020.

Conflicts of Interest: The authors declare no conflict of interest.

References

1. Eskola, M.; Kos, G.; Elliott, C.T.; Hajšlová, J.; Mayar, S.; Krska, R. Worldwide contamination of food-crops with mycotoxins: Validity of the widely cited 'FAO estimate' of 25%. *Crit. Rev. Food Sci. Nutr.* **2019**, *0*, 1–17. [CrossRef] [PubMed]
2. Soto, J.B.; Fernández-Franzón, M.; Ruiz, M.J.; Juan-García, A. Presence of ochratoxin a (OTA) mycotoxin in alcoholic drinks from southern european countries: Wine and beer. *J. Agric. Food Chem.* **2014**, *62*, 7643–7651. [CrossRef] [PubMed]
3. Malir, F.; Ostry, V.; Pfohl-Leszkowicz, A.; Malir, J.; Toman, J. Ochratoxin A: 50 years of research. *Toxins* **2016**, *8*, 191. [CrossRef]
4. Duarte, S.C.; Pena, A.; Lino, C.M. Human ochratoxin A biomarkers-from exposure to effect. *Crit. Rev. Toxicol.* **2011**, *41*, 187–212. [CrossRef] [PubMed]
5. Gifford, F.J.; Gifford, R.M.; Eddleston, M.; Dhaun, N. Endemic Nephropathy around the World. *Kidney Int. Rep.* **2017**, *2*, 282–292. [CrossRef] [PubMed]
6. Jadot, I.; Declèves, A.E.; Nortier, J.; Caron, N. An integrated view of aristolochic acid nephropathy: Update of the literature. *Int. J. Mol. Sci.* **2017**, *18*, 297. [CrossRef] [PubMed]
7. Ostry, V.; Malir, F.; Toman, J.; Grosse, Y. Mycotoxins as human carcinogens—The IARC Monographs classification. *Mycotoxin Res.* **2017**, *33*, 65–73. [CrossRef]
8. Aresta, A.; Palmisano, F.; Vatinno, R.; Zambonin, C.G. Ochratoxin A determination in beer by solid-phase microextraction coupled to liquid chromatography with fluorescence detection: A fast and sensitive method for assessment of noncompliance to legal limits. *J. Agric. Food Chem.* **2006**, *54*, 1594–1598. [CrossRef]
9. Juan, C.; Mañes, J.; Font, G.; Juan-García, A. Determination of mycotoxins in fruit berry by-products using QuEChERS extraction method. *LWT Food Sci. Technol.* **2017**, *86*, 344–351. [CrossRef]
10. Juan, C.; Moltó, J.C.; Lino, C.M.; Mañes, J. Determination of ochratoxin A in organic and non-organic cereals and cereal products from Spain and Portugal. *Food Chem.* **2008**, *107*, 525–530. [CrossRef]
11. Anli, E.; Alkis, İ.M. Ochratoxin A and Brewing Technology: A Review. *J. Inst. Brew.* **2010**, *116*, 23–32. [CrossRef]
12. Běláková, S.; Benešová, K.; Mikulíková, R.; Svoboda, Z. Determination of ochratoxin A in brewing materials and beer by ultra performance liquid chromatography with fluorescence detection. *Food Chem.* **2011**, *126*, 321–325. [CrossRef]
13. Bertuzzi, T.; Rastelli, S.; Mulazzi, A.; Donadini, G.; Pietri, A. Mycotoxin occurrence in beer produced in several European countries. *Food Control* **2011**, *22*, 2059–2064. [CrossRef]
14. Kawashima, L.M.; Vieira, A.P.; Valente Soares, L.M. Fumonisin B 1 and ochratoxin A in beers made in Brazil Fumonisina B 1 e ocratoxina A em cervejas fabricadas no Brasil. *Ciência E Tecnol. Aliment.* **2007**, *27*, 317–323. [CrossRef]
15. Medina, Á.; Jiménez, M.; Gimeno-Adelantado, J.V.; Valle-Algarra, F.M.; Mateo, R. Determination of ochratoxin A in beer marketed in Spain by liquid chromatography with fluorescence detection using lead hydroxyacetate as a clean-up agent. *J. Chromatogr. A* **2005**, *1083*, 7–13. [CrossRef] [PubMed]
16. Park, J.W.; Chung, S.H.; Kim, Y.B. Ochratoxin a in Korean food commodities: Occurrence and safety evaluation. *J. Agric. Food Chem.* **2005**, *53*, 4637–4642. [CrossRef] [PubMed]

17. Tangni, E.K.; Ponchaut, S.; Maudoux, M.; Rozenberg, R.; Larondelle, Y. Ochratoxin A in domestic and imported beers in Belgium: Occurence and exposure assessment. *Food Addit. Contam.* **2002**, *19*, 1169–1179. [CrossRef]
18. Odhav, B.; Naicker, V. Mycotoxins in South African traditionally brewed beers. *Food Addit. Contam.* **2002**, *19*, 55–61. [CrossRef]
19. Lhotská, I.; Šatínský, D.; Havlíková, L.; Solich, P. A fully automated and fast method using direct sample injection combined with fused-core column on-line SPE-HPLC for determination of ochratoxin A and citrinin in lager beers. *Anal. Bioanal. Chem.* **2016**, *408*, 3319–3329. [CrossRef]
20. Rubert, J.; Soler, C.; Marín, R.; James, K.J.; Mañes, J. Mass spectrometry strategies for mycotoxins analysis in European beers. *Food Control* **2013**, *30*, 122–128. [CrossRef]
21. Prelle, A.; Spadaro, D.; Denca, A.; Garibaldi, A.; Gullino, M.L. Comparison of clean-up methods for ochratoxin a on wine, beer, roasted coffee and chili commercialized in Italy. *Toxins* **2013**, *5*, 1827–1844. [CrossRef] [PubMed]
22. Mahdavi, R.; Khorrami, S.A.H.; Jabbari, V. Evaluation of ochratoxin A contamination in non alcoholic beers in Iran. *Res. J. Biol. Sci.* **2007**, *2*, 546–550.
23. Kabak, B. Ochratoxin A in cereal-derived products in Turkey: Occurrence and exposure assessment. *Food Chem. Toxicol.* **2009**, *47*, 348–352. [CrossRef] [PubMed]
24. Wu, J.; Tan, Y.; Wang, Y.; Xu, R. Occurrence of ochratoxin a in wine and beer samples from China. *Food Addit. Contam. B Surveill.* **2011**, *4*, 52–56. [CrossRef] [PubMed]
25. Tamura, M.; Uyama, A.; Mochizuki, N. Development of a Multi-mycotoxin Analysis in Beer-based Drinks by a Modified QuEChERS Method and Ultra-High-Performance Liquid Chromatography Coupled with Tandem Mass Spectrometry. *Anal. Sci.* **2011**, *27*, 629–635. [CrossRef] [PubMed]
26. Reinsch, M.; Töpfer, A.; Lehmann, A.; Nehls, I.; Panne, U. Determination of ochratoxin A in beer by LC-MS/MS ion trap detection. *Food Chem.* **2007**, *100*, 312–317. [CrossRef]
27. Novo, P.; Moulas, G.; França Prazeres, D.M.; Chu, V.; Conde, J.P. Detection of ochratoxin A in wine and beer by chemiluminescence-based ELISA in microfluidics with integrated photodiodes. *Sens. Actuators B Chem.* **2013**, *176*, 232–240. [CrossRef]
28. Ostry, V.; Malir, F.; Dofkova, M.; Skarkova, J.; Pfohl-Leszkowicz, A.; Ruprich, J. Ochratoxin a dietary exposure of ten population groups in the czech republic: Comparison with data over the world. *Toxins* **2015**, *7*, 3608–3635. [CrossRef]
29. European Commission. Commission Regulation (EC) No 1881/2006. *Off. J. Eur. Union* **2006**, *49*, 5–24.
30. EFSA. Opinion of the Scientific Panel on Contaminants in the food Chain on a Request from the Commission Related to Ochratoxin A in Food. *Efsa J.* **2006**, *365*, 1–56. [CrossRef]
31. European Commission. Commission Regulation (EC) No 401/2006 of 23 February 2006 laying down the methods of sampling and analysis for the official control of the levels of mycotoxins in foodstuffs. *Off. J. Eur. Union* **2006**, *L70*, 12–34.
32. Harcz, P.; Tangni, E.K.; Wilmart, O.; Moons, E.; Van Peteghem, C.; De Saeger, S.; Schneider, Y.J.; Larondelle, Y.; Pussemier, L. Intake of ochratoxin A and deoxynivalenol through beer consumption in Belgium. *Food Addit. Contam.* **2007**, *24*, 910–916. [CrossRef] [PubMed]
33. Pascari, X.; Ramos, A.J.; Marín, S.; Sanchís, V. Mycotoxins and beer. Impact of beer production process on mycotoxin contamination. A review. *Food Res. Int.* **2018**, *103*, 121–129. [CrossRef] [PubMed]
34. Mateo, R.; Medina, Á.; Mateo, E.M.; Mateo, F.; Jiménez, M. An overview of ochratoxin A in beer and wine. *Int. J. Food Microbiol.* **2007**, *119*, 79–83. [CrossRef] [PubMed]
35. Mastanjević, K.; Šarkanj, B.; Krska, R.; Sulyok, M.; Warth, B.; Mastanjević, K.; Šantek, B.; Krstanović, V. From malt to wheat beer: A comprehensive multi-toxin screening, transfer assessment and its influence on basic fermentation parameters. *Food Chem.* **2018**, *254*, 115–121. [CrossRef]
36. Peters, J.; Van Dam, R.; Van Doorn, R.; Katerere, D.; Berthiller, F.; Haasnoot, W.; Nielen, M.W.F. Mycotoxin profiling of 1000 beer samples with a special focus on craft beer. *PLoS ONE* **2017**, *12*, e0185887. [CrossRef]
37. Bertuzzi, T.; Rastelli, S.; Mulazzi, A.; Donadini, G.; Pietri, A. Known and Emerging Mycotoxins in Small- and Large-Scale Brewed Beer. *Beverages* **2018**, *4*, 46. [CrossRef]
38. Silva, A.P.; Jager, G.; Zyl, H.; Van Voss, H.; Hogg, T.; Graaf, C.; De Patricia, A.; Jager, G.; Zyl, H.; Van Voss, H. Cheers, proost, saúde: Cultural, contextual and psychological factors of wine and beer consumption in Portugal and in the Netherlands. *Crit. Rev. Food Sci. Nutr.* **2017**, *57*, 1340–1349. [CrossRef]

39. The Brewers of Europe. *The Contribution Made by Beer to the European Economy*; The Brewers of Europe: Brussels, Belgium, 2016.
40. De Nijs, M.; Mengelers, M.J.B.; Boon, P.E.; Heyndrickx, E.; Hoogenboom, L.A.P.; Lopez, P.; Mol, H.G.J. Strategies for estimating human exposure to mycotoxins via food. *World Mycotoxin J.* **2016**, *9*, 831–845. [CrossRef]
41. Anselme, M.; Tangni, E.K.; Pussemier, L.; Motte, J.C.; Van Hove, F.; Schneider, Y.J.; Van Peteghem, C.; Larondelle, Y. Comparison of ochratoxin A and deoxynivalenol in organically and conventionally produced beers sold on the Belgian market. *Food Addit. Contam.* **2006**, *23*, 910–918. [CrossRef]
42. IPCS. Dietary exposure assessment of chemicals in food. In *Principles and Methods for the Risk Assessment of Chemicals in Food*; International Programme on Chemical Safety; WHO: Geneve, Switzerland, 2009; p. 98.
43. INE Statistics Portugal. *Balança Alimentar Portuguesa 2012–2016*; INE Statistics Portugal: Lisbon, Portugal, 2017.
44. Arezes, P.M.; Barroso, M.P.; Cordeiro, P.; Costa, L.G.; Miguel, A.S. *Estudo Antropométrico da População Portuguesa*, 1st ed.; Instituto para a Segurança, Higiene e Saúde no Trabalho: Lisboa, Portugal, 2006.

toxins MDPI

Article

Using Cholinesterases and Immobilized Luminescent Photobacteria for the Express-Analysis of Mycotoxins and Estimating the Efficiency of Their Enzymatic Hydrolysis

Elena Efremenko [1,2,*], Olga Maslova [1], Nikolay Stepanov [1,2] and Anvar Ismailov [3]

[1] Faculty of Chemistry, Lomonosov Moscow State University, Lenin Hills 1/3, 119991 Moscow, Russia; olga-still@mail.ru (O.M.); na.stepanov@gmail.com (N.S.)
[2] N.M. Emanuel Institute of Biochemical Physics RAS, Kosigina str., 4, 119334 Moscow, Russia
[3] Faculty of Biology, Lomonosov Moscow State University, Lenin Hills 1/12, 119234 Moscow, Russia; anvaris@list.ru
* Correspondence: elena_efremenko@list.ru; Tel.: +7-495-939-3170

Abstract: Novel sensitive analytical agents that can be used for simple, affordable, and rapid analysis of mycotoxins are urgently needed in scientific practice, especially for the screening of perspective bio-destructors of the toxic contaminants. We compared the characteristics of a rapid quantitative analysis of different mycotoxins (deoxynivalenol, ochratoxin A, patulin, sterigmatocystin, and zearalenone) using acetyl-, butyrylcholinesterases and photobacterial strains of luminescent cells in the current study. The best bioindicators in terms of sensitivity and working range (μg/mL) were determined as follows: *Photobacterium* sp. 17 cells for analysis of deoxynivalenol (0.8–89) and patulin (0.2–32); *Photobacterium* sp. 9.2 cells for analysis of ochratoxin A (0.4–72) and zearalenone (0.2–32); acetylcholinesterase for analysis of sterigmatocystin (0.12–219). The cells were found to be more sensitive than enzymes. The assayed strains of photobacterial cells ensured 44%–83% lower limit of detection for deoxynivalenol and sterigmatocystin as compared to the previously known data for immobilized luminescent cells, and the range of working concentrations was extended by a factor of 1.5–3.5. Calibration curves for the quantitative determination of patulin using immobilized photobacteria were presented in this work for the first time. This calibration was applied to estimate the enzyme efficiency for hydrolyzing mycotoxins using zearalenone and His_6-tagged organophosphorus hydrolase as examples.

Keywords: mycotoxins; bioluminescent bacteria; immobilized cells; cholinesterase-based analysis; analytical characteristics; enzymatic detoxification

Key Contribution: The express-evaluation of enzymatic degradation efficiency of mycotoxins can be undertaken using inhibition of activity of cholinesterases or bioluminescence of immobilized photobacterial cells. The comparison of bioanalytical characteristics of the express analysis of several mycotoxins was performed.

Citation: Efremenko, E.; Maslova, O.; Stepanov, N.; Ismailov, A. Using Cholinesterases and Immobilized Luminescent Photobacteria for the Express-Analysis of Mycotoxins and Estimating the Efficiency of Their Enzymatic Hydrolysis. *Toxins* **2021**, *13*, 34. https://doi.org/10.3390/toxins13010034

Received: 30 November 2020
Accepted: 4 January 2021
Published: 6 January 2021

1. Introduction

Studying mycotoxins is topical and relevant for ensuring food and biological safety [1–3]. Analytical approaches to the detection and identification of mycotoxins [4] are being actively developed, and so are strategies for mycotoxin control and detoxification [5–8].

These are currently the most actively pursued areas: (i) elucidating the mechanisms of toxic effects of mycotoxins on living organisms [5]; (ii) development and testing of effective selective and sensitive analytical methods for the detection of mycotoxins in food, agricultural feed, and raw materials for the pharmaceutical industry [9,10]; (iii) search for sorbents capable of removing mycotoxins from raw materials [11]; (iv) the search for new methods for the destruction of mycotoxins, especially those involving bio-destructors [12,13]. The last of the above directions is especially important today, since it implies the development of means, including combined action, that eliminate mycotoxins not only due to their sorption, but also due to their catalytic decomposition. Various enzymes are considered as such biocatalytic detoxifiers [13,14].

In fundamental and applied research in the field of mycotoxins, liquid chromatography (LC) and enzyme-linked immunosorbent assay (ELISA) are most widely used today. An LC run is followed by mass spectrometry (MS), sensitive fluorescence detection (FLD), or ultraviolet (UV) detection [9,10,12]. High analytical accuracy and selectivity are the main advantages of the abovementioned methods. However, in this case, the duration and complexity of the sample preparation are obvious limiting factors for the express use of LC. ELISA kits allow for express analysis; however, they are distinguished by their high cost, since special antibodies are required for each mycotoxin.

When developing approaches to detoxification of mycotoxins using biocatalysts, selectivity and accuracy are not always priority indicators at the stage of screening and selection of primary candidates. Analytical express methods are more popular at this stage, because they allow the rapid assessment the residual toxicity of the test samples after their enzymatic or cellular treatment. Thus, ineffective candidates can be quickly eliminated from the study, whereas more promising biocatalysts can be chosen for a deeper study of their characteristics using more accurate analytical instruments based on LC or ELISA.

The initial choice of perspective biocatalysts for in-depth study is based on the published data. For example, it is known that enzymes of some classes, including hexahistidine-tagged organophosphorus hydrolase (His_6-OPH), exhibit destructive activity towards various mycotoxins [3,9,10,13–17]. Computer design, and, in particular, the molecular docking method [18,19], is yet another technique which has been proved useful for the initial selection of promising potential candidates from a number of enzymes for the decomposition of mycotoxins. The next stages of research already imply practical experimental research.

To quickly screen out candidates selected as a result of docking, but which do not efficiently detoxify mycotoxins, luminescent photobacterial cells can be successfully used for the rapid assessment of the toxicity of samples [17]. These cells sensitively react to the presence of mycotoxins via changing the level of their bioluminescence. It is important that when the cells are used in an immobilized form, such analyzes become possible both in discrete and continuous modes and the analytical signal is stable enough [17,20]. It appears possible to find ways of increasing the sensitivity of mycotoxin detection with this technique by varying the strains of photobacteria immobilized by the same method. We have not identified such comparative studies conducted earlier.

The search for other sensitive analytical agents that can be used for affordable rapid analysis essential for controlling mycotoxins is of obvious scientific and practical importance. In particular, cholinesterases can be considered among the promising candidates, which have proven themselves well in the rapid analysis of many other toxic compounds [21]. Our previous results showing mycotoxins docking to the surface of cholinesterases [13] indicated that inactivation of these enzymes under the action of mycotoxins is feasible. Therefore, cholinesterases (acetyl- (AChE) and/or butyrylcholinesterase (BChE)) can be used for assessing the concentrations of mycotoxins and the effectiveness of the action of destructors on these substances. However, we were unable to find any reports on systematic studies of the inhibition of the cholinesterases by various mycotoxins and on the possibility of implementing an analytical technique based on this effect.

The aim of the present work was to compare the characteristics of cholinesterases and luminescent photobacterial strains for use in rapid quantitative analysis of mycotoxins using cholinesterases and luminescent photobacterial strains. We also studied the applicability of this technique for assessing the effectiveness of mycotoxin biodegradation in the case of zearalenone and the His_6-OPH.

2. Results

2.1. The Quantitative Express-Analysis of Mycotoxins in Liquid Media Involving Cholinesterases or Immobilized Bioluminescent Photobacterial Cells

It was shown with sufficiently good reproducibility, that cholinesterases and immobilized luminescent photobacterial cells can be successfully used to perform the quantitative express-analysis of at least one of five mycotoxins (deoxynivalenol, ochratoxin A, patulin, sterigmatocystin, and zearalenone) in liquid media in discrete mode (Table 1 and Figures 1–3).

Table 1. Analytical characteristics of different mycotoxins' assay (Figures 1–3) based on application of cholinesterases (Figures 1 and 2) or immobilized luminescent cells (Figure 3) and linearization equations (R^2 is adjusted coefficient of determination).

Mycotoxin	Coefficients of the Linearization Equation		R^2	Working Range, µg/mL	Limit of Quantification (LOQ), µg/mL	Limit of Detection (LOD), µg/mL
	a	b				
	AChE					
Deoxynivalenol [1]	97.9 ± 0.1	4.0 ± 0.1	0.998	≥1698	1698	563
Ochratoxin A [1]	64.9 ± 5.4	180.9 ± 9.9	0.979	30−354	30	10
Patulin [1]	98.9 ± 0.1	4.0 ± 0.1	0.998	≥2951	2951	984
Sterigmatocystin [1]	65.3 ± 0.2	21.5 ± 6.0	0.999	0.12−219	0.12	0.04
Zearalenone [2]	111.5 ± 0.9	0.9 ± 0.01	0.999	29−103	29	10
	BChE					
Deoxynivalenol [2]	101.0 ± 0.1	0.05 ± 0.001	0.999	320−1720	320	105
Ochratoxin A [2]	102.0 ± 0.1	0.1 ± 0.01	0.999	170−870	170	56
Patulin [1]	104.0 ± 0.4	6.0 ± 0.2	0.997	≥1548	1548	511
Sterigmatocystin [1]	101.0 ± 0.1	0.5 ± 0.01	0.999	32−172	32	11
Zearalenone [1]	108.0 ± 0.2	45.9 ± 0.1	0.999	3−107	3	1
	Photobacterium sp. 9.2 cells					
Deoxynivalenol [1]	84.1 ± 1.2	38.0 ± 0.6	0.999	1−66	1	0.3
Ochratoxin A [1]	73.6 ± 10.2	31.5 ± 5.5	0.923	0.4−72	0.4	0.13
Patulin [1]	57.1 ± 1.3	45.2 ± 1.4	0.999	0.3−8	0.3	0.1
Sterigmatocystin [1]	71.8 ± 6.3	33.0 ± 3.9	0.981	0.4−52	0.4	0.13
Zearalenone [1]	57.6 ± 9.0	28.2 ± 5.6	0.934	0.2−32	0.2	0.07
	Photobacterium sp. 17 cells					
Deoxynivalenol [1]	82.1 ± 2.6	34.4 ± 1.4	0.995	0.8−89	0.8	0.27
Ochratoxin A [1]	87.0 ± 13.3	35.8 ± 7.1	0.925	1.1−102	1.1	0.37
Patulin [1]	60.2 ± 10.1	29.9 ± 6.4	0.912	0.2−32	0.4	0.07
Sterigmatocystin [1]	63.8 ± 10.2	34.7 ± 6.1	0.941	0.3−25	0.4	0.1
Zearalenone [1]	70.5 ± 11.6	33.0 ± 7.4	0.905	0.4−48	0.4	0.13

[1] Activity = a − bx lg (concentration, µg/mL); [2] Activity = a − bx (concentration, µg/mL).

Calibration plots for quantitative analysis are presented in Figures 1–3 in the coordinates, in which the obtained data can be successfully linearized. Enzymes were found to be less sensitive than photobacteria to the presence of mycotoxins. In general, a shift in the range of working concentrations upward was noted for enzymes. Both enzymes showed lower sensitivity to the presence of patulin as compared to cells.

AChE was more sensitive to ochratoxin A and sterigmatocystin and less sensitive to DON as compared to BChE. According to the results obtained, the adjusted coefficient of determination (R^2) for both enzymes was close to 1 (Table 1), whereas for luminescent bacterial cells, mainly for the *Photobacterium* sp. 17, the values of R^2 below 0.97 were obtained. Note that calculated R^2 values exceeding 0.9 indicate the possibility of using the corresponding tool (both enzymes and photobacteria in our case) for analytical purposes.

The results obtained allow the selection of the most acceptable analytical method for an express analysis of each mycotoxin in terms of the working concentration range and the lower limit of detection (LOD) value.

Thus, *Photobacterium* sp. 17 cells provide the lowest LOD and a fairly wide working concentration range for the analysis of deoxynivalenol, whereas *Photobacterium* sp. 9.2 ensure the best set of parameters for ochratoxin A and zearalenone detection, *Photobacterium* sp. 17 cells are optimal for patulin, and AChE is the instrument of choice for sterigmatocystin.

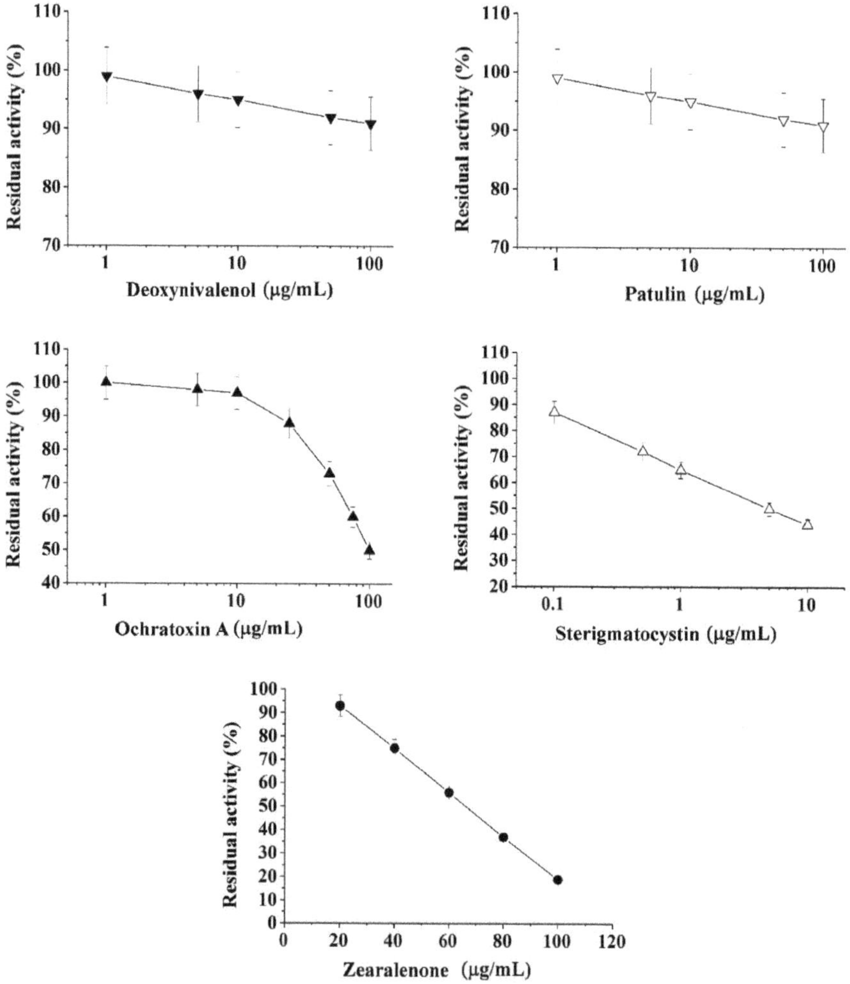

Figure 1. Inhibition effect of deoxynivalenol, patulin, ochratoxin A, sterigmatocystin, and zearalenone on acetylcholinesterase (AChE) activity. Activity was measured by Ellman assay with acetylthiocholine iodide as substrate in 0.1 M phosphate buffer (pH 8.0).

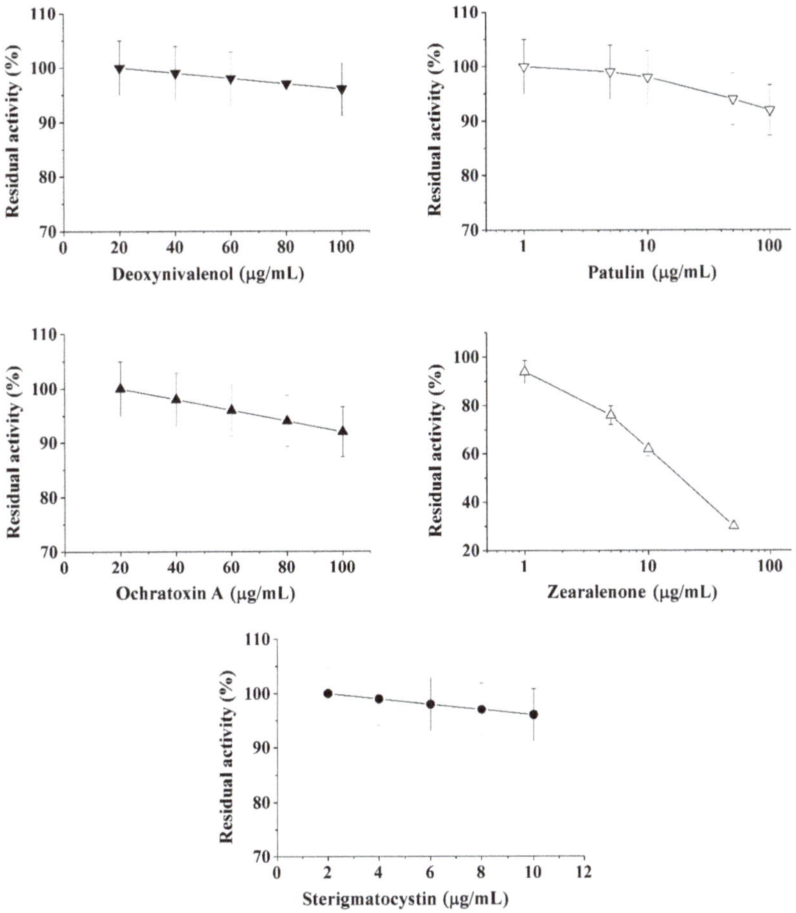

Figure 2. Inhibition effect of deoxynivalenol, patulin, ochratoxin A, zearalenone, and sterigmatocystinon on butyrylcholinesterase (BChE) activity. Activity was measured by Ellman assay with butyrylthiocholine iodide as substrate in 0.1 M phosphate buffer (pH 8.0).

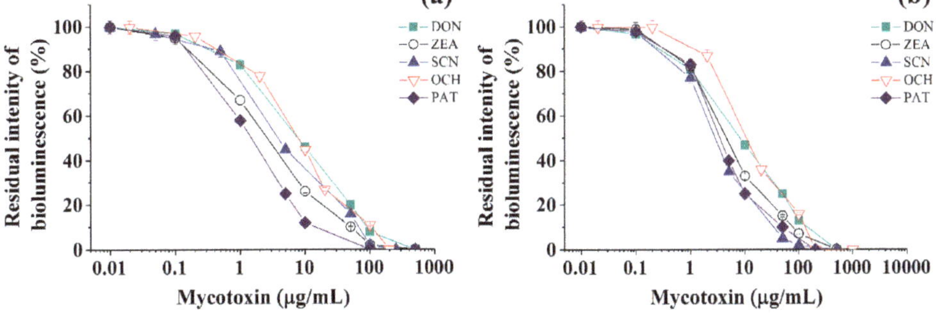

Figure 3. Residual intensity of luminescence of immobilized *Photobacterium* sp. 9.2 (**a**) and *Photobacterium* sp. 17 (**b**) cells in the presence of various mycotoxins (DON—deoxynivalenol, ZEA—zearalenone, SCN—sterigmatocystin, OCH—ochratoxin A, PAT—patulin) in discrete analysis.

2.2. Assessment of Toxicity of the Reaction Medium Obtained after Hydrolysis of Zearalenone by His_6-OPH in the Media with Different pH

Using acetyl-cholinesterases, photobacterial cells, and ELISA Test Kit as analytical tools, we have proven the possibility of zearalenone destruction under the action of His_6-OPH in a liquid medium at different pH values at an initial mycotoxin concentration of 65 ± 3 μg/mL (Table 2). The results of this study agree with those we obtained earlier [17]. It was noted that the low sensitivity of enzymes allowed the detection of only the initial concentration of mycotoxin in the test solution. The residual concentration of zearalenone after the action of His_6-OPH in the case of enzymatic analytical agents could only be determined using BChE for a sample with pH 7.4 (Table 2). Photobacterial cells, however, ensured accuracy high enough to reliably assess the degree of zearalenone destruction under the action of His_6-OPH for different medium pH values. The accuracy of mycotoxin detection with photobacteria was in fact found to be at least as high as that ensured with the ELISA Test Kit.

Table 2. The residual zearalenone concentrations in the media with hexa-histidine-tagged organophosphorus hydrolase (His_6-OPH) after 1 h of enzymatic treatment. The initial zearalenone concentration was 65 ± 3 μg/mL.

Analytical Method *	Zearalenone, μg/mL		* DH, %	Reference
	pH 7.4	pH 8.5	pH 8.5	
BChE	3.8 ± 0.1	-	-	This work
Photobacterium sp. 9.2	4.3 ± 0.1	0.67 ± 0.03	98.8 ± 0.9	This work
Photobacterium sp. 17	4.5 ± 0.1	0.63 ± 0.03	99.0 ± 0.9	This work
MaxSignal® Zearalenone ELISA Test Kit	3.8 ± 0.1	0.58 ± 0.02	99.1 ± 0.9	This work
	3.9 ± 0.2	-	-	[17]
Photobacterium phosphoreum B-1717	4.1 ± 0.2	-	-	[17]

* DH is the degree of zearalenone hydrolysis = the percentage of the hydrolyzed zearalenone concentration in relation to its initial level; -: samples were not analyzed.

2.3. Zearalenone Biodegradation in Feed Grain Mixture under the Action of the Enzyme His_6-OPH

In a model experiment using enzymes, photobacterial cells, and ELISA Test Kit as analytical agents, it was possible for the first time to assess detoxification of food raw materials (feed grain mixture) initially contaminated with zearalenone at a concentration of 10 mg/kg. Feed was treated with His_6-OPH enzyme to push the toxin concentration below the levels specified in the generally accepted quality standards, so that the resulting contaminant concentration was below 1 mg/kg (Table 3).

Table 3. Residual concentrations of zearalenone in the feed grain mixture (initial contamination of feed grain mixture by zearalenone was 10 mg/kg) after its treatment with enzyme His_6-OPH (ED) during 12 h and without it (NE).

Analytical Method	Zearalenone, mg/kg Feed		* R, %	** D, %
	NE	ED		
BChE	8.5 ± 0.3	***	85 ± 4	***
Photobacterium sp. 9.2	8.1 ± 0.3	0.82 ± 0.04	81 ± 4	89.9 ± 4.1
Photobacterium sp. 17	8.2 ± 0.3	0.85 ± 0.05	82 ± 4	89.6 ± 4.2
MaxSignal® Zearalenone ELISA Test Kit	7.9 ± 0.3	0.77 ± 0.03	79 ± 4	90.3 ± 4.1

* R is the degree of zearalenone recovery; the percentage of the NE zearalenone concentration to its initial concentration; ** D is the level of zearalenone detoxification in feed; the percentage of the change in zearalenone concentration in feed grain mixture as the result of enzymatic destruction (NE-ED) to the non-enzymatic degradation (NE); *** There was no inhibition of BChE activity.

In the case of enzymatic analytical agents, only BChE allowed the determination of the concentration of zearalenone in the analytical sample of the raw material with the maximum concentration of zearalenone (Table 3). The use of biological analytical agents resulted in slightly higher values of toxicant concentration than in case of using the ELISA Test Kit. This was probably due to the presence of substances other than zearalenone, which reduce the activity of enzymes in the analytical samples. These substances could have originated from the feedstock and been transferred together with zearalenone during the extraction stage. It is important that the calculated detoxification degree was similar in the case of photobacterial cells and ELISA Test Kit (Table 3).

Thus, photobacteria can be efficiently used as analytical agents for evaluating the detoxification of real raw materials. They can greatly facilitate the search for bio-destructors of any target mycotoxin, as well as the assessment of the efficiency of detoxification using various biological agents. It was shown that an acetonitrile-based extractant can be recommended for the extraction of zearalenone from the feedstock during sample preparation. This extractant provides a high degree of recovery of this toxicant (Table 3), which is consistent with the previously published data [22,23].

3. Discussion

The development of new express analytical methods that could reduce the time and cost of research is very topical. Novel efficient techniques are urgently needed both for selecting the potential bio-destructors of mycotoxins and for assessing the effectiveness of their action under various conditions. It was shown that cholinesterases and immobilized luminescent cells of photobacteria give a stable analytical signal in the presence of common mycotoxins (Table 1).

The key points for choosing a biological analytical agent for the determination of mycotoxins are LOD and working range. The availability of equipment, the duration of the analysis, the volume of the sample, the need to use additional reagents, and the range of analyzed mycotoxins should also be taken into account. The duration of the analysis (with calibration graph available) was ca. 2–5 min in the case of using enzymes in this work, and 30 min in that of photobacterial cells.

The volume of mycotoxin-containing sample sufficient for the contaminant determination was 10 μL and 4 μL in the cases of cholinesterases or luminescent bacteria, respectively. The analysis of mycotoxins was carried out using generally available laboratory equipment: a spectrophotometer (in the case of enzymes) or a luminometer (in the case of photobacteria). In contrast to the case of luminescent bacteria, the enzyme-based analysis required the use of additional reagents: acetylthiocholine iodide or butyryl-thiocholine iodide was used as substrate and 5,5′-dithiobis-(2-nitrobenzoic acid) was used as indicator.

The enzymes were found to be less sensitive to the presence of mycotoxins in the analyzed samples. This was probably due to the fact that in the luminescent cells, in addition to the main analytical luminescent system, there is a large number of interconnected enzymatic systems that are sensitive to the toxicant. Thus, in general, under the conditions of the experiments, the enzymatic analytical systems based on AChE and BChE are somewhat inferior in terms of significant parameters to the cells of photobacteria (Table 1).

Among the studied bacterial strains, despite the high degree of phylogenetic homology, the best analytical characteristics corresponded to *Photobacterium* sp. 9.2 cells (Table 1). The luminescent *Photobacterium* sp. 9.2 and *Photobacterium* sp. 17 cells ensured 44%–83% lower LOD values for zearalenone determination compared to the case of *Photobacterium phosphoreum* B-1717 [17], and for deoxynivalenol and sterigmatocystin the range of working concentrations was 1.5–3.5 times greater in this study. Calibration curves for the quantitative determination of patulin by using photobacterial cells immobilized in poly(vinyl alcohol) cryogel are presented in this work for the first time (Table 1).

The use of the studied biological analytical agents (enzymes and cells) specifically for the direct quantitative determination of mycotoxins in feed is most likely to be inappropriate. The reason is that the solvents that are used to extract mycotoxins into an analytical sample and ensure a high degree of contaminant recovery can themselves be toxic to living cells and enzymes. For an accurate quantitative analysis, in this case, complex sample preparation and standardization for the secondary toxicant are required; in this case, preference is given to liquid chromatography and ELISA [10].

It was shown in this work that the most expedient way to use the photobacteria is the express analysis of mycotoxins, which is an important stage in the assessment of the degree of detoxification of analytical samples due to the destruction of mycotoxins. The analytical samples often contain component toxic to cells other than mycotoxin, e.g., methanol or acetonitrile which are commonly used as extractants-solvents of mycotoxins. In this case it is necessary to account for these additional toxicants when carrying out the calculations, e.g., by appropriate normalization, which was also done in this work.

Despite their somewhat lower sensitivity, enzymes could be used in searching for effective bio-destructors of some mycotoxins. In this case the destruction products are the most predictable, and additional agents can be introduced (if necessary) into the reaction system for directed detoxification of the toxic intermediates of enzymatic mycotoxins' decomposition [5].

The expediency of using the His_6-OPH for the destruction of lactone-containing mycotoxins, like zearalenone, was confirmed in the work (Tables 2 and 3). Using immobilized cells of photobacteria as analytical agents, it was shown for the first time that a shift in the pH of the medium from 7.4 to 8.5 when using His_6-OPH makes it possible to improve the degree of zearalenone destruction from 93%–94% to 98%–99% (Table 2).

In general, the results obtained are consistent with the literature data on the relatively high hydrolytic activity of lactonases in relation to zearalenone in neutral and slightly alkaline media [17]; the catalytic activity of the enzyme decreases when the pH is lowered [12,18]. The established regularity, allows us to draw certain conclusions about the prospects of creating food supplements based on His_6-OPH. The controlled release of this enzyme in the digestive system in the areas with alkaline pH values can ensure efficient decomposition of mycotoxins that enter the body of animals with nutrition under the action of His_6-OPH. His_6-OPH can be potentially introduced into the feed contaminated with zearalenone, as in the case of recombinant lactonohydrolase [12], for mycotoxin detoxification. Additionally, using His_6-OPH in a medium at pH 8.5 provided up to five times faster degradation of zearalenone as compared to recombinant lactonohydrolase expressed in *Penicillium canescence*. This was also demonstrated in this work for the first time.

There is a general consensus that bioanalytical agents such as cholinesterases and photobacterial cells are not selective in their inhibition reactions with various toxins. However, in this work, some obvious preferences were found for bacterial strains, possessing close phylogenetic relations, and cholinesterases in reactions with the same mycotoxins. The best bioindicators in terms of sensitivity and working range (μg /mL) were determined as follows: *Photobacterium* sp. 17 cells for analysis of deoxynivalenol (0.8–89) and patulin (0.2–32); *Photobacterium* sp. 9.2 cells-for analysis of ochratoxin A (0.4–72) and zearalenone (0.2–32); AChE for analysis of sterigmatocystin (0.12–219). Cholinesterases were found to be less sensitive than cells. Calibrations for quantitative determination of patulin using immobilized photobacteria are presented in this work for the first time.

Generally, the use of luminescent cells can significantly reduce the time and financial costs when conducting primary evaluative analyzes of the mycotoxin content in samples during laboratory studies. The efficiency of enzymatic destructors in reactions with mycotoxins can be adequately evaluated using simple equipment and a well-known approach. The information obtained regarding the preferences of bioanalytical agents used for the analysis of a particular mycotoxin will be useful for those researchers who are engaged in the scientific search for bio-destructors of mycotoxins, and simplifies their laboratory screening.

4. Materials and Methods

4.1. Chemicals and Strains

Mycotoxins (ochratoxin A, sterigmatocystin, zearalenone, deoxynivalenol, and patulin); cholinesterase enzymes (AChE and BChE); 5,5′-dithiobis (2-nitrobenzoic acid), acetylthiocholine iodide, and butyrylthiocholine iodide were purchased from Sigma-Aldrich (St. Louis, MO, USA). For the experiments, concentrated solutions of mycotoxins in methanol were preliminarily prepared. Solutions of mycotoxins of the required concentration were prepared by diluting the original stock solutions of mycotoxins in methanol.

In the analysis, the quenching of the bioluminescence of the immobilized luminous bacteria under the action of the methanol present in the reaction medium was taken into account. Poly(vinyl alcohol) 16/1 (M.w. 84 kDa) was purchased from Sinopec Corp (Beijing, China); peptone and yeast extract were purchased from Difco (Becton, Dickinson and Company, Franklin Lakes, NJ, USA); inorganic salts for Farghaly growth medium and other reagents were purchased from Chimmed (Moscow, Russia). *Photobacterium* sp. 9.2 and *Photobacterium* sp. 17 were provided by A.D. Ismailov (Lomonosov Moscow State University, Moscow, Russia).

4.2. *Growth Cells Conditions, Immobilization and Luminescence Measurements*

Phosphoreum sp. cells were grown in the Farghaly growth medium and maintained in a submerged culture at 18 °C at 60 rpm (IRC-1-U temperature-controlled shaker, Adolf Kuhner AG Apparatebau, Switzerland). The optical density of the culture medium was determined by spectrophotometry at 660 nm (Agilent UV-853 spectrophotometer, Agilent Technologies, Waldbronn, Germany), and the cells were cultivated for 22 h to an optical density of 0.73 ± 0.05, separated from the culture medium by centrifugation (5000 rpm, 15 min, J2 21 centrifuge, Beckman, Brea, CA, USA), and cell biomass used in the immobilization procedure. The procedure for immobilizing the bioluminescent cells in poly (vinyl alcohol) (PVA) cryogel was described previously [20]. The cell biomass was mixed with a 10% (*w*/*v*) aqueous PVA solution to obtain a 10% (*w*/*w*) concentration of bacterial cells. This mixture was pipetted into 96-well microplates (0.2 mL/well), which were placed in a freezer at −20 °C for 24 h and then thawed at +4 °C. The cylinder granules of PVA cryogel (d = 6.6 ± 0.1 mm, h = 4.8 ± 0.1 mm) formed in this way contained cells immobilized by inclusion. The average wet weight of one granule was 0.172 ± 0.001 g.

Luminescence of immobilized bacteria was measured using a 3560 microluminometer (New Horizons Diagnostics Co, Columbia, MD, USA). Luminescence detection was performed in aqueous media based on a 2% NaCl solution at 10 ± 1 °C. The maximum level of luminescence (I_0) was determined for 10 s at 10 °C after thermal equilibration of the flow-through system. For practical purposes, the residual intensity of luminescence was used (I/I_0), which was expressed as a percentage of the baseline signal (I_0). The residual intensity of luminescence (I/I_0) was analyzed in a discrete test after the exposure of the cells to a certain mycotoxin for 0.5 h after its addition to medium containing the analytical agent. The assays were performed in triplicate.

4.3. *Mycotoxins Analyses with Cholinesterase Enzymes (AChE and BChE)*

The activity of cholinesterases was determined using the Ellman method [24]. Briefly, 0.96 mL of 0.1 M phosphate buffer (pH 8.0) in a spectrophotometric cell was supplemented with 10 μL of 20 mM 5,5′-dithiobis (2-nitrobenzoic acid) in a 0.1 M phosphate buffer (pH 7.0), containing 1.5 g/L Na_2CO_3. Then, 10 μL of 0.01 mg/mL AChE or 0.2 mg/mL BChE followed by a 10 μL of 0–10 mg/mL mycotoxin in methanol or ethanol was added and vigorously mixed. Reaction was initiated by addition of 10 μL of 50 mM acetylthiocholine iodide or 200 mM butyrylthiocholine iodide for AChE or BChE, respectively.

The rate of formation of 2-nitro-5-thiobenzoic acid at λ = 412 nm was determined using the Agilent 8453 UV-visible spectroscopy system (Agilent Technologies, Waldbronn, Germany). All enzymes, substrates, mycotoxins, and other reagents were freshly prepared before use.

Enzyme activity without any toxins or solvents was monitored, and results were adjusted accordingly. One unit of AChE or BChE activity was defined as the enzyme amount that hydrolyzed 1 μmol of substrate per min at 25 °C. The experiments were realized in triplicate.

4.4. *Hydrolysis of Zearalenone in Medium with Different pH under the Action of the His$_6$-OPH*

For the experiment, the initial concentration of zearalenone in the reaction medium based on phosphate buffer (pH 7.4 or 8.5) was 65 ± 3 mg/L. The initial toxicity of this solution was evaluated under the conditions indicated above. The solution of the His_6-OPH (0.1 mg/mL) with an activity of 200 U/mL was added to zearalenone solution.

The treatment of the mycotoxin was carried out for 1 h at room temperature without agitation, and the residual toxicity of the obtained solution was verified using immobilized luminescent cells or cholinesterases in a discrete mode of analysis (Table 2).

4.5. Hydrolysis of Zearalenone in Feed Grain Mixture under the Action of the His_6-OPH

Using 0.1 M phosphate buffer (pH 7.5), a solution of zearalenone with concentration 2 g/L was prepared from its concentrated methanol stock solution. The preparation was injected (in the form of a spray) into the feed grain mixture for rats using Classic TiTBiT (Dmitrov, Moscow Region, Russia) at the rate of 10 mg of zearalenone per 1 kg of grain mixture. After that, one half of the grain mixture containing zearalenone was sprayed with a solution of His_6-OPH, prepared based on 0.1 M phosphate buffer (pH 7.5), at a dose of 4000 U/kg of the grain mixture, after which the mixture was mechanically stirred and kept for 12 h at 25 °C.

The procedure for enzyme production and purification was detailed previously [25]. The activity of His_6-OPH was determined as described previously [26], with 7.8 mM aqueous Paraoxon stock solution at 405 nm using the Agilent 8453 UV-visible spectroscopy system (Agilent Technology, Waldbronn, Germany) equipped with a thermostated analytical cell.

After 12 h, the zearalenone concentration was determined in the feed samples with zearalenone, pretreated with the enzyme or without the pretreatment, as well as in the control sample, without any additives. 15 g of each feed grain mixture sample was ground into powder in a laboratory mill and was subject to triple extraction with 40 mL of 84% acetonitrile aqueous solution (*v*/*v*) by mechanical shaker for 15 min. Fractions obtained from each sample were pooled. Then the extract was filtered through paper filters and evaporated to dryness under nitrogen flow. The obtained weighed portion was dissolved in 300 µL of methanol. A total of three samples of methanol stock solution from grain mixture samples were obtained (Table 3). Next, the required dilution of samples was carried out using aqueous buffer solutions to a methanol content of no more than 2%–4%, and the concentration of zearalenone in the samples was determined using cholinesterase enzymes, luminescent cells, or ELISA kit (Table 3).

4.6. Determination of Zearalenone by Enzyme-Linked Immunosorbent Assay (ELISA) Test Kit

Analyses were carried out using MaxSignal® Zearalenone ELISA Test Kit (Bio Scientific Corp, Austin, TX, USA) with sensitivity 0.3 ng/mL Samples were prepared according to the instructions provided by the manufacturers of the ELISA kits. Optical density was measured at 450 nm using a microplate reader iMark (Bio-Rad Laboratories, Inc., Hercules, CA, USA).

4.7. Calculations

The data were linearized in various plots with OriginPro (ver. 9.4.2, OriginLab Corporation, Northhampton, MA, USA) and the most suitable coordinates were selected. The limit of detection (LOD) and limit of quantification (LOQ) for enzymes and photobacterial cells were calculated as a minimal mycotoxin concentration which is distinguishable from the blank measurement (i.e., enzymes or cells without inhibitors) by more than three sigmas and ten sigmas (standard deviation, σ) in at least, six independent measurements), respectively. All measurements with MaxSignal® Zearalenone ELISA Test Kit were repeated three times, and the results were analyzed with the Microplate Manager® 6, version 6.3.

The data are presented as means $\pm$ standard deviation ($\pm\sigma$) unless otherwise stated.

5. Patents

RU Patent #2394910 Luminescent biocatalyst for the determination of toxicants.

RU Patent #2255975 Recombinant plasmid DNA pTES-His-OPH and producer of oligo-histidine containing organophosphate hydrolase.

Author Contributions: Conceptualization, E.E.; methodology, E.E., A.I.; validation, O.M. and N.S.; formal analysis, O.M.; investigation, O.M. and N.S.; data curation, N.S.; writing—original draft preparation, O.M. and N.S.; writing—review and editing, E.E.; visualization, O.M. and N.S.; supervision, E.E.; project administration, E.E.; funding acquisition, E.E. All authors have read and agreed to the published version of the manuscript.

Funding: This work was financially supported by Russian Science Foundation (grant 16-14-00061).

Institutional Review Board Statement: Not applicable.

Informed Consent Statement: Not applicable.

Data Availability Statement: The data presented in this study are available in this article.

Acknowledgments: This research was performed according to the Development program of the Interdisciplinary Scientific and Educational School of Lomonosov Moscow State University "The future of the planet and global environmental change". The authors thank Ilya Lyagin (Chemistry Faculty, Lomonosov MSU, Moscow, Russia) for his valuable comments on calibration plots obtained with cholinesterases.

Conflicts of Interest: The authors declare no conflict of interest E.E. and A.I. are co-inventors and patent holders of the RU patent #2394910; E.E. is inventor of RU patent #2255975 which involves producer of His_6-OPH and the plasmid with gene encoding synthesis of the enzyme as a base active compound.

References

1. Kluczkovski, A.M. Fungal and mycotoxin problems in the nut industry. *Curr. Opin. Food Sci.* **2019**, *29*, 56–63. [CrossRef]
2. Janik, E.; Niemcewicz, M.; Ceremuga, M.; Stela, M.; Saluk-Bijak, J.; Siadkowski, A.; Bijak, M. Molecular aspects of mycotoxins—A serious problem for human health. *Int. J. Mol. Sci.* **2020**, *21*, 8187. [CrossRef] [PubMed]
3. Mamo, F.T.; Abate, B.A.; Tesfaye, K.; Nie, C.; Wang, G.; Liu, Y. Mycotoxins in Ethiopia: A review on prevalence, economic and health impacts. *Toxins* **2020**, *12*, 648. [CrossRef] [PubMed]
4. Kunz, B.M.; Wanko, F.; Kemmlein, S.; Bahlmann, A.; Rohn, S.; Maul, R. Development of a rapid multi-mycotoxin LC-MS/MS stable isotope dilution analysis for grain legumes and its application on 66 market samples. *Food Control* **2020**, *109*, 106949. [CrossRef]
5. Tran, V.N.; Viktorová, J.; Ruml, T. Mycotoxins: Biotransformation and bioavailability assessment using caco-2 cell monolayer. *Toxins* **2020**, *12*, 628. [CrossRef]
6. Agriopoulou, S.; Stamatelopoulou, E.; Varzakas, T. Advances in occurrence, importance, and mycotoxin control strategies: Prevention and detoxification in foods. *Foods* **2020**, *9*, 137. [CrossRef]
7. Li, P.; Su, R.; Yin, R.; Lai, D.; Wang, M.; Liu, Y.; Zhou, L. Detoxification of mycotoxins through biotransformation. *Toxins* **2020**, *12*, 121. [CrossRef]
8. Adebiyi, J.A.; Kayitesi, E.; Adebo, O.A.; Changwa, R.; Njobeh, P.B. Food fermentation and mycotoxin detoxification: An African perspective. *Food Control* **2019**, *106*, 106731. [CrossRef]
9. Narváez, A.; Rodríguez-Carrasco, Y.; Castaldo, L.; Izzo, L.; Ritieni, A. Ultra-high-performance liquid chromatography coupled with quadrupole Orbitrap high-resolution mass spectrometry for multi-residue analysis of mycotoxins and pesticides in botanical nutraceuticals. *Toxins* **2020**, *12*, 114. [CrossRef]
10. Wu, Y.; Yu, J.; Li, F.; Li, J.; Shen, Z. A calibration curve implanted enzyme-linked immunosorbent assay for simultaneously quantitative determination of multiplex mycotoxins in cereal samples, soybean and peanut. *Toxins* **2020**, *12*, 718. [CrossRef]
11. Lucci, P.; David, S.; Conchione, C.; Milani, A.; Moret, S.; Pacetti, D.; Conte, L. Molecularly imprinted polymer as selective sorbent for the extraction of zearalenone in edible vegetable oils. *Foods* **2020**, *9*, 1439. [CrossRef] [PubMed]
12. Shcherbakova, L.; Rozhkova, A.; Osipov, D.; Zorov, I.; Mikityuk, O.; Statsyuk, N.; Sinitsyna, O.; Dzhavakhiya, V.; Sinitsyn, A. Effective zearalenone degradation in model solutions and infected wheat grain using a novel heterologous lactonohydrolase secreted by recombinant *Penicillium canescens*. *Toxins* **2020**, *12*, 475. [CrossRef] [PubMed]
13. Lyagin, I.; Efremenko, E. Enzymes for detoxification of various mycotoxins: Origins and mechanisms of catalytic action. *Molecules* **2019**, *24*, 2362. [CrossRef] [PubMed]
14. Ben Taheur, F.; Kouidhi, B.; Al Qurashi, Y.M.A.; Ben Salah-Abbès, J.; Chaieb, K. Review: Biotechnology of mycotoxins detoxification using microorganisms and enzymes. *Toxicon* **2019**, *160*, 12–22. [CrossRef] [PubMed]
15. Valera, E.; García-Febrero, R.; Elliott, C.T.; Sánchez-Baeza, F.; Marco, M.P. Electrochemical nanoprobe-based immunosensor for deoxynivalenol mycotoxin residues analysis in wheat samples. *Anal. Bioanal. Chem.* **2019**, *411*, 1915–1926. [CrossRef]

16. Stadler, D.; Berthiller, F.; Suman, M.; Schuhmacher, R.; Krska, R. Novel analytical methods to study the fate of mycotoxins during thermal food processing. *Anal. Bioanal. Chem.* **2020**, *412*, 9–16. [CrossRef]
17. Senko, O.; Stepanov, N.; Maslova, O.; Akhundov, R.; Ismailov, A.; Efremenko, E. Immobilized luminescent bacteria for the detection of mycotoxins under discrete and flow-through conditions. *Biosensors* **2019**, *9*, 63. [CrossRef]
18. Lin, M.; Tan, J.; Xu, Z.; Huang, J.; Tian, Y.; Chen, B.; Wu, Y.; Tong, Y.; Zhu, Y. Computational design of enhanced detoxification activity of a zearalenone lactonase from *Clonostachysrosea* in acidic medium. *RSC Adv.* **2019**, *9*, 31284–31295. [CrossRef]
19. Chen, J.; Ye, J.; Zhang, Y.; Shuai, C.; Yuan, Q. Computer-aid molecular docking technology in cereal mycotoxin analysis. *J. Food Sci. Eng.* **2019**, *9*, 244–253. [CrossRef]
20. Efremenko, E.N.; Maslova, O.V.; Kholstov, A.V.; Senko, O.V.; Ismailov, A.D. Biosensitive element in the form of immobilized luminescent photobacteria for detecting ecotoxicants in aqueous flow–through systems. *Luminescence* **2016**, *31*, 1283–1289. [CrossRef]
21. Varfolomeev, S.D.; Efremenko, E.N. *Organophosphorus Neurotoxins: Monograph*; RIOR Publisher: Moscow, Russia, 2020; p. 380. [CrossRef]
22. Göbel, R.; Lusky, K. Simultaneous determination of aflatoxins, ochratoxin A, and zearalenone in grains by new immunoaffinity column/liquid chromatography. *J. AOAC Int.* **2004**, *87*, 411–416. [CrossRef] [PubMed]
23. Huang, B.; Han, Z.; Cai, Z.; Wu, Y.; Ren, Y. Simultaneous determination of aflatoxins B1, B2, G1, G2, M1 and M2 in peanuts and their derivative products by ultra-high-performance liquid chromatography–tandem mass spectrometry. *Anal. Chim. Acta* **2010**, *662*, 62–68. [CrossRef] [PubMed]
24. Ellman, G.L.; Courtney, K.D.; Andres, V., Jr.; Feather-Stone, R.M. A new and rapid colorimetric determination of acetylcholinesterase activity. *Biochem. Pharmacol.* **1961**, *7*, 88–95. [CrossRef]
25. Efremenko, E.; Votchitseva, Y.; Plieva, F.; Galaev, I.; Mattiasson, B. Purification of His_6-organophosphate hydrolase using monolithic supermacroporous polyacrylamide cryogels developed for immobilized metal affinity chromatography. *Appl. Microbiol. Biotechnol.* **2006**, *70*, 558–563. [CrossRef]
26. Votchitseva, Y.A.; Efremenko, E.N.; Aliev, T.K.; Varfolomeyev, S.D. Properties of hexahistidine-tagged organophosphate hydrolase. *Biochemistry* **2006**, *71*, 167–172. [CrossRef]

toxins

MDPI

Article

Biomonitoring of Enniatin B1 and Its Phase I Metabolites in Human Urine: First Large-Scale Study

Yelko Rodríguez-Carrasco [1,*,†], Alfonso Narváez [2,†], Luana Izzo [2], Anna Gaspari [2], Giulia Graziani [2] and Alberto Ritieni [2]

1 Department of Food Chemistry and Toxicology, University of Valencia, Av/Vicent A. Estellés s/n, 46100 Valencia, Spain

2 Department of Pharmacy, Università di Napoli Federico II, Via D. Montesano, 49-80131 Napoli, Italy; alfonsonsimon@gmail.com (A.N.); luana.izzo@unina.it (L.I.); annagaspari@virgilio.it (A.G.); gulia.graziani@unina.it (G.G.); alberto.ritieni@unina.it (A.R.)

* Correspondence: yelko.rodriguez@uv.es; Tel.: +34-963-544-117; Fax: +34-963-544-954

† These authors contributed equally to this work.

Received: 17 May 2020; Accepted: 17 June 2020; Published: 22 June 2020

Abstract: Enniatins (Enns) are mycotoxins produced by *Fusarium* spp. which are a fungus widely spread throughout cereals and cereal-based products. Among all the identified enniatins, Enn B1 stands as one of the most prevalent analogues in cereals in Europe. Hence, the aim of this study was to evaluate for the first time the presence of Enn B1 and its phase I metabolites in 300 human urine samples using an ultrahigh-performance liquid chromatography high resolution mass spectrometry (UHPLC-Q-Orbitrap HRMS) methodology. Enn B1 was detected in 94.3% of samples ranging from 0.007 to 0.429 ng/mL (mean value: 0.065 ng/mL). In accordance with previous in vitro and in vivo analysis, hydroxylated metabolites (78.0% samples) and carbonylated metabolites (66.0% samples) were tentatively identified as the major products. Results from this biomonitoring study point to a frequent intake of Enn B1 in the studied population, suggesting that in-depth toxicological studies are needed in order to understand the potential effects in humans.

Keywords: Enniatin B1; biomonitoring; in vivo; metabolomics; high resolution mass spectrometry (HRMS)

Key Contribution: The occurrence of the *Fusarium* mycotoxin Enn B1 and its phase I metabolites was evaluated for the first time in 300 human urine samples throughout ultrahigh-performance liquid chromatography high resolution mass spectrometry (UHPLC-Q-Orbitrap HRMS).

1. Introduction

Mycotoxins are toxic secondary metabolites mainly produced by the genera *Fusarium*, *Aspergillus*, *Penicillium*, *Claviceps*, and *Alternaria*. These compounds can be found in food and feed commodities, and consuming contaminated products can lead to adverse health effects in humans and animals. *Fusarium* fungi are frequent pathogens of cereal grains and maize, with a large impact in temperate regions of America and Europe [1]. Considering occurrence, toxicity, and consumption data, maximum limits have been set in foodstuffs for several mycotoxins alongside tolerable daily intakes (TDI) or provisional TDIs by a Joint Food and Agriculture Organization and World Health Organization (FAO/WHO) Expert Committee on Food Additives [2]. During the last few years attention has been put into emerging *Fusarium* mycotoxins, such as enniatins (Enns). Its core structure consists of a cyclohexadepsipeptide with alternating residues of three *N*-methyl amino acids and three hydroxyisovaleric acid [3]. To date, 29 different enniatins have been isolated as single compounds or as mixtures of homologues, being Enn B, Enn B1, Enn A1, and Enn A, being the most relevant in that order [4]. These Enns have been reported in cereal samples from Mediterranean and Scandinavian countries in concentration levels ranging from μg/kg to mg/kg [5,6] and also Enns carry-over potential from feedstuffs to animals has been suggested [7,8]. However, no maximum limits have been set for Enns in foodstuffs yet. In 2014, the European Food Safety Authority (EFSA) released a scientific opinion on the risk related to the occurrence of Enns in food and feed, concluding that there might be a concern about chronic exposure but the lack of toxicological studies hampers the risk assessment of dietary exposure [9]. To date, data is still being collected [10].

The toxicity of Enns is based on its ionophoric properties, being able to integrate themselves in biological membranes forming cation selective pores. Transport of mono and divalent cations through these pores disrupts normal physiological concentrations, leading to a wide range of toxicological effects. In vitro studies have reported phytotoxic, insecticidal, antibacterial, enzyme inhibition, antifungal, and immuno-modulatory activities. Besides, cytotoxic effects have been observed in several animal and cell lines at a low micromolar range [4,11]. Nevertheless, Enns have shown low toxicity in vivo, and rapid metabolization and elimination of Enns might be the main reason [12].

Regarding bioavailability, the Enn analogue with the highest oral absorption is Enn B [13,14]. There might also exist a specie-dependent relation, since absolute Enn B1 bioavailability in pigs (91%) is in strong contrast with the one observed in broiler chicken (5%) after single oral application [12,14]. Referring to metabolism, transformation of Enn B1 predominantly occurs via cytochrome P-450 3A-dependent oxidation reaction. Therefore, only phase I products seem relevant, since no phase II metabolites have been found yet. After incubation of Enn B1 with human and pig liver microsomes, 11 different metabolites were structurally characterized using liquid chromatography coupled to: iontrap mass spectrometry (ITMS), multiple-stage mass fragmentation (MS^n), and high resolution mass spectrometry (HRMS) coupled to an Orbitrap mass spectrometer [15,16]. Biotransformation processes of Enn B1 consisted in carbonylation, carboxylation, hydroxylation, and *N*-demethylation, following the same pattern observed for Enn B except for carbonylation [15,17].

There is scarce literature referring to the detection of enniatins and its resultant metabolites in biological samples, making it harder to assess the risk related to enniatins. Recently, the occurrence of Enn B and its tentative phase I metabolites in human urine was evaluated, finding the parental toxin and some of its tentative metabolites at a concentration of a few ng/mL [18]. Nevertheless, to date, there is no data available concerning the occurrence of Enn B1 and its tentative phase I metabolites in human biological fluids. In order to obtain a risk evaluation precisely, mycotoxins potentially present in foods and its metabolites have to be included in biological studies since the overall toxic profile could be influenced. Therefore, the aim of the present study was to evaluate for the first time the presence of Enn B1 and Enn B1 phase I metabolites in 300 urine samples from volunteers residing in southern Italy using ultrahigh-performance liquid chromatography coupled to high resolution Orbitrap mass spectrometry (UHPLC-Q-Orbitrap HRMS) and to tentatively identify the main Enn B1 metabolic pathway for producing scientific evidence on the pharmacokinetics process of this toxin.

2. Results and Discussion

2.1. Evaluation of UHPLC-Q-Orbitrap HRMS Conditions

The Enn B1-dependent tandem mass spectrometry (MS/MS) parameters were optimized by injection of 1 μg/mL of Enn B1-analytical standard into the UHPLC-Q-Orbitrap instrument. Results revealed a peak at 8.06 min in full scan mass spectrometry (MS), which showed a stable and abundant ammonium adduct $(M + NH_4)^+$ at *m/z* 671.45986 under positive electrospray ionization (ESI) mode corresponding to Enn B1. The mass error of the observed *m/z* was less than 2.5 ppm indicating exceptional agreement with the calculated *m/z*. In addition, product ions (*m/z* 558, 549, 458, 214 and 196) were generated by collision-induced dissociation of the Enn B1 ammonium adduct. These ions correspond to the loss of one or various *N*-methyl-valine, *N*-methyl-isoleucine, and hydroxyisovaleryl residues leading to the formation of main Enn B1 fragments.

Apart from the parent compound, in literature, up to 11 metabolic products were detected and their structures tentatively characterized through high-performance liquid chromatographic/mass spectrometric analyses. In this work, the ammonium adducts of the reported molecular masses were targeted in the Q-Orbitrap HRMS to evaluate the occurrence of the enniatin B1 metabolites in human urine samples. Therefore, a qualitative procedure was developed for detecting theoretical masses of the metabolites previously reported, whereas the same chromatographic gradient was used since all the investigated compounds were able to elute in that short run time.

Data for retention times, observed ion mass, and mass accuracy for Enn B1 and its metabolites are shown in Table 1.

Table 1. Retention times, observed mass, and mass accuracy of Enn B1 and its phase I metabolites.

Compound	Retention Time (min)	Molecular Formula	Observed Mass $(M + NH_4)^+$	Accuracy (Δppm)
Enn B1	5.75	$C_{34}H_{59}N_3O_9$	671.4591	−0.60
M1	4.76	$C_{33}H_{55}N_3O_{11}$	687.4175	−0.78
M2	5.44	$C_{34}H_{59}N_3O_{10}$	687.4532	−1.78
M3	5.5		687.4535	−1.34
M4	5.55		687.4536	−1.19
M5	5.6		687.4540	−0.61
M6	5.61	$C_{34}H_{57}N_3O_{10}$	685.4380	−1.12
M7	5.64		685.4384	−0.54
M8	5.67		685.4378	−1.42
M9	4.1	$C_{34}H_{57}N_3O_{11}$	701.4328	−1.26
M10	4.77		701.4335	−0.26
M11	4.79		701.4333	−0.55

2.2. Method Performance

Method results referring to matrix effects, linearity, trueness, repeatability, within-lab reproducibility, limit of quantification (LOQ), and limit of detection (LOD) were obtained following the guidelines set at Commission Decision 2002/ 657/EC [19] are shown in Table 2. A matrix influence was observed, leading to a signal suppression effect (63%) for Enn B1 in the urine samples. Hence, matrix-matched calibration was chosen for quantitative purposes. A coefficient of linearity (R^2) of 0.9997 was obtained within the range from 0.001 to 5 ng/mL. In order to evaluate the carry-over, a blank sample (n = 10) was analyzed just after the highest calibration sample. Since no peaks eluted in the same Enn B1 retention time area, no carry-over was assumed. Acceptable recoveries, ranging from 78% at 0.5 ng/mL to 95% at 5 ng/mL of spiking levels, were obtained. The RSD_r and RSD_R were ≤12% for all the concentrations studied, remarking the satisfactory precision of the developed method. LOQ and LOD values were extracted from matrix-matched solutions, being 0.0005 and 0.001 ng/mL, respectively. The developed method allowed a reliable detection and quantification of Enn B1 at low ppt range (Table 3).

Table 2. Method performance.

Parameters	R^2	SSE (%)	Recovery, % (RSD_R, %; n = 9)				LOD (ng/mL)	LOQ (ng/mL)
			5 ng/mL	1 ng/mL	0.5 ng/mL	0.1 ng/mL		
Enn B1	0.9997	63	95 (7)	88 (6)	78 (7)	84 (12)	0.0005	0.001

R^2, coefficient of correlation; RSD_R, inter-day relative standard deviation; LOD, limit of detection; LOQ, limit of quantification.

Table 3. Available methods for measurement of Enn B1 in human urine.

Urine Samples (*n*)	Origin	Positives Pamples (*n*, (%))	Sample Preparation	Determination			Reference
				Range (ng/mL)	Sensitivity (LOQ, ng/mL)	Detection Method	
10	Italy	1 (10)	SPE	<LOQ	0.005	QQQ (Thermo Fisher Scientific) ESI+ SRM mode	Serrano et al. (2015) [20]
10	Spain	6 (60)	DLLME	<LOQ–0.34	0.1	QQQ (Applied Biosystems) ESI+ SRM mode	Escrivá et al. (2017) [21]
60	China	0 (0)	SPE	-	0.0002	QQQ (AB SCIEX) ESI+ MRM mode	Liu et al. (2020) [22]
300	Italy	283 (94)	SALLE	<LOQ–0.429	0.001	Q-Orbitrap (Exactive, Thermo Fisher Scientific) ESI+ HRMS	This work

ESI+, positive ion mode; HRMS, high-resolution MS; SRM, selected reaction monitoring transition; MRM, multiple reaction monitoring transition; LOQ, limit of quantification; QQQ, triple quadrupole; SPE, solid phase extraction; DLLME, dispersive liquid-liquid microextraction; SALLE, salting-out liquid-liquid extraction.

2.3. *Occurrence of Enniatin B1 in Human Urines*

Enn B1 has been detected in 283 out of 300 urine (94.3%) ranging from <LOQ to 0.429 ng/mL (mean value: 0.065 ng/mL; Table 4). In a previous study, Escrivá et al. [21] evaluated the presence of Enn B1 in urine samples from the Spanish population, reporting occurrence in six samples (60%, $n = 10$), but only two samples could be quantified (0.1–0.34 ng/mL) due to analytical limitations (LOQ = 0.1 ng/mL). Serrano et al. [20] detected Enn B1 in one urine sample (10%, $n = 10$) collected from Italian volunteers, despite having high instrumental sensitivity (LOQ = 0.005 ng/mL). Differences showed among the mentioned studies could be due to the limited sampling. A more recent work, conducted by Liu et al. [22], analyzed 60 urine sample from the Chinese population, reporting the absence of Enn B1 (LOQ = 0.0002 ng/mL). The variation between the Chinese population urinary patterns of Enn B1 and the obtained results could be explained either by dietary habits or the quality of foodstuffs. Wheat has been reported as one of the most susceptible cereals for *Fusarium* spp. contamination [1] and, according to the data reported by FAO [23], the per capita annual consumption of wheat and wheat-based products during 2017 in Italy (146.22 kg) was more than double the consumption in China (62.75 kg). Following the same line, the urinary excretion pattern of Enn B, a structurally similar mycotoxin, was also reported to vary depending on geographical areas with different dietary habits [18]. Recently, strong associations to some cereals and to dietary fiber was reported for Enn B urinary concentration in Sweden [24]. These authors also reported associations to other *Fusarium* mycotoxins, such as deoxynivalenol, in these food categories; nonetheless, Enn B association to rice was negative but strong, which indicates that rice was not as contaminated as the other cereals (e.g., wheat). Hence, if rice consumption was increased in the diet, as in the case of the Asiatic people, the occurrence of Enns in biological fluids would consequently be reduced, which is in line with previous studies [22]. Therefore, the occurrence of Enn B1 in the majority of Italian cereals and cereal-based products analyzed by previous studies [25–27] alongside the high consumption of cereals (45–60% kcal per day for an Italian adult) [23] may account for the high incidence reported in the obtained results.

A statistical study for the evaluation of the occurrence of Enn B1 in urines from the three different population groups was conducted. The highest Enn B1 concentration was observed within the low-age group (age ≤ 30 years, mean = 0.071 ng/mL); however, no significant differences were found between occurrence of Enn B1 and age groups ($p = 0.93$). Similarly, gender did not show any correlation referring to Enn B1 concentrations ($p = 0.85$) in accordance with previous mycotoxins monitoring studies in urine [28–30].

Table 4. Occurrence of Enn B1 and Enn B1 metabolites in the analyzed human urine samples ($n = 300$).

Compound/Group	Incidence (%)	Range (ng/mL)	Mean [a] (ng/mL)
	Parent Compound		
Enn B1	94.3	0.007–0.429	0.069
	Enn B1 Biotransformation Products		
M1	5.3	0.007–0.177	0.035
Demethylated and hydroxylated (M1)	5.3	0.007–0.177	0.035
M2	11.0	0.006–0.019	0.010
M3	50.0	0.005–0.076	0.023
M4	18.0	0.002–0.143	0.025
M5	77.3	0.006–0.186	0.047
Hydroxylated group (M2–M5)	78.0	0.006–0.233	0.069
M6	40.0	0.012–1.511	0.105
M7	30.7	0.008–0.510	0.085
M8	48.0	0.042–1.310	0.128
Carbonylated group (M6–M8)	66.0	0.012–1.763	0.196
M9	0.7	0.019–0.045	0.032
M10	21.0	0.008–0.241	0.047
M11	14.0	0.002–0.451	0.053
Carboxylated group (M9–M11)	26.3	0.008–0.656	0.066

[a] Mean values are based in positive samples only.

2.4. Urinary Excretion Pattern of Enn B1 Phase I Metabolites

To date, there is scarce literature regarding Enn B1 metabolism. In vivo studies have been carried out in pigs and broiler chickens fed with Enn B1 contaminated feed, reporting the presence up to 11 tentative major Enn B1 metabolites in plasma and showing a good correlation with previous in vitro studies [14,15]. In a recent investigation conducted by Ivanova et al. [16], the same tentative metabolites were detected in vitro after the incubation of human liver microsomes with Enn B1. These metabolites are products of oxidative demethylation (M1), hydroxylation (M2–M5), carbonylation (M6–M8), and carboxylation (M9–M11) reactions. From a chromatographic point of view, all the identified metabolites eluted before the parental compound in reversed-phase chromatography since they became more hydrophilic after going through phase I metabolism pathways (Table 1). Nevertheless, the lack of standards of Enn B1 metabolites avoid an accurate quantification. To overcome that, the matrix-matched calibration curve from the parent compound was used as an approach in order to quantify its metabolites. The results obtained are shown in Table 4. The most prevalent groups were the hydroxylated and carbonylated Enn B1 metabolites, ranging from 0.006 to 0.233 ng/mL (78% samples) and from 0.012 to 1.763 ng/mL (66% samples), respectively. The carboxylated metabolites were found between 0.008 and 0.656 ng/mL (26.3% samples) and the demethylated products ranged from 0.007 to 0.177 ng/mL (5.3% samples). Within the hydroxylated group, the main metabolites were M5 > M3 > M4 > M2, in this order, with M5 representing 68% of all the hydroxylated metabolites quantified. Significant differences were found among concentration values of each metabolite ($p \leq 0.05$). Similarly, the main carbonylated metabolites were M8 > M6 > M7, and statistical analysis revealed significant differences among them ($p \leq 0.05$), with M8 being 48% of the total carbonylated metabolites. Whereas results reported by Ivanova et al. [16] showed a similar trend for hydroxylated compounds with M5 as the major one, the most relevant carbonylated product was M6, differing from the here-analyzed samples in which M6 only represented a 32% of the carbonylated products. The most important Enn B1 carboxylated metabolites were M10 and M11, whereas M9 showed very low incidence (0.7%). Ivanova et al. [15] detected M9 and M11 only in in vitro samples of pig liver microsomes, whereas the occurrence of M10 was restricted to in vivo samples. However, the results highlight M11 as another important product of carboxylation pathways in human. Differences observed between this work and in vitro Enn B1 biotransformation assays stand as additional evidence of potential pre-systemic metabolism. The demethylated metabolite M1 appeared to be irrelevant and the multiple reactions needed to generate this product may account for the low incidence showed (5.3%). Figure 1 shows the chromatograms of a sample contaminated with Enn B1 at 0.036 ng/mL; hydroxylated Enn B1 metabolites (M3: 0.053 ng/mL; M5: 0.174 ng/mL); carbonylated Enn B1 metabolites (M6: 0.034 ng/mL; M8: 0.045 ng/mL); and carboxylated Enn B1 metabolites (M10: 0.028 ng/mL; M11: 0.017 ng/mL).

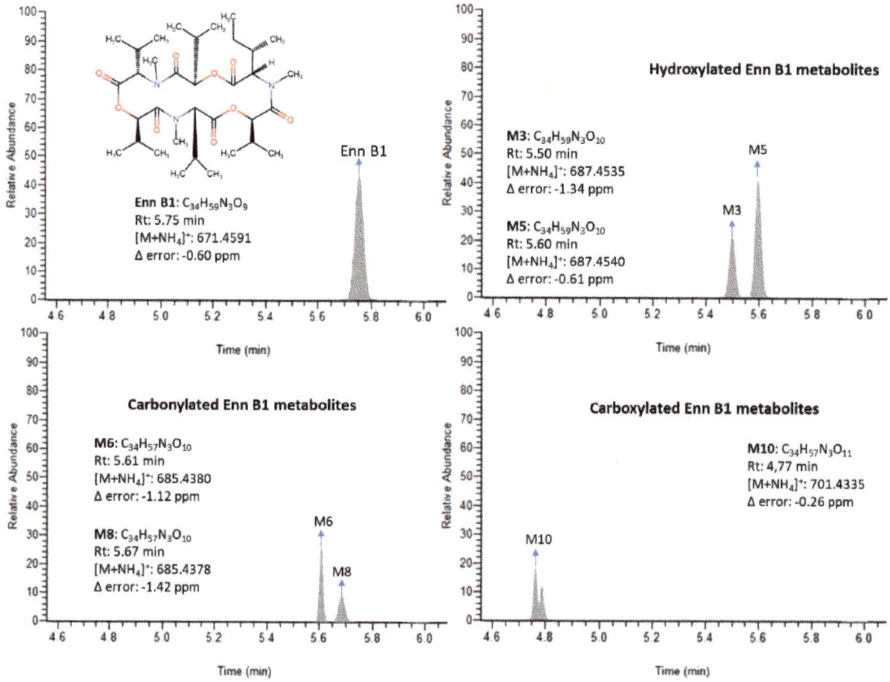

Figure 1. Chromatograms of a human urine sample containing Enn B1 at 0.036 ng/mL; hydroxylated Enn B1 metabolites (M3: 0.053 ng/mL; M5: 0.174 ng/mL); carbonylated Enn B1 metabolites (M6: 0.034 ng/mL; M8: 0.045 ng/mL); and carboxylated Enn B1 metabolites (M10: 0.028 ng/mL; M11: 0.017 ng/mL).

Referring to the samples with no Enn B1 contamination (5.7%, n = 17), only 1.3% (n = 4) did not show any Enn B1 metabolite, whereas at least two different metabolites were found in the 4.3% (n = 13) of the remaining samples, pointing to a complete biotransformation. The results reported above showed that the metabolization of Enn B1 in humans mainly occurs via hydroxylation and carbonylation reactions. Although cytochrome P450 3A4 (CYP3A4) is the main enzyme in the metabolism of Enn B and Enn B1, additional enzymes are also involved; CYP1A2 and CYP2C19 are present in Enn B pathway, whereas CYP3A4/5 is responsible for carbonylated products of Enn B1 as evidenced by Fæste et al. [31] and Ivanova et al. [16]. In fact, a previous work conducted by Rodríguez-Carrasco et al. [18] remarked the hydroxylated and demethylated products as the most relevant Enn B metabolites, whereas demethylated Enn B1 metabolite (M1) showed very low incidence in the present study. Despite a similar pattern of metabolic pathways for Enn B1 and Enn B has been reported in in vitro assays, major metabolites found in human urine are different for each mycotoxin. In the here analyzed samples, major metabolites frequently co-occurred with minor metabolites from the same group; M5 was found alongside any other hydroxylated metabolite in 99% (n = 232) of the positive samples (n = 234). Referring to carbonylated products, the presence of M8 combined with at least one different metabolite was detected in 52% (n = 103) of the positive samples (n = 198). Finally, co-occurrence was detected in 34% (n = 28) of samples containing carboxylated metabolites (n = 79).

3. Conclusions

In this study, the occurrence of the *Fusarium* mycotoxin Enn B1 and its phase I metabolites was evaluated in 300 human urine samples throughout ultrahigh-performance liquid chromatography high resolution mass spectrometry (UHPLC-Q-Orbitrap HRMS). Results confirmed the presence of Enn B1 in 94.3% of samples ranging from 0.007 to 0.429 ng/mL (mean value: 0.065 ng/mL). Furthermore, the occurrence of Enn B1 metabolites previously found in in vitro and in vivo analysis was evaluated for the first time in human urine samples. In accordance with literature, demethylated and oxidated metabolite (5.3% samples, mean content = 0.035 ng/mL), hydroxylated metabolites (78.0% samples, mean content = 0.069 ng/mL), carbonylated metabolites (66.0% samples, mean content = 0.196 ng/mL), and carboxylated metabolites (26.3%, mean content = 0.066 ng/mL) were tentatively identified. Statistical analysis confirmed hydroxylated and carbonylated products as the most prevalent metabolites of Enn B1 in human urine. Differences observed between this work and in vitro Enn B1 biotransformation assays stand as additional evidence of potential pre-systemic metabolism. The characterization of metabolites derived from food contaminants is an important issue when performing safety and risk evaluations, and according to the here-obtained results a frequent exposure to Enn B1 is highlighted in Italian population.

4. Materials

4.1. Chemicals, Reagents and Materials

Methanol (MeOH), acetonitrile (AcN), and water for liquid chromatography (LC) mobile phase (HPLC grade) were purchased from Merck (Darmstadt, Germany). Ammonium formate and formic acid were acquired from Fluka (Milan, Italy). Sodium chloride and C18 were provided from Sigma–Aldrich (Milan, Italy). Syringe filters with polytetrafluoroethylene membrane (PTFE; 15 mm, diameter 0.2 μm) were purchased from Phenomenex (Castel Maggiore, Italy). Analytical standard of Enn B1 (>95% HPLC purity) was obtained from Sigma–Aldrich (Milan, Italy). A stock solution (1 mg/mL in MeOH) was prepared and working standard solutions were built by serial dilution of the stock and stored at −20 °C.

4.2. Sampling

During January and February 2018, 300 Italian volunteers residing in Campania region (southern Italy) provided first-spot morning urine samples. The following exclusion criteria were considered for the study: (i) only one member per family allowed; (ii) people with severe issues in liver, kidney, or bile were not allowed due to potential interferences in the metabolic processes related to mycotoxins; (iii) people exposed to high amounts of mycotoxins in a different way from food, such as farmers and veterinarians, were not allowed. The use of medication was not an exclusion criterion due to the lack of information available about interferences with mycotoxins. Urine was stored in plastic containers at −20 °C within 2 h after collection. All volunteers signed informed consent following the Helsinki Declaration on ethical principles for medical research when humans are involved. The present study was accepted by the University of Valencia Institutional human research Committee and the procedures and purposes were properly justified and approved. The numerosity of the sampling (n = 300) is in accordance with the International Federation of Clinical Chemists (IFCC) recommendations [32].

Volunteers were asked to specify their age and gender on their own container, in order to classify the sample. The sampling tried to keep the gender parity (male: 45.7%, female: 54.3%). According to the age of participants, three different groups were considered for statistical analysis: ≤30 years old (n = 94), from 31 to 59 years old (n = 72), and ≥60 years old (n = 134). Samples with undetected levels of the analytes of interest were chosen as "blank" and used in spiking and recovery studies. The consumption data were set according to age and gender, following the Guidelines for Healthy Italian Food Supply reported by the National Institute for Food Research and Nutrition [33].

4.3. *Sample Preparation*

The sample was processed following a previous procedure slightly modified [34]. Briefly, 1.5 mL of sample was placed into a 2 mL Eppendorf Safe-Lock Microcentrifuge tube and centrifuged for 3 min at 4000 rpm. After that, 1 mL of the supernatant was transferred to a 15 mL screw cap test tube with conical bottom and 1 mL of acetonitrile was added. The mixture was vortexed for 30 s and subsequently 30 mg of C18 sorbent and 0.3 g sodium chloride were incorporated to minimize interference from matrix. The solution was vortexed again for 30 s and centrifuged for 3 min at 4000 rpm and 4 °C. Then, the upper layer was collected, evaporated under gentle nitrogen stream in a water bath at 45 °C, reconstituted with 0.5 mL of MeOH/H_2O (70:30 *v*/*v*) and filtered through a 0.2 µm filter before to UHPLC-Q-Orbitrap HRMS analysis.

4.4. *UHPLC-Q-Orbitrap HRMS Analysis*

Quantitative and qualitative profiles of Enn B1 and Enn B1 phase I metabolites were acquired through Ultra High Pressure Liquid Chromatograph (UHPLC; Thermo Fisher Scientific, Waltham, MA, USA) equipped with an auto sampler device, a degassing system, a thermostated (T = 30 °C) Luna Omega 1.6 µm (50 × 2.1 µm) column, a Dionex Ultimate 3000 a Quaternary UHPLC pump working at 1250 bar.

The eluent consisted of two different phases, both H_2O (phase A) and MeOH (phase B) containing 0.1% formic acid and 5 mM ammonium formate. The gradient elution program for LC prior to Orbitrap HRMS analysis was developed as follows: 0–1 min–0% of phase B, 2 min–95% of phase B, 2.5 min–95% of phase B, 5 min–75% of phase B, 6 min–60% of phase B, 6.5 min–0% of phase B, and 1.5 min–0% phase B for equilibrating the column. The flow rate was set at 0.4 mL/min. A total of 5 µL of the sample was injected. Detection was performed using a Q-Exactive mass spectrometer. Data were acquired through full scan in positive mode at a resolving power of 70,000 FWHM at *m/z* 200. Ion source parameters in positive (ESI+) mode were: sheath gas (N_2 > 95%) 35, auxiliary gas (N_2 > 95%) 10, spray voltage 4 kV, capillary temperature 290 °C, auxiliary gas heater temperature 305 °C, S-lens RF level 50. Data analysis and processing were carried-out using the Xcalibur software, v. 3.1.66.10 (Thermo Fisher Scientific, Waltham, MA, USA). A scan range of *m/z* 100–800 was set for the compounds of interest; the injection time was set to 200 ms and the automatic gain control (AGC) was selected at 1×10^6. Scan-rate was set at 2 scans/s.

4.5. *Metabolomic Data Processing*

Data processing and data pretreatment were performed to allow the putative identification of significant metabolites. Screening was done by investigating spectral data collected using a mycotoxin spectral library (version 1.1 for Library View Software, AB Sciex, Framingham, MA, USA) containing spectral data for 245 mycotoxins and other fungal/bacterial metabolites and 236 full MS/MS spectral library entries. The features, defined by their m/z and retention time, and their intensities in different samples were used to carry out the statistical analysis. Then, samples were grouped to perform the statistical analysis.

4.6. *Method Validation*

An in-house validation study was conducted according to the Commission Decision 2002/657/EC [19]. The parameters measured included linearity, matrix effect, trueness, precision, LOQ, and LOD. Linearity was evaluated using solvent and matrix-matched calibration curves, analyzing in triplicate six concentration levels ranging between 0.001–5 ng/mL. The matrix-matched calibration curves were prepared spiking aliquots of the corresponding matrices with Enn B1 at similar concentrations than the calibration curve made in solvent. Signal suppression or enhancement effect due to matrix co-elution interferences, was evaluated through a comparison between the slope of pure standard curve with the slope of matrix-matched standard curve following the next equation:

SSE (%) = Slope matrix-matched calibration/Slope standard in solvent × 100. Trueness and precision were assessed using recovery studies since no suitable reference material was available. Recovery measurements were performed by spiking blank urines with the standard working solution of Enn B1 at the levels of 0.1, 0.5, 1, and 5 ng/mL. Intra-day (RSD_r, %) and inter-day precision (RSD_R, %) were expressed as the relative standard deviation after repeating three measurements per concentration level on the same day and in three non-consecutive days, respectively. LOD was established as the minimum concentration at which the molecular ion can be identified (mass error < 5 ppm) and the LOQ as the lowest concentration of the analyte at which the concentration can be determined with accuracy and precision ≤20%.

4.7. Statistical Analysis

Statistical analysis of data was carried out using IBM SPSS version 25 statistical software package (SPSS, Chicago, IL, USA). For comparison of categorical data, the Pearson chi-square and Fisher exact tests were evaluated in order to assess whether Enn B1 occurrence in several subgroups (age, gender, cereal consumption) were significantly different. A non-parametric Kruskal–Wallis test was used to evaluate significant differences in Enn B1 metabolites concentrations. A confidence level of 95 % was assumed for examining data, whereas a p-value below 0.05 was considered as significant.

Author Contributions: Conceptualization, Y.R.-C. and A.R.; methodology, L.I. and A.N.; software, A.G. and G.G.; validation, L.I. and Y.R.-C.; formal analysis, L.I., A.N. and Y.R.-C.; data curation, A.G. and G.G.; writing—original draft preparation, A.N.; writing-review and editing, Y.R.-C.; supervision, Y.R.-C and A.R. All authors have read and agreed to the published version of the manuscript.

Funding: This research received no external funding.

Acknowledgments: Authors also acknowledge the technical support of Chiara Piemonte.

Conflicts of Interest: The authors declare no conflict of interest.

References

1. Ferrigo, D.; Raiola, A.; Causin, R. Fusarium toxins in cereals: Occurrence, legislation, factors promoting the appearance and their management. *Molecules* **2016**, *21*, 627. [CrossRef]
2. Commission Regulation (EC) No 1881/2006 of 19 December 2006 setting maximum levels for certain contaminants in foodstuffs. *Off. J. Eur. Union* **2006**, *364*, 324–365.
3. Prosperini, A.; Berrada, H.; Ruiz, M.J.; Caloni, F.; Coccini, T.; Spicer, L.J.; Perego, M.C.; Lafranconi, A. A review of the mycotoxin enniatin B. *Front. Public Health* **2017**, *5*, 304. [CrossRef]
4. Fraeyman, S.; Croubels, S.; Devreese, M.; Antonissen, G. Emerging Fusarium and Alternaria mycotoxins: Occurrence, toxicity and toxicokinetics. *Toxins* **2017**, *9*, 228. [CrossRef]
5. Meca, G.; Zinedine, A.; Blesa, J.; Font, G.; Mañes, J. Further data on the presence of Fusarium emerging mycotoxins enniatins, fusaproliferin and beauvericin in cereals available on the Spanish markets. *Food Chem. Toxicol.* **2010**, *48*, 1412–1416. [CrossRef]
6. Gruber-Dorninger, C.; Novak, B.; Nagl, V.; Berthiller, F. Emerging mycotoxins: Beyond traditionally determined food contaminants. *J. Agric. Food Chem.* **2016**, *65*, 7052–7070. [CrossRef] [PubMed]
7. Jestoi, M.; Rokka, M.; Jarvenpaa, E.; Peltonen, K. Determination of Fusarium mycotoxins beauvericin and enniatins (A, A1, B, B1) in eggs of laying hens using liquid chromatography–tandem mass spectrometry (LC–MS/MS). *Food Chem.* **2009**, *115*, 1120–1127. [CrossRef]
8. Johny, A.; Fæste, C.; Bogevik, A.S.; Berge, G.M.; Fernandes, J.M.O.; Ivanova, L. Development and Validation of a Liquid Chromatography High-Resolution Mass Spectrometry Method for the Simultaneous Determination of Mycotoxins and Phytoestrogens in Plant-Based Fish Feed and Exposed Fish. *Toxins* **2019**, *11*, 222. [CrossRef] [PubMed]
9. EFSA. Scientific Opinion on the risks to human and animal health related to the presence of beauvericin and enniatins in food and feed. *EFSA J.* **2014**, *12*, 3802. [CrossRef]
10. Maranghi, F.; Tassinari, R.; Narciso, L.; Tait, S.; Rocca, C.L.; Felice, G.D.; Butteroni, C.; Corinti, S.; Barletta, B.; Cordelli, E.; et al. In vivo toxicity and genotoxicity of beauvericin and enniatins. Combined approach to study

in vivo toxicity and genotoxicity of mycotoxins beauvericin (BEA) and enniatin B (ENNB). *EFSA Support. Publ.* **2018**, *15*, 1406E. [CrossRef]

11. Huang, C.H.; Wang, F.T.; Chan, W.H. Enniatin B1 exerts embryotoxic effects on mouse blastocysts and induces oxidative stress and immunotoxicity during embryo development. *Environ. Toxicol.* **2019**, *34*, 48–59. [CrossRef] [PubMed]
12. Devreese, M.; Broekaert, N.; De Mil, T.; Fraeyman, S.; De Backer, P.; Croubels, S. Pilot toxicokinetic study and absolute oral bioavailability of the Fusarium mycotoxin enniatin B1 in pigs. *Food Chem. Toxicol.* **2014**, *63*, 161–165. [CrossRef] [PubMed]
13. Devreese, M.; De Baere, S.; De Backer, P.; Croubels, S. Quantitative determination of the Fusarium mycotoxins beauvericin, enniatin A, A1, B and B1 in pig plasma using high performance liquid chromatography-tandem mass spectrometry. *Talanta* **2013**, *106*, 212–219. [CrossRef] [PubMed]
14. Fraeyman, S.; Devreese, M.; Antonissen, G.; De Baere, S.; Rychlik, M.; Croubels, S. Comparative Oral Bioavailability, Toxicokinetics, and Biotransformation of Enniatin B1 and Enniatin B in Broiler Chickens. *J. Agric. Food Chem.* **2016**, *64*, 7259–7264. [CrossRef] [PubMed]
15. Ivanova, L.; Uhlig, S.; Devreese, M.; Croubels, S.; Fæste, C.K. Biotransformation of the mycotoxin enniatin B1 in pigs: A comparative in vitro and in vivo approach. *Food Chem. Toxicol.* **2017**, *105*, 506–517. [CrossRef] [PubMed]
16. Ivanova, L.; Denisov, I.G.; Grinkova, Y.V.; Sligar, S.G.; Fæste, C. Biotransformation of the Mycotoxin Enniatin B1 by CYP P450 3A4 and Potential for Drug-Drug Interactions. *Metabolites* **2019**, *9*, 158. [CrossRef]
17. Ivanova, L.; Fæste, C.; Uhlig, S. In vitro phase I metabolism of the depsipeptide enniatin B. *Anal. Bioanal. Chem.* **2011**, *400*, 2889–2901. [CrossRef]
18. Rodríguez-Carrasco, Y.; Izzo, L.; Gaspari, A.; Graziani, G.; Mañes, J.; Ritieni, A. Urinary levels of enniatin B and its phase I metabolites: First human pilot biomonitoring study. *Food Chem. Toxicol.* **2018**, *118*, 454–459. [CrossRef]
19. European Commission. Commission Decision of 12 August 2002 implementing Council Directive 96/23/EC concerning the performance of analytical methods and the interpretation of results. *Off. J. Eur. Communities* **2002**, *221*, 8–36.
20. Serrano, A.B.; Capriotti, A.L.; Cavaliere, C.; Piovesana, S.; Samperi, R.; Ventura, S.; Laganà, A. Development of a Rapid LC-MS/MS Method for the Determination of Emerging Fusarium mycotoxins Enniatins and Beauvericin in Human Biological Fluids. *Toxins* **2015**, *7*, 3554–3571. [CrossRef]
21. Escrivá, L.; Manyes, L.; Font, G.; Berrada, H. Mycotoxin Analysis of Human Urine by LC-MS/MS: A Comparative Extraction Study. *Toxins* **2017**, *9*, 330. [CrossRef] [PubMed]
22. Liu, Z.; Zhao, X.; Wu, L.; Zhou, S.; Gong, Z.; Zhao, Y.; Wu, Y. Development of a Sensitive and Reliable UHPLC-MS/MS Method for the Determination of Multiple Urinary Biomarkers of Mycotoxin Exposure. *Toxins* **2020**, *12*, 193. [CrossRef] [PubMed]
23. FAO. Food Balance Sheets. Available online: http://www.fao.org/faostat/en/#data/ (accessed on 24 March 2020).
24. Lemming, E.W.; Montes, A.M.; Schmidt, J.; Cramer, B.; Humpf, H.-U.; Moraeus, L.; Olsen, M. Mycotoxins in blood and urine of Swedish adolescents-possible associations to food intake and other background characteristics. *Mycotoxin Res.* **2020**, *36*, 193–206. [CrossRef] [PubMed]
25. Jestoi, M.; Somma, M.; Kouva, M.; Veijalainen, P.; Rizzo, A.; Ritieni, A.; Peltonen, K. Levels of mycotoxins and sample cytotoxicity of selected organic and conventional grain-based products purchased from Finnish and Italian markets. *Mol. Nutr. Food Res.* **2004**, *48*, 299–307. [CrossRef]
26. Wallin, S.; Gambacorta, L.; Kotova, N.; Warensjö Lemming, E.; Nälsén, C.; Solfrizzo, M.; Olsen, M. Biomonitoring of concurrent mycotoxin exposure among adults in Sweden through urinary multi-biomarker analysis. *Food Chem. Toxicol.* **2015**, *83*, 133–139. [CrossRef]
27. Ciasca, B.; Pascale, M.; Altieri, V.; Longobardi, F.; Suman, M.; Catellani, D.; Lattanzio, V. In house validation and small scale collaborative study to evaluate analytical performances of multi-mycotoxin screening methods based on liquid chromatography-high resolution mass spectrometry: Case study on Fusarium toxins in wheat. *J. Mass. Spectrom.* **2018**, *53*, 743–752. [CrossRef]
28. Rodríguez-Carrasco, Y.; Moltó, J.C.; Mañes, J.; Berrada, H. Development of a GC–MS/MS strategy to determine 15 mycotoxins and metabolites in human urine. *Talanta* **2014**, *128*, 125–131. [CrossRef]

29. Ali, N.; Degen, G.H. Urinary biomarkers of exposure to the mycoestrogen zearalenone and its modified forms in German adults. *Arch. Toxicol.* **2018**, *92*, 2691–2700. [CrossRef]
30. Li, C.; Deng, C.; Zhou, S.; Zhao, Y.; Wang, D.; Wang, X.; Gong, Y.Y.; Wu, Y. High-throughput and sensitive determination of urinary zearalenone and metabolites by UPLC-MS/MS and its application to a human exposure study. *Anal. Bioanal. Chem.* **2018**, *410*, 5301–5312. [CrossRef]
31. Fæste, C.K.; Ivanova, L.; Uhlig, S. In Vitro Metabolism of the Mycotoxin Enniatin B in Different Species and Cytochrome P450 Enzyme Phenotyping by Chemical Inhibitors. *Drug Metab. Dispos.* **2011**, *39*, 1768–1776. [CrossRef]
32. Pérez, R.; Domenech, E.; Coscollà, C.; Yusa, V. Human Biomonitoring of food contaminants in Spanish children: Design, sampling and lessons learned. *Int. J. Hyg. Environ. Health* **2017**, *220*, 1768–1776. [CrossRef] [PubMed]
33. INRAN. *Dietary Guidelines for Healthy Eating*; Revision 2018; National Institute for Food Research and Nutrition: Rome, Italy, 2018.
34. Rodríguez-Carrasco, Y.; Moltó, J.C.; Mañes, J.; Berrada, H. Development of microextraction techniques in combination with GC–MS/MS for the determination of mycotoxins and metabolites in human urine. *J. Sep. Sci.* **2017**, *40*, 1572–1582. [CrossRef] [PubMed]

toxins

MDPI

Article

Individual and Combined Effect of Zearalenone Derivates and Beauvericin Mycotoxins on SH-SY5Y Cells

Fojan Agahi, Guillermina Font, Cristina Juan * and Ana Juan-García

Laboratory of Food Chemistry and Toxicology, Faculty of Pharmacy, University of Valencia, Av. Vicent Andrés Estellés s/n, 46100 Burjassot, València, Spain; agahifozhan@gmail.com (F.A.); crisjua3@uv.es (G.F.); ana.juan@uv.es (A.J.-G.)

* Correspondence: Cristina.juan@uv.es

Received: 9 February 2020; Accepted: 25 March 2020; Published: 27 March 2020

Abstract: Beauvericin (BEA) and zearalenone derivatives, α-zearalenol (α-ZEL), and β-zearalenol (β-ZEL), are produced by several *Fusarium* species. Considering the impact of various mycotoxins on human's health, this study determined and evaluated the cytotoxic effect of individual, binary, and tertiary mycotoxin treatments consisting of α-ZEL, β-ZEL, and BEA at different concentrations over 24, 48, and 72 h on SH-SY5Y neuronal cells, by using the MTT assay (3-(4,5-dimethylthiazol-2-yl)-2,5diphenyltetrazoliumbromide). Subsequently, the isobologram method was applied to elucidate if the mixtures produced synergism, antagonism, or additive effects. Ultimately, we determined the amount of mycotoxin recovered from the media after treatment using liquid chromatography coupled with electrospray ionization–quadrupole time-of-flight mass spectrometry (LC–ESI–qTOF-MS). The IC_{50} values detected at all assayed times ranged from 95 to 0.2 μM for the individual treatments. The result indicated that β-ZEL was the most cytotoxic mycotoxin when tested individually. The major effect detected for all combinations assayed was synergism. Among the combinations assayed, α-ZEL + β-ZEL + BEA and α-ZEL + BEA presented the highest cytotoxic potential with respect to the IC value. At all assayed times, BEA was the mycotoxin recovered at the highest concentration in individual form, and β-ZEL + BEA was the combination recovered at the highest concentration.

Keywords: SH-SY5Y cells; zearalenone derivates; beauvericin; MTT; qTOF–MS/MS

Key Contribution: β-ZEL alone presented the highest cytotoxicological potency than α-ZEL and BEA on SH-SY5Y neuronal cells; α-ZEL + β-ZEL + BEA and α-ZEL + BEA presented the highest cytotoxic potential with respect to the IC value.

---

1. Introduction

Mycotoxins represent one of the most important categories of biologically produced natural toxins with potential effects on human and animal health. The worldwide contamination by these natural products of food, feed, and environment, represents a health risk for animals and humans [1].

Several *Fusarium* species produce toxic substances of considerable concern to livestock and poultry producers. The mycotoxins beauvericin (BEA) and zearalenone (ZEN) and their derivatives (α-zearalenol (α-ZEL), β-zearalenol (β-ZEL), zeranol, taleranol, and zearalanone) can be produced by several *Fusarium* species (mainly *Fusarium graminearum*, but also *Fusarium culmorum*, *Fusarium cerealis*, *Fusarium equiseti*, and *Fusarium semitectum*) that grow on crops in temperate and warm-climate zones [2]. These fungi are present in almost all continents, can grow under poor storage conditions, and mainly contaminate cereal grains, such as maize, wheat, oats, soybeans, and their derived food products [3,4].

It has been proved that ZEN and α-ZEL bind to human estrogen receptors and elicit permanent reproductive tract alterations, and consequently, chronical exposure to ZEN present contaminated food can be a cause of female reproductive changes as a result of its powerful estrogenic activity [5–8]. It has been also reported that ZEN induces genotoxic effects by induction of DNA adducts, DNA fragmentation, and apoptosis [9,10]. As reported by Dong et al. (2010) [5], metabolic conversion of ZEN mycotoxin to α-ZEL and β-ZEL was found in almost all tissues and occurred more efficiently to α-ZEL than to β-ZEL; these mycotoxins are endocrine disruptors which affect steroid hormones such as progesterone [7]. In 2016, EFSA (European food Safety Authorities) indicated that there is a high uncertainty associated with the exposure to ZEN and its modified forms and so that it would rather overestimate than underestimate any risk associated with exposure to modified ZEN [8]. Also, recent studies have indicated that ZEN is immunotoxic [4,11,12] and cytotoxic in various cell lines by inhibiting cell proliferation and increasing ROS (reactive oxygen species) generation [13–15].

On the other hand, BEA causes cytotoxic effects by reducing cell proliferation in a time- and concentration-dependent manner [16,17]. Moreover, it can increase ROS generation and lipid peroxidation and produces oxidative stress and depletion of antioxidant cellular mechanisms [14,18,19].

Neurotoxicological testing is mainly based on experimental animal models, but several cell lines and tissue culture models have been developed to study the mechanism of neurotoxicity. In general, cells of human origin are attractive alternatives to animal models for the exploration of toxicity to humans. Nonetheless, there are few studies about the effect of mycotoxins at the neuronal level [6,20–22].

Regarding the important role of the food industry in human health, studying the impact of mycotoxins and their combinations in feed and food commodities has gained attention over the last few years, due to the ability of most *Fusarium* spp. to simultaneously produce different mycotoxins [23–25]. Hence, EFSA has recently published a draft guidance document where a harmonized risk assessment methodology for combined exposure to multiple chemicals in all relevant areas is described [26].

Due to the importance of dietetic exposure to various mycotoxins and their impacts on human's health, there is an increasing concern about the hazard of co-occurrence of mycotoxins produced by *Fusarium* and of co-exposure to them through diet. Many studies have been conducted on the toxicity of individual mycotoxins; however, few studies have been dedicated to the toxicological interaction of mycotoxins when present in double and triple combinations on different cell lines [16–18,27–29].

The objective of the present study was to investigate the cytotoxicological interactions between α-ZEL, β-ZEL, and BEA mycotoxins in human neuroblastoma SH-SY5Y cells, via the MTT assay. The effects of combinations of two and three mycotoxins were evaluated by isobologram analysis [30] to determine whether their interaction was synergistic, additive, or antagonistic, as well as to understand how mycotoxins can act at the cellular level.

2. Results

2.1. Cytotoxicity Assay of Individual and Combined Mycotoxins

The cytotoxicity effects of α-ZEL, β-ZEL, and BEA mycotoxins on SH-SY5Y cells were evaluated by the MTT assays over 24, 48, and 72 h. Figure 1 shows the time- and concentration-dependent decrease in cell viability after exposure to each mycotoxin individually, while IC_{50} values are shown in Table 1. After 24 h, the IC_{50} value could be calculated only for β-ZEL and was 94.3 ± 2.0 μM; after 48 h of exposure, the IC_{50} values were 20.8 ± 0.5 μM for α-ZEL and 9.1 ± 1.8 μM for β-ZEL. After 72 h of exposure, the IC_{50} values were 14.0 ± 1.8 μM, 7.5 ± 1.2 μM. and 2.5 ± 0.2 μM for α-ZEL, β-ZEL, and BEA, respectively. According to the IC_{50} values obtained at 72 h, BEA showed the highest cytotoxic effect on SH-S5Y5 cells (Table 1).

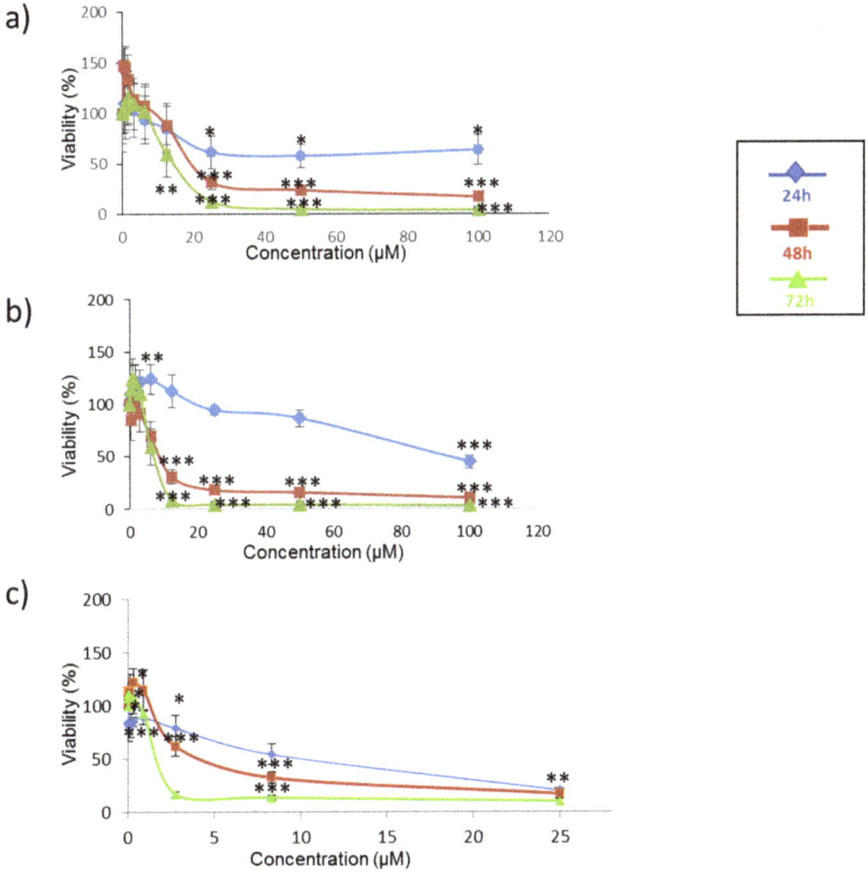

Figure 1. Cytotoxicity of the mycotoxins α-ZEL (**a**), β-ZEL (**b**), and BEA (**c**) individually at 24 h, 48 h, and 72 h. All values are the results of three independent experiments with eight replicates and are expressed as mean ± SD; $p \leq 0.05$ (*), $p \leq 0.01$ (**), $p \leq 0.001$ (***).

Table 1. Medium inhibitory concentration (IC_{50} ± SD) of α-zearalenol (α-ZEL), β-zearalenol (β-ZEL), and beauvericin (BEA) for SH-SY5Y cells after 24, 48, and 72 h of exposure, determined by the MTT assay. Three independent experiments were performed with eight replicates each.

Mycotoxin	IC_{50} (μM) ± SD		
	24 h	**48 h**	**72 h**
α-ZEL	n.a	20.8 ± 0.5	14.0 ± 1.8
β-ZEL	94.3 ± 2.0	9.1 ± 1.8	7.5 ± 1.2
BEA	n.a	n.a	2.5 ± 0.2

n.a: not available.

The cytotoxic effect of binary and tertiary combinations of α-ZEL, β-ZEL, and BEA on SH-SY5Y cells was evaluated by the MTT assays over 24, 48, and 72 h. The dose–response curves of the two- and three-mycotoxin combinations are shown in Figures 2 and 3, which demonstrate higher cytotoxicity of the combinations compared with individual mycotoxin. Figure 2 shows the concentration-dependent decrease in SH-SY5Y cell viability upon combined treatment with α-ZEL + BEA (5:1) (Figure 2a), β-ZEL + BEA (5:1) (Figure 2b), α-ZEL + β-ZEL (1:1) (Figure 2c); Figure 3 shows the results for α-ZEL + β-ZEL + BEA (5:5:1).

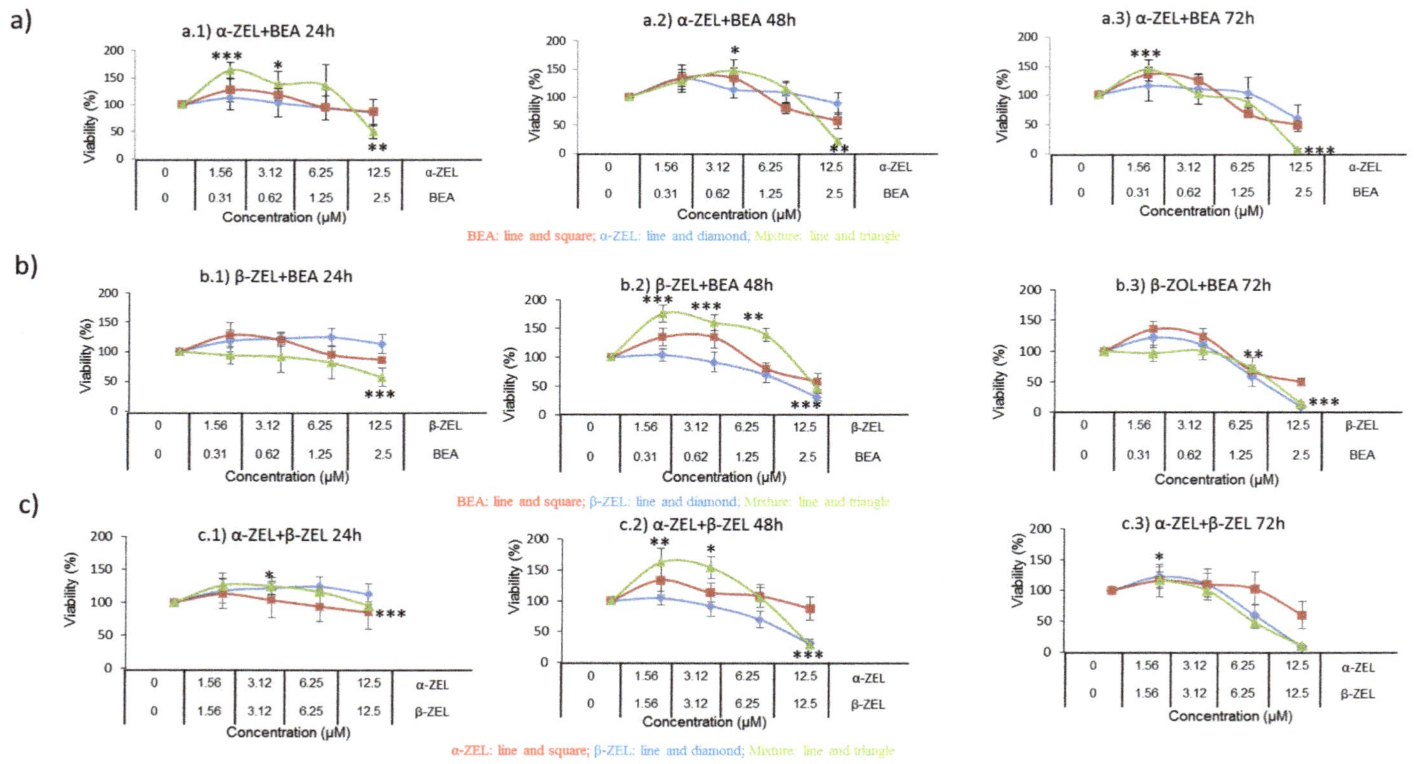

Figure 2. Cytotoxicity of the mycotoxin combinations of α-ZEL + BEA (5:1) (**a**), β-ZEL + BEA (5:1) (**b**), and α-ZEL + β-ZEL (1:1) (**c**) at 24 h (a.1, b.1, and c.1), 48 h (a.2, b.2, and c.2) and 72 h (a.3, b.3, and c.3). All values are the results of three independent experiments with eight replicates and are expressed as mean ± SD; $p \leq 0.05$ (*), $p \leq 0.01$ (**), $p \leq 0.001$ (***).

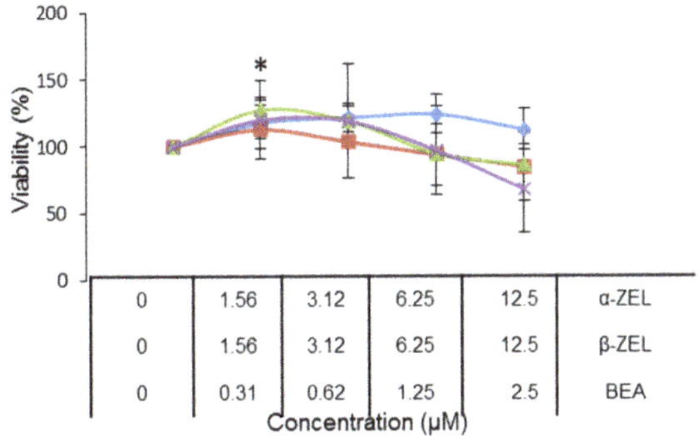

(**a**)

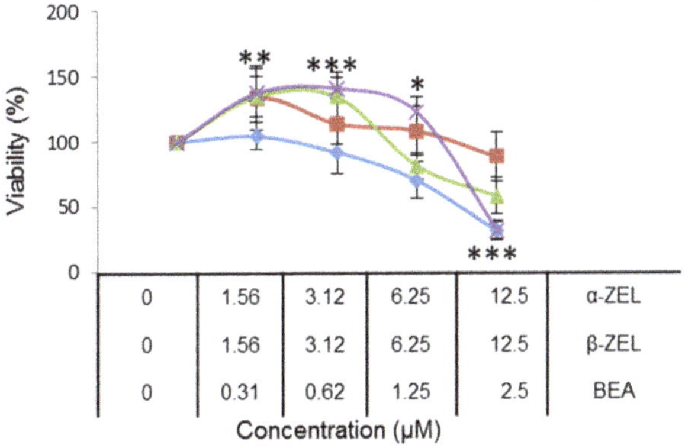

(**b**)

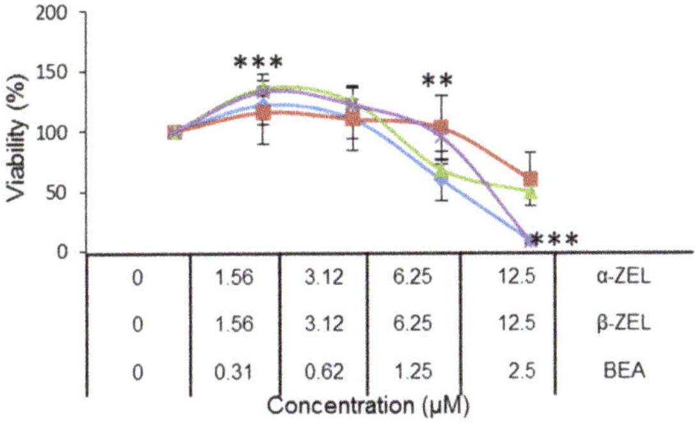

(**c**)

Figure 3. Cytotoxicity of the mycotoxin combination of α-ZEL + β-ZEL + BEA (5:5:1) at 24 h (**a**), 48 h, (**b**) and 72 h (**c**). All values are the results of three independent experiments with eight replicates and are expressed as mean ± SD; $p \leq 0.05$ (*), $p \leq 0.01$ (**), $p \leq 0.001$ (***). BEA: line and square; β-ZEL: line and diamond; α-ZEL: line and triangle; Mixture: line and ×.

The α-ZEL + BEA combination at the highest concentration induced a decrease in cell proliferation at 24 h of exposure (Figure 2a) of 35% with respect to the effect α-ZEL tested individually and of 37% with respect to the effect BEA. After 48 h of exposure, the decrease in cell proliferation was 67% with respect to that measured for α-ZEL and 36% with respect to that measured for BEA. After 72 h of exposure, the viability decreased 53% with respect to α-ZEL and 43% with respect to BEA. After 24 h of exposure, the β-ZEL + BEA combination (Figure 2b) decreased cell proliferation by about 55% and 29% at the highest concentration with respect to β-ZEL and BEA tested individually, respectively. After 48 h of exposure, the highest concentration of the combination reduced cell proliferation by 11% with respect to BEA tested individually. Also, at 72 h of exposure, the combination decreased cell proliferation by approximately 36% with respect to BEA individually tested. Such effect was not noticed after 48 and 72 h with respect to b-ZEL. In Figure 2c, the α-ZEL + β-ZEL combination after 24 h of exposure showed 17% of decrease in cell proliferation compared to β-ZEL individually assayed. After 48 and 72 h of exposure, the highest concentration of the combination reduced cell proliferation by 60% and 50%, respectively, compared to α-ZEL tested alone, whereas, this did not happen with respect to β-ZEL after 48 and 72 h of exposure. Figure 3 shows the dose–response curves for the tertiary combination of α-ZEL, β-ZEL, and BEA at 24, 48, and 72 h of exposure in SH-SY5Y cells. At 24 h of exposure, cell proliferation decreased by 16%, 44%, and 18% compared to cells exposed to α-ZEL, β-ZEL, and BEA alone. After 48 and 72 h of exposure, a significant reduction in cell proliferation, corresponding to 57% and 51%, was observed with respect to α-ZEL alone, and a reduction of 26% and 41% was observed with respect to BEA alone, while such effect was not observed with respect to β-ZEL alone.

The isobologram analysis was used to determine the type of interaction between α-ZEL, β-ZEL, and BEA. The values of the parameters *Dm*, *m*, and *r* of the double and triple combinations, as well as of the mean combination index (CI) are shown in Table 2. The IC_{50}, IC_{75}, and IC_{90} are the doses required to inhibit proliferation at 25%, 50%, 75%, and 90%, respectively. These CI values were calculated automatically by the computer software CalcuSyn. The CI fractional effect (*fa*) curves for α-ZEL, β-ZEL, and BEA combinations in SH-SY5Y cells are shown in Figure 4. Synergism for all concentration of the α-ZEL + BEA (5:1) mixture after 24 and 48 h of exposure was demonstrated; however, after 72 h of exposure, an additive effect for the α-ZEL + BEA combination was observed (Figure 4a, Table 2). The β-ZEL + BEA (5:1) mixture showed synergism after 24 h of exposure; however, after 48 and 72 h it showed antagonism at high concentrations and moderate synergism at low concentrations (Figure 4b, Table 2). The mixture of α-ZEL + β-ZEL showed antagonism after 24 h of exposure at all concentrations assayed but at 48 and 72 h, it showed antagonism at high concentration and a moderate synergism at low concentration (Figure 4c, Table 2). The tertiary mixture, after 24 h of exposure, showed antagonism at high concentration and synergism at low concentration, while after 48 h, it showed synergism and after 72 h, antagonism at all concentrations assayed (Figure 4d, Table 2).

Cytotoxicity after 24 h of incubation decreased in this order: α-ZEL + BEA > β-ZEL + BEA > α-ZEL + β-ZEL + BEA > α-ZEL + β-ZEL. After 48 and 72 h of incubation, the ranking was α-ZEL + BEA > β-ZEL + BEA >α-ZEL + β-ZEL > α-ZEL + β-ZEL + BEA.

2.2. *α-ZEL, β-ZEL, and BEA Present in Cell Medium after Treatment in Binary and Tertiary Combination*

The medium of SH-SY5Y cells containing α-ZEL, β-ZEL, and BEA after treatments (individual and combined after 24, 48, and 72h) was collected from each well. The amount of each mycotoxin remaining in the medium was calculated as a percentage with respect to the respective amount used in the exposure assays. In this sense, we determined whether the amounts were above or below 50% of those used for treatment (Figure 5). In individual exposures, the amounts of BEA and β-ZEL in the medium were below 50% at 48 and 72 h (Figure 5b,c), while, at 24 h, their concentrations tended to be higher and >50% for both mycotoxins. For α-ZEL, the concentration in the medium was maintained above 50% at all times studied (Figure 5a). This evidenced that a lower amount of α-ZEL exerted the examined effect compared to the amount necessary for BEA and β-ZEL, as higher amounts of α-ZEL were detectable in the medium at all times and concentrations.

In the binary combination α-ZEL + BEA (5:1), the amounts of each mycotoxin after 24 and 48 h were below 50% (Figure 5d.1,d.2), although the amount of BEA was higher than that of α-ZEL once the concentration assayed overpassed 0.62 μM for BEA and 3.12 μM for α-ZEL, revealing that the effects exerted by this mixture in neuroblastoma cells depended on both mycotoxins and were due more to α-ZEL than to BEA. This tendency at 72 h was more accentuated, as the amount of BEA in the medium was above 50% for all concentrations, while that of α-ZEL was below 50% (Figure 5d.3).

Also, for the combination β-ZEL + BEA (5:1), the mycotoxin's percentage remaining in the media was the same as that found for α-ZEL + BEA; however, β-ZEL was detected in higher amount than BEA in all scenarios, revealing that the effect of this mixture and was due more to BEA than to β-ZEL (Supplementary Figure S1A). On the other hand, for the binary combination of ZEN metabolites, α-ZEL + β-ZEL (1:1), the amounts of mycotoxins recovered were below 50%, and slightly superior for α-ZEL than for β-ZEL. This revealed that both mycotoxins contributed to the effect of this mixture in SH-SY5Y cell line (Supplementary Figure S1B). For the tertiary combination (α-ZEL + β-ZEL + BEA, (5:5:1)), the mycotoxins' percentages detected were also below 50% of the administered concentration, and this percentage was higher for higher concentrations administered and lower time of exposure (Figure 5e). This revealed that high amounts of α-ZEL and β-ZEL accessed the neuroblastoma cells, and the effect was due more to β-ZEL at 48 and 72 h, according to the results in Figures 3 and 5.

Table 2. The parameters *Dm*, *m*, and *r* are the antilog of x-intercept, the slope, and the linear correlation of the median-effect plot, which means the shape of the dose–effect curve, the potency (IC_{50}), and the conformity of the data to the mass action law, respectively [30,31]. *Dm* and *m* values are used for calculating the combination index (CI) value (CI < 1, =1, and >1 indicate synergism (Syn), additive (Add) effect, and antagonism (Ant), respectively. IC_{50}, IC_{75}, and IC_{90} are the doses required to inhibit proliferation at 50%, 75%, and 90%, respectively. CalcuSyn software automatically provided theses values.

Mycotoxin	Time (h)	Dm (μM)	m	r	IC Values					
					IC_{50}		IC_{75}		CI_{90}	
α-ZEL	24	66.10	1.36	0.9679						
	48	31.59	1.82	0.9726						
	72	15.24	2.02	0.9873						
β-ZEL	24	171.33	1.28	0.9709						
	48	12.46	1.26	0.9715						
	72	11.65	2.28	0.9464						
BEA	24	21.65	0.98	0.9763						
	48	3.68	1.24	0.9945						
	72	2.59	1.40	0.9805						
α-ZEL+BEA	24	3.05	1.36	0.9736	0.37 ± 0.33	Syn	0.34 ± 0.35	Syn	0.31 ± 0.38	Syn
	48	1.16	1.56	0.9933	0.50 ± 0.24	Syn	0.47 ± 0.26	Syn	0.44 ± 0.29	Syn
	72	1.34	1.54	0.94708	0.96 ± 0.86	Add	1.00 ± 0.51	Add	1.20 ± 1.30	Ant
β-ZEL+BEA	24	3.78	1.20	0.9698	0.29 ± 0.19	Syn	0.26 ± 0.21	Syn	0.24 ± 0.24	Syn
	48	4.81	3.04	0.7744	3.24 ± 0.42	Ant	1.94 ± 0.32	Ant	1.00 ± 0.14	Add
	72	1.89	3.14	0.7585	1.35 ± 0.51	Ant	1.00 ± 0.12	Add	0.60 ± 0.52	Syn
α-ZEL+β-ZEL	24	133.46	1.73	0.7782	2.80 ± 1.01	Ant	2.32 ± 0.51	Ant	1.92 ± 0.62	Ant
	48	19.12	3.40	0.7782	2.14 ± 0.23	Ant	1.35 ± 0.18	Ant	0.30 ± 0.14	Syn
	72	7.89	5.01	0.9409	2.60 ± 0.90	Ant	1.42 ± 0.63	Ant	0.45 ± 0.42	Syn
α-ZEL+β-ZEL+BEA	24	3.74	3.14	0.9478	0.57 ± 0.30	Syn	0.32 ± 0.20	Syn	0.19 ± 0.14	Syn
	48	0.01	0.43	0.7465	0.23 ± 0.06	Syn	0.15 ± 0.07	Syn	0.18 ± 0.10	Syn
	72	7.47	2.30	0.8966	8.54 ± 0.77	Ant	7.60 ± 0.85	Ant	6.88 ± 0.95	Ant

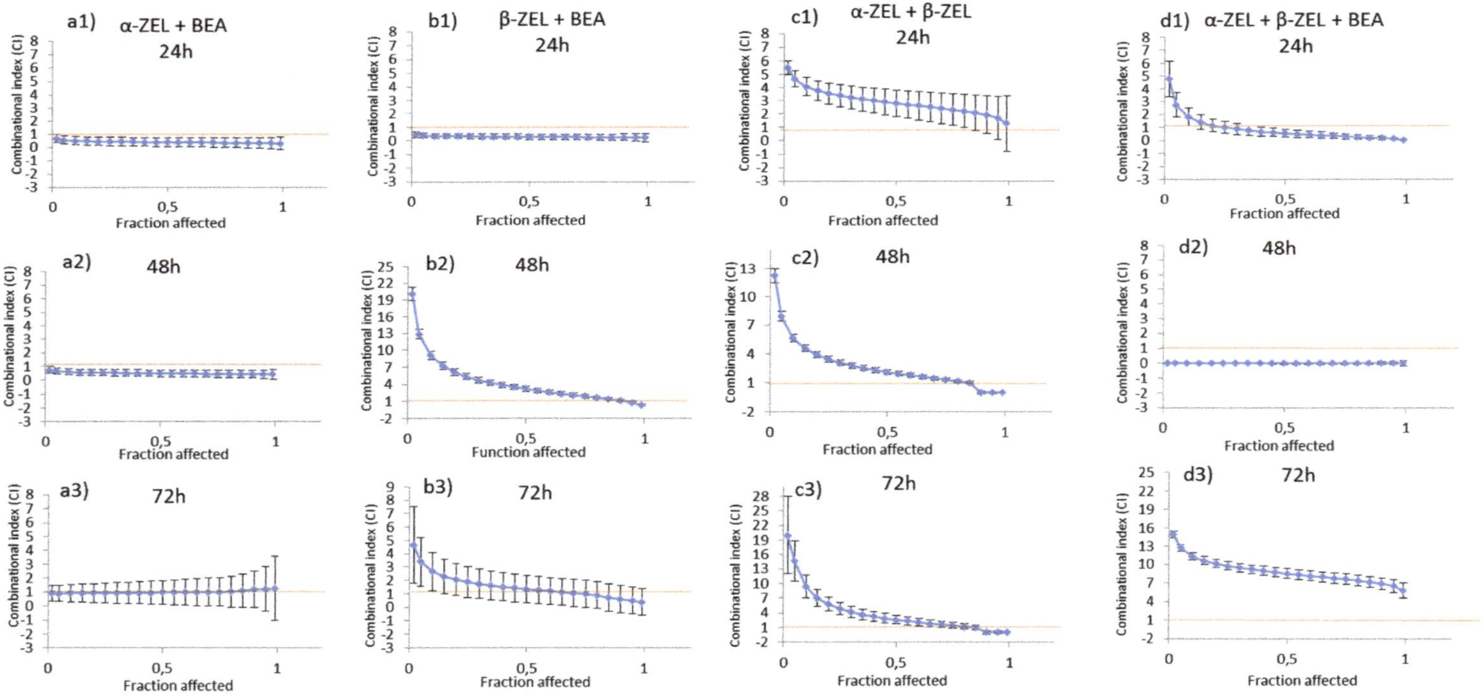

Figure 4. CI vs. fractional effect curve, as described by Chou and Talalay, for SH-SY5Y cells exposed to α-ZEL, β-ZEL, and BEA in binary and tertiary combinations. Each point represents the CI ± SD at a fractional effect as determined in our experiments. The line (CI = 1) indicates additivity, the area under this line indicates synergism, and the area above the line indicates antagonism. SH-SY5Y cells were exposed for 24, 48, and 72 h to α-ZEL + BEA and β-ZEL + BEA at a molar ratio of 5:1 (equimolar proportion), to α-ZEL + β-ZEL at a molar ratio of 1:1, and to α-ZEL + β-ZEL + BEA at a molar ratio of 5:5:1.

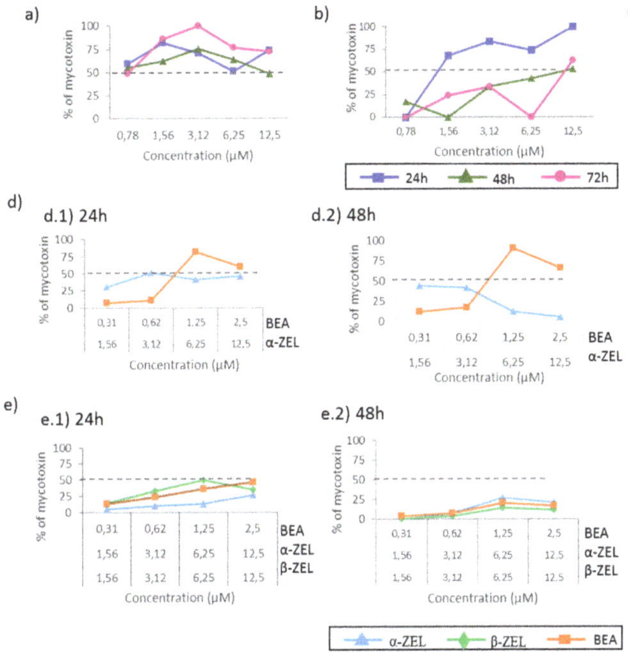

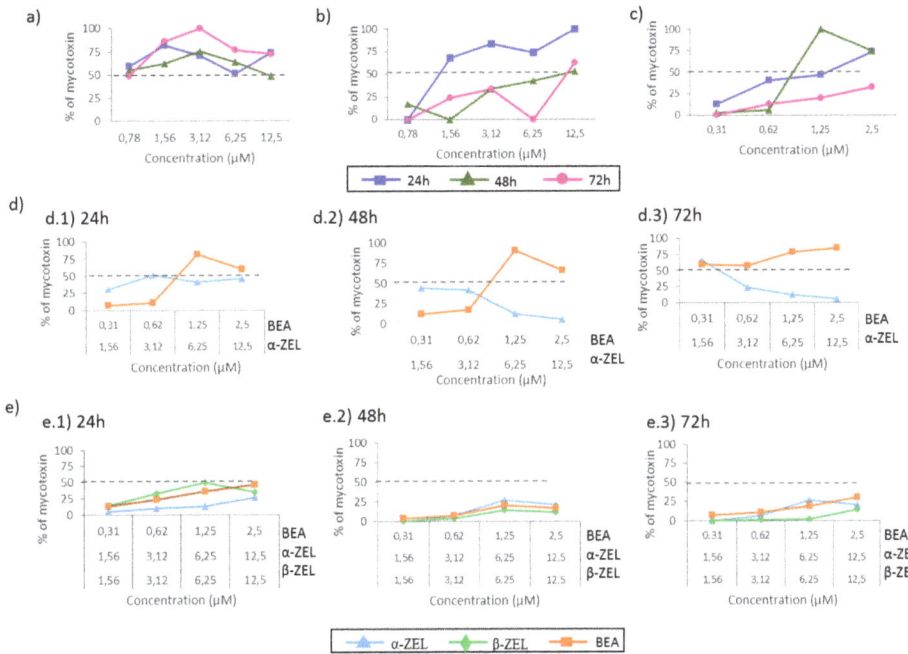

Figure 5. Percentage of α-ZEL, β-ZEL, and BEA remaining in the medium of SH-SY5Y cells after treatment for 24, 48, and 72 h at different concentrations individually or in combination by LC–ESI–qTOF-MS. (**a**) α-ZEL; (**b**) β-ZEL; (**c**) BEA; (**d**) α-ZEL + BEA and (**e**) α-ZEL + β-ZEL + BEA.

3. Discussion

Several studies have discussed the cytotoxic and an anti-proliferative effect of ZEN mycotoxin and its metabolites in various cell lines, such as Caco-2 [11], HepG2 cells [13], CHO-K1 cells [32], and SH-SY5Y [6], and hose of BEA mycotoxin in Caco [14], CHO-K1 [19], and Hep G2 cells [17]. However, there are no reports on the effect of ZEN metabolites and BEA in neuronal cells. In the present study, we proved the toxicity of ZEN metabolites (α-ZEL and β-ZEL) and BEA in human neuroblastoma SH-SY5Y cells in relation to exposure time, mycotoxin concentration, and mixture of mycotoxins.

According to the IC_{50} values of single mycotoxins, β-ZEL was the most cytotoxic mycotoxin compared to the other mycotoxins assayed individually, which is in accordance with Marin et al. (2019) [33] who studied the cytotoxicity of ZEN and its metabolites in HepG2 cells, individually and in double combinations. On the contrary, Tatay et al. (2014) [32] demonstrated that α-ZEL was the most cytotoxic among three mycotoxins tested (α-ZEL, β-ZEL, and ZEN) in CHO-K1 cells. Regarding to double combinations, it was revealed that presence of two mycotoxins increased the cytotoxic potential in SH-SY5Y cells, as shown by the lower IC_{50} values. According to Figure 2a, IC50 for α-ZEL and BEA was not reached in individual treatment however, binary combination α-ZEL + BEA (5:1) inhibited cell proliferation from up to 50 to 90% for all times studied. For the β-ZEL + BEA (5:1) binary combination, as it can be observed in Figure 2b, the IC_{50} values at 48 and 72 h were lower than that of β-ZEL. This was also observed when β-ZEL was combined with α-ZEL, for which combination (α-ZEL + β-ZEL (1:1)), the IC_{50} value was the same as that found for β-ZEL alone. This result was not achieved by Tatay et al. (2014) [31] in CHO-K1 cells, although the mycotoxin concentrations studied in binary assays in that work were two times higher than the concentrations assayed in our study. The proliferation of CHO-K1 cells treated with the α-ZEL + β-ZEL mixture at the highest concentration decreased only by 20% with respect to the values found when each mycotoxin was tested alone. In addition, in that study, the IC_{50} value was never reached for binary mixtures, whereas in our study in SH-SY5Y cells, after 48 and 72 h, the α-ZEL + β-ZEL combination inhibited cell proliferation up to 70% and 90%, respectively (Figure 2c). For the triple combination (α-ZEL + β-ZEL + BEA, (5:5:1)), cell proliferation inhibition was lower than when β-ZEL was assayed individually, and the same result was found for β-ZEL + BEA after 48 and 72 h and for α-ZEL + β-ZEL after 48 h in SH-SY5Y cells. This is in contrast with the results obtained for the tertiary combination of α-ZEL + β-ZEL + ZEN in CHO-K1 cells, as this combination was more cytotoxic than each mycotoxin tested alone [30].

As the co-occurrence of mycotoxins in food and feed is very common, some studies evaluated the toxicity and cytotoxicity of several mycotoxins, both individually and in combination, in different cell lines, using the isobologram model. In these experiments, HepG2 cells were exposed to ochratoxin A (OTA) and BEA [16], to double and triple combinations of alternariol, 3-acetyl-deoxynivalenol, and 15-acetyl-deoxynivalenol [28], and to combinations of ZEN and OTA or α-ZEL (tested also individually) [33], CHO-K1 cells in vitro were used to examine the interactions between the mycotoxins beauvericin, deoxynivalenol (DON), and T-2 toxin [26] as well as the combination of BEA, patulin, and ZEN [17], whereas Caco-2 cells were exposed to DON, ZEN, and Aflatoxin B1 [34]. It is important to understand whether the interaction between mycotoxins shows synergism, additive effects, and/or antagonism concerning cell viability.

In SH-SY5Y cells, almost all the combinations tested reduced cell viability more than the individual mycotoxins, except the β-ZEL + BEA (5:1), α-ZEL + β-ZEL (1:1), and α-ZEL + β-ZEL + BEA (5:5:1) combinations, for which the reduction in cell viability was not significantly different from that obtained when β-ZEL was assayed individually. According to Dong et al. (2010) [5], ZEN is degraded more efficiently to α-ZEL than to β-ZEL in almost all tissues, whereas it is converted more efficiently to β-ZEL than to α-ZEL in liver and lungs. Some studies demonstrated that β-ZEL is more cytotoxic than α-ZEL [31,35,36], whereas other studies found that α-ZEL is more cytotoxic [30,35]. Hence, there is a necessity to clarify the cytotoxicity of these two mycotoxins with studies of the toxicity mechanisms involved.

The IC_{50} values obtained by the MTT assay and the amount of mycotoxin detected in the media by LC–ESI–qTOF-MS were determined and translated into percentage values as an attempt to calculate the amount of each mycotoxin involved in the cytotoxic effect and in the type of interaction effect. Hence, the percentage of mycotoxin present in the media was considered in accordance to the IC_{50} value obtained from the MTT assay (Table 1). The results showed that among the individual mycotoxins assayed, the amount of α-ZEL that remained in the culture medium was above 50% of the administered quantity at all times assayed (Figure 5a). This can be related to the effect in Figure 1a, which shows that the viability was above 100% for the doses reported in Figure 5. This can be justified by the chemical structure of this compound, which might impede its access in the cell. Our results suggest that the availability and capacity of the tested mycotoxins to get into cells were greater than those of α-ZEL, and as a consequence, the amounts of these mycotoxins detected in the media were lower than that of α-ZEL. To notice that the higher the amount of mycotoxin in the medium (at 24 h), the higher the cell viability, which might be related to the lower amount of mycotoxin affecting the live cells. On the contrary, BEA seemed to have easier access the cells, as its percentage in the medium was generally below 50%, but cell viability was maintained above 50% for the doses assayed, indicating the lower potential toxicity of BEA in SH-SY5Y cells compared to ZEN metabolites. In fact, among all three mycotoxins tested, BEA reached the IC_{50} values after long exposures times (72 h) (Table 1 and Figure 1c), highlighting again the mild toxic effect of BEA in SHY-SY5Y cells compared to ZEN metabolites.

According to this and when analyzing combinations, the amounts of ZEN metabolites found in the medium were in most cases below BEA's amounts, indicating easier access of these compounds in SH-SY5Y compared to BEA. In detail, for the α-ZEL + BEA combination (Figure 2a), it can be observed that the lower the amount of α-ZEL in the medium over time (Figure 5d), the lower the viability of SH-SY5Y cells, in particular at 72h. For triple mixtures, the cytotoxic effect was weaker at all times and for all mixtures compared with that of binary combinations; however, the amounts of each mycotoxin detected were all below 50%, and the cytotoxic effect seemed to be bearable for SH-SY5Y cells for doses administered in the first and second mixture but not for those of the third mixture (6.25 + 6.26 + 1.25) μM (α-ZEL + β-ZEL + BEA, 5:5:1), specifically at 48 and 72 h. We suggest that cytotoxicity is due to the stimulation of different biochemical mechanisms that, after a certain level of stimulation, cannot be controlled and cause cell death. Therefore, it is necessary to study in detail the mechanisms of action implicated in the cytotoxic effects that occur when several mycotoxins are present in the same food or diet.

4. Conclusions

In conclusion, the treatment with β-ZEL alone presented the highest cytotoxicological potency compared to treatments with the other mycotoxins assayed (α-ZEL and BEA). The main type of interaction detected between mycotoxins for all combinations assayed was synergism. The potential interaction effects between combinations in this study are difficult to explain since α-ZEL + BEA for binary and α-ZEL + β-ZEL + BEA for tertiary combination were found more in favor of synergic effect respect to CI value, compared with other combinations, which could be related to the concentration range studied, ratio in each mixture, exposure time assayed and cell line studied. Moreover, among all mycotoxins assayed, α-ZEL appeared to remain in the culture medium at the highest concentration and was less abile to get into SH-SY5Y cells compared to BEA and β-ZEL. In combinations, such effect observed for BEA reaching the highest in α-ZEL + BEA.

5. Materials and Methods

5.1. Reagents

The reagent-grade chemicals and cell culture components used, Dulbecco's Modified Eagle's Medium- F12 (DMEM/F-12), fetal bovine serum (FBS), and phosphate-buffered saline (PBS) were supplied by Thermofisher, Gibco ™ (Paisley, UK). Methanol (MeOH, HPLC LS/MS grade), was obtained from VWR International (Fontenay-sous-Bois, France). Dimethyl sulfoxide was obtained from Fisher Scientific Co, Fisher BioReagnts ™ (Geel, Belgium). The compound (3-(4,5-dimethylthiazol-2-yl)-2,5-diphenyltetrazolium bromide) (MTT) for the MTT assay, penicillin, streptomycin, and Trypsin–EDTA were purchased from SigmaAldrich (St. Louis, MO, USA). Deionized water (<18, MΩcm resistivity) was obtained in the laboratory using a Milli-QSP® Reagent Water System (Millipore, Beadford, MA, USA). Standard BEA (MW: 783.95 g/mol), α-ZEL, and β-ZEL (MW: 320.38 g/mol) were purchased from SigmaAldrich (St. Louis Mo. USA) (Figure 6). Stock solutions of mycotoxins were prepared in MeOH (α-ZEL and β-ZEL) and DMSO (BEA) and maintained at −20 °C in the dark. The final concentration of either methanol or DMSO in the medium was ≤1% (v/v) as previously established. All other reagents were of standard laboratory grade.

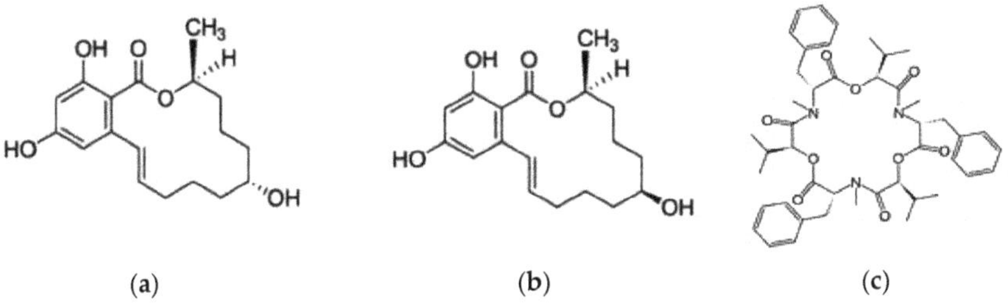

(a) (b) (c)

Figure 6. Chemical structures of the mycotoxins (**a**) α-ZEL, (**b**) β-ZEL, and (**c**) BEA.

5.2. *Cell Culture*

The human neuroblastoma cell line SH-SY5Y was obtained from the American Type Culture Collection (ATCC, Manassas, VA, USA) and cultured in Dulbecco's Modified Eagle's Medium/F12 (DMEM/F-12), supplemented with 10% FBS, 100 U/mL penicillin, and 100 mg/mL streptomycin. The cells were sub-cultivated after trypsinization once or twice a week and suspended in complete medium in a 1:3 split ratio. The cells were maintained as monolayers in 150 cm^2 cell culture flasks with filter screw caps (TPP, Trasadingen, Switzerland). Cell cultures were incubated at 37 °C, 5% CO_2 atmosphere.

5.3. *Mycotoxin Exposure*

Concentration of the mycotoxins and exposure time are two factors that were considered to in this study. The cells were exposed to α-ZEL, β-ZEL, and BEA mycotoxins individually for 24, 48, and 72 h at a concentration in the ranges of 0.39 to 100 μM for α-ZEL and β-ZEL and 0.009 to 25 μM for BEA, all with 1:2 dilution (Table 3). Also, the mycotoxins were assayed in combination in the following mixtures: α-ZEL + BEA, β-ZEL + BEA, α-ZEL + β-ZEL, and α-ZEL + β-ZEL + BEA at three exposure times 24, 48, and 72 h. The concentrations ranged from 1.87 to 25 μM for the binary combinations were studied and from 3.43 to 27.5 μM for the tertiary combination, including four dilutions of each mycotoxin: BEA (0.31, 0.62, 1.25, and 2.5 μM), α-ZEL and β-ZEL (1.56, 3.12, 6.25 and 12.5 μM) (Table 3). The dilution ratios of the concentrations for the binary combinations were 5:1 for α-ZEL + BEA and β-ZEL + BEA, 1:1 for α-ZEL + β-ZEL, and 5:5:1 for the tertiary combination (β-ZEL + α-ZEL + BEA) (Table 3).

Table 3. Concentration range (μM) of mycotoxins studied individually and in combinations. The dilution ratios were 5:1 for the combinations α-ZEL + BEA and β-ZEL + BEA, 1:1 for α-ZEL + β-ZEL, and 5:5:1 for α-ZEL + β-ZEL + BEA.

Combination Tested	Concentration Range (μM)
α-ZEL	(0.39–00)
β-ZEL	(0.39–100)
BEA	(0.009–25)
α-ZEL + BEA	(1.56–2.5) + (0.31–2.5)
β-ZEL + BEA	(1.56–2.5) + (0.31–2.5)
α-ZEL + β-ZEL	(1.56–12.5) + (1.56–12.5)
α-ZEL + β-ZEL + BEA	(1.56–12.5) + (1.56–12.5) + (0.31–2.5)

5.4. *MTT Assay*

Cytotoxicity was examined by the MTT assay, performed as described by Ruiz et al. (2006) [37], with few modifications. The assay consists in measuring the viability of cells by determining the reduction of the yellow soluble tetrazolium salt only in cells that are metabolically active via a mitochondrial reaction to an insoluble purple formazan crystal. Cells were seeded in 96-well culture plates at 2 × 96 cells/well and allowed to adhere for 18–24 h before mycotoxin additions. Serial dilutions of α-ZEL, β-ZEL, and BEA at 1:2 dilutions were prepared with supplemented medium and added to the respective plates (Table 3). Culture medium without mycotoxins and with 1% MeOH or DMSO was used as a control. After treatment, the medium was removed, and each well received 200 μL of fresh medium containing 50 μL of MTT solution (5 mg/mL; MTT powder dissolved in phosphate-buffered saline). After an incubation time of 4 h at 37 °C in the darkness, the MTT-containing medium was removed, and 200 μL of DMSO and 25 μL of Sorensen's solution were added to each well before reading the optical density at 620 nm with the ELISA plate reader Multiskan EX (Thermo Scientific, MA, USA). Each mycotoxin combination plus a control were tested in three independent experiments. Mean inhibition concentration (IC_{50}) values were calculated from full dose–response curves.

5.5. Experimental Design and Combination Index

The isobologram analysis (Chou–Talalay model) was used to determine the type of interaction (synergism, additive effect, and antagonism) that occurred when the mycotoxins studied were in combination. This model allows characterizing the interactions induced by combinations of mycotoxins in different cell lines and with different mycotoxins but it does not allow the elucidation of the mechanisms by which these types of interaction are produced. The median effect/combination index (CI) isobologram equation by Chou (2006) [31] and Chou and Talalay (1984) [30] permitted analyzing drug combination effects. The isobologram analysis involves plotting the dose–effect curves for each compound and its combinations in multiple diluted concentrations. Parameters such as *Dm* (median effect dose), *fa* (fraction affected by concentration), and *m* (coefficient signifying the shape of the dose–effect relationship) are relevant in the equation [30]. Therefore, the method considers both potency (*Dm*) and shape (*m*) parameters.

Chou and Talalay (1984) [30] introduced the term combination index (CI). CI values <1, =1, and >1 indicate synergism, additive effects, and antagonism of the combination, respectively. CalcuSyn software version 2.1. (Biosoft, Cambridge, UK, 1996–2007) was used to study the types of interactions assessed by the isobologram analysis. The IC_{25}, IC_{50}, IC_{75}, and IC_{90} are the doses required to produce toxicity at 25%, 50%, 75%, and 90%, respectively.

5.6. Extraction of α-ZEL, β-ZEL, and BEA from the Culture Media

To determine the intracellular accumulation of the mycotoxins studied, an extraction procedure of the culture media was carried out following the method described by Juan-García et al. (2015 and 2016) [27,28], with several modifications. Briefly, 0.8 mL of culture medium was collected and transferred into a polypropylene tube, 1.5 mL of ethyl acetate was added, and the mixture was shaken for 2 min with an Ultra-Turrax Ika T18 basic (Staufen, Germany). Afterwards, the mixture as sonicated in an ultrasound cleaning bath (VWR, USC1700TH) for 10 min. Finally, the mixture was centrifuged at ~5600× *g* for 5 min at 22 °C (Centrifuge 5810R, Eppendorf, Germany). The supernatant phase was collected. The liquid–liquid extraction process was repeated three times. Finally, the total volume obtained (approx. 4.5 mL) was evaporated to dryness at 45 °C in an N2 stream with a TurboVap-LV (Zymark, Allschwil, Switzerland) and then re-dissolved in 0.25 mL of a mixture of methanol and water (70:30, v/v) by vortexing vigorously (15 s), before being transferred into a vial for LC–ESI–qTOF-MS injection.

5.7. Determination of BEA, β-ZEL, and α-ZEL by LC–ESI–qTOF-MS

The analysis was performed using an LC–ESI–qTOF-MS system, consisting of an LC Agilent 1200-LC system (Agilent Technologies, Palo Alto, CA, USA) equipped with a vacuum degasser, an autosampler, and a binary pump. The columns were a Gemini NX-C18 column (150 × 2 mm, i.d. 3 μm, Phenomenex, Torrance, California) and a guard column C18 (4 × 2 mm, i.d. 3 μM).

Mobile phases consisted of milli-Q water with 0.1% of formic acid as solvent system A and acetonitrile and 0.1% of formic acid as solvent system B, with the following gradient elution: 3 min, 70% B; in 2 min 70–80% B; in 1 min get 90% of B, maintained 4 min; 90–100% B 4 min and maintained 2 min; in 2 min decrease to 50% B; in 2 min 90% B, maintained 2 min. The flow rate used was 0.250 mL min^{-1}, and the total run time was 22 min. The sample volume injected was 20 μL.

MS analysis was carried out using a 6540 Agilent Ultra- High-Definition Accurate-Mass q-TOF-MS, equipped with an Agilent Dual Jet Stream electrospray ionization (Dual AJS ESI) interface in negative and positive ionization modes. Operation conditions were as follows: sheath gas temperature 350 °C at a flow rate of 8 L/min, capillary voltage 3500 V, nebulizer pressure 45 psig, drying gas 10 L/min, gas temperature 300 °C, skimmer voltage 65 V, octopole RF peak 750 V, and fragmentor voltage 130 V. Analyses were performed using AutoMS/MS mode with fixed collision energy (10, 20 and 30) and in mass range of 50–1700 *m*/*z*. Acquisition rate was 3 spectra/second. Acquisition data were processed with Agilent MassHunter Workstation software.

5.8. Statistical Analysis

Statistical analysis of data was carried out using IBM SPSS Statistic version 23.0 (SPSS, Chicago, Il, USA) statistical software package. Data are expressed as mean ± SD of three independent experiments. The statistical analysis of the results was performed by student's T-test for paired samples. Difference between groups were analyzed statistically with ANOVA followed by the Tukey HDS post-hoc test for multiple comparisons. The level of $p \leq 0.05$ was considered statistically significant.

Supplementary Materials: The following are available online at http://www.mdpi.com/2072-6651/12/4/212/s1, Figure S1. Percentage of α-ZEL, β-ZEL, and BEA remaining in the medium of SH-SY5Y cells after treatment during 24, 48, and 72 h at different concentrations and combinations by LC–ESI–qTOF-MS. (**A**) β-ZEL+ BEA and (**B**) α-ZEL + β-ZEL.

Author Contributions: Data curation, F.A.; Formal analysis, C.J. and A.J.-G.; Funding acquisition, G.F., C.J., and A.J.-G.; Investigation, F.A., C.J., and A.J.-G.; Methodology, A.J.-G.; Supervision, C.J. and A.J.-G.; Writing—original draft, F.A, C.J. and A.J.-G.; Writing—review & editing, C.J. and A.J.-G. All authors have read and agreed to the published version of the manuscript.

Funding: This research was supported by the Spanish Ministry of Economy and Competitiveness AGL2016-77610-R and the Generalitat Valencian GVPROMETEO2018-126.

Conflicts of Interest: The authors declare no conflict of interest.

References

1. Zain, M.E. Impact of mycotoxins on humans and animals. *J. Saudi Chem. Soc.* **2011**, *15*, 129–144. [CrossRef]
2. Mally, A.; Solfrizzo, M.; Degen, G.H. Volume Biomonitoring of the mycotoxin Zearalenone: Current state-of-the art and application to human exposure assessment. *Arch. Toxicol.* **2016**, *90*, 1281–1292. [CrossRef] [PubMed]
3. Richard, J.L. Some major mycotoxins and their mycotoxicoses—An overview. *Int. J. Food Microbiol.* **2007**, *119*, 3–10. [CrossRef] [PubMed]
4. Hueza, I.M.; Raspantini, P.C.; Raspantini, L.E.; Latorre, A.O.; Górniak, S.L. Zearalenone, an estrogenic mycotoxin, is an immunotoxic compound. *Toxins* **2014**, *6*, 1080–1095. [CrossRef]
5. Dong, M.; Tulayakul, P.; Li, J.-Y.; Dong, K.-S.; Manabe, N.; Kumagai, S. Metabolic Conversion of Zearalenone to α-Zearalenol by Goat Tissues. *J. Vet. Med. Sci.* **2010**, *72*, 307–312. [CrossRef]
6. Venkataramana, M.; Chandra Nayaka, S.; Anand, T.; Rajesh, R.; Aiyaz, M.; Divakara, S.T.; Murali, H.S.; Prakash, H.S.; Lakshmana Rao, P.V. Zearalenone induced toxicity in SHSY-5Y cells: The role of oxidative stress evidenced by N-acetyl cysteine. *Food Chem. Toxicol.* **2014**, *65*, 335–342. [CrossRef]
7. Gajecka, M.; Zielonka, L.; Gajecki, M. The effect of low monotonic doses of zearalenone on selected reproductive tissues in pre-pubertal female dogs-a review. *Molecules* **2015**, *20*, 20669–20687. [CrossRef]
8. EFSA CONTAM Panel (EFSA Panel on Contaminants in the Food Chain). Scientific opinion on the appropriateness to set a group health-based guidance value for zearalenone and its modified forms. *EFSA J.* **2016**, *14*, 4425.
9. Wang, J.J.; Wei, Z.K.; Han, Z.; Liu, Z.Y.; Zhu, X.Y.; Li, X.W.; Wang, K.; Yang, Z.T. Zearalenone Induces Estrogen-Receptor-Independent Neutrophil Extracellular Trap Release in Vitro. *J. Agric. Food Chem.* **2019**, *67*, 4588–4594. [CrossRef]
10. El-Makawy, A.; Hassanane, M.S.; Abd Alla, E.S.A.M. Genotoxic evaluation for the estrogenic mycotoxin zearalenone. *Reprod. Nutr. Dev* **2001**, *41*, 79–89. [CrossRef]
11. Abid-Essefi, S.; Baudrimont, I.; Hassen, W.; Ouanes, Z.; Mobio, T.A.; Anane, R.; Creppy, E.E.; Bacha, H. DNA fragmentation, apoptosis and cell cycle arrest induced by zearalenone in cultured DOK, Vero and Caco-2 cells: Prevention by Vitamin E. *Toxicology* **2003**, *192*, 237–248. [CrossRef]
12. Cai, G.; Pan, S.; Feng, N.; Zou, H.; Gu, J.; Yuan, Y.; Liu, X.; Liu, Z.; Bian, J. Zearalenone inhibits T cell chemotaxis by inhibiting cell adhesion and migration related proteins. *Ecotox. Environ. Safe* **2019**, *175*, 263–271. [CrossRef]
13. Hassen, W.; El Golli, E.; Baudrimont, I.; Mobio, A.T.; Ladjimi, M.M.; Creppy, E.E.; Bacha, H. Cytotoxicity and Hsp70 induction in HepG2 cells in response to zearalenone and cytoprotection by sub-lethal heat shock. *Toxicology* **2005**, *207*, 293–301. [CrossRef] [PubMed]

14. Prosperini, A.; Juan-García, A.; Font, G.; Ruiz, M.J. Beauvericin induced cytotoxicity via ROS production and mitochondrial damage in Caco-2 cells. *Toxicol. Lett.* **2013**, *222*, 204–211. [CrossRef] [PubMed]
15. Zhang, K.; Tan, X.; Li, Y.; Liang, G.; Ning, Z.; Ma, Y.; Li, Y. Transcriptional profiling analysis of Zearalenone-induced inhibition proliferation on mouse thymic epithelial cell line 1. *Ecotox. Environ. Safe* **2018**, *153*, 135–141. [CrossRef]
16. Zouaoui, N.; Mallebrera, B.; Berrada, H.; Abid-Essefi, S.; Bacha, H.; Ruiz, M.J. Cytotoxic effects induced by patulin, sterigmatocystin and beauvericin on CHO–K1 cells. *Food Chem. Toxicol.* **2016**, *89*, 92–103. [CrossRef]
17. Juan-García, A.; Tolosa, J.; Juan, C.; Ruiz, M.J. Cytotoxicity, Genotoxicity and Disturbance of Cell Cycle in HepG2 Cells Exposed to OTA and BEA: Single and Combined Actions. *Toxins* **2019**, *11*, 341. [CrossRef]
18. Ferrer, E.; Juan-García, A.; Font, G.; Ruiz, M.J. Reactive oxygen species induced by beauvericin, patulin and zearalenone in CHO-K1 cells. *Toxicol. In Vitro* **2009**, *23*, 1504–1509. [CrossRef]
19. Mallebrera, B.; Font, G.; Ruiz, M.J. Disturbance of antioxidant capacity produced by beauvericin in CHO-K1 cells. *Toxicol. Lett.* **2014**, *226*, 337–342. [CrossRef]
20. Stockmann-Juvala, H.; Mikkola, J.; Naarala, J.; Loikkanen, J.; Elovaara, E.; Savolainen, K. Oxidative stress induced by fumonisin B1 in continuous human and rodent neural cell cultures. *Free Radic. Res.* **2004**, *38*, 933–942. [CrossRef]
21. Zhang, X.; Boesch-Saadatmandi, C.; Lou, Y.; Wolffram, S.; Huebbe, P.; Rimbach, G. Ochratoxin A induces apoptosis in neuronal cells. *Genes Nutr.* **2009**, *4*, 41–48. [CrossRef]
22. Zingales, V.; Fernández-Franzón, M.; Ruiz, M.J. Sterigmatocystin-induced cytotoxicity via oxidative stress induction in human neuroblastoma cells. *Food Chem. Toxicol.* **2020**, *136*, 110956. [CrossRef]
23. Stanciu, O.; Juan, C.; Miere, D.; Loghin, F.; Mañes, J. Occurrence and co-occurrence of Fusarium mycotoxins in wheat grains and wheat flour from Romania. *Food Control.* **2017**, *73*, 147–155. [CrossRef]
24. Juan, C.; Berrada, H.; Mañes, J.; Oueslati, S. Multi-mycotoxin determination in barley and derived products from Tunisia and estimation of their dietary intake. *Food Chem. Toxicol.* **2017**, *103*, 148–156. [CrossRef] [PubMed]
25. Oueslati, S.; Berrada, H.; Mañes, J.; Juan, C. Presence of mycotoxins in Tunisian infant foods samples and subsequent risk assessment. *Food Control.* **2017**, *84*, 362–369. [CrossRef]
26. EFSA. Guidance on harmonised methodologies for human health, animal health and ecological risk assessment of combined exposure to multiple chemicals. *EFSA J.* **2019**, *17*, 5634. [CrossRef]
27. Ruiz, M.J.; Franzova, P.; Juan-García, A.; Font, G. Toxicological interactions between the mycotoxins beauvericin, deoxynivalenol and T-2 toxin in CHO-K1 cells in vitro. *Toxicon* **2011**, *58*, 315–326. [CrossRef] [PubMed]
28. Juan-García, A.; Juan, C.; König, S.; Ruiz, M.J. Cytotoxic effects and degradation products of three mycotoxins: Alternariol, 3-acetyl-deoxynivalenol and 15-acetyl-deoxynivalenol in liver hepatocelular carcinoma cells. *Toxicol. Lett.* **2015**, *235*, 8–16. [CrossRef]
29. Juan-García, A.; Juan, C.; Manyes, L.; Ruiz, M.J. Binary and tertiary combination of alternariol, 3-acetyl-deoxynivalenol and 15-acetyl-deoxynivalenol on HepG2 cells: Toxic effects and evaluation of degradation products. *Toxicol. In Vitro* **2016**, *34*, 264–273. [CrossRef]
30. Chou, T.C.; Talalay, P. Quantitative analysis of dose-effect relationships: The combined effects of multiple drugs or enzyme inhibitors. *Adv. Enzyme Regul.* **1984**, *22*, 27–55. [CrossRef]
31. Chou, T.C. Theoretical basis, experimental design, and computerized simulation of synergism and antagonism in drug combination studies. *Pharmacol. Rev.* **2006**, *58*, 621–681. [CrossRef] [PubMed]
32. Tatay, E.; Meca, G.; Font, G.; Ruiz, M.J. Interactive effects of zearalenone and its metabolites on cytotoxicity and metabolization in ovarian CHO-K1 cells. *Toxicol. In Vitro* **2014**, *28*, 95–103. [CrossRef] [PubMed]
33. Marin, D.E.; Pistol, G.C.; Bulgaru, C.V.; Taranu, I. Cytotoxic and inflammatory effects of individual and combined exposure of HepG2 cells to zearalenone and its metabolites. *N-S. Arch. Pharmacol.* **2019**, *392*, 937–947. [CrossRef] [PubMed]
34. Zheng, N.; Gao, Y.N.; Liu, J.; Wang, H.W.; Wang, J.Q. Individual and combined cytotoxicity assessment of zearalenone with ochratoxin A or α-zearalenol by full factorial design. *Food Sci. Biotechnol.* **2018**, *27*, 251–259. [CrossRef] [PubMed]
35. Jia, J.; Wang, Q.; Wud, H.; Xiaa, S.; Guoa, H.; Blaženovićc, I.; Zhanga, Y.; Suna, X. Insights into cellular metabolic pathways of the combined toxicity responses of Caco-2 cells exposed to deoxynivalenol, zearalenone and Aflatoxin B1. *Food Chem. Toxicol.* **2019**, *126*, 106–112. [CrossRef] [PubMed]

36. Abid, S.; Bouaziz, C.E.; Golli-Bennour, E.; Ouanes Ben Othmen, Z.; Bacha, H. Comparative study of toxic effects of zearalenone and its two major metabolites α-zearalenol and β-zearalenol on cultured human Caco-2 cells. *J. Biochem. Mol. Toxic.* **2009**, *23*, 233–243. [CrossRef] [PubMed]
37. Ruiz, M.J.; Festila, L.E.; Fernandez, M. Comparison of basal cytotoxicity of seven carbamates in CHO-K1 cells. *Environ. Toxicol. Chem.* **2006**, *88*, 345–354. [CrossRef]

toxins MDPI

Article

Efficacy of Potentially Probiotic Fruit-Derived *Lactobacillus fermentum*, *L. paracasei* and *L. plantarum* to Remove Aflatoxin M_1 In Vitro

Paloma Oliveira da Cruz [1], Clarisse Jales de Matos [1], Yuri Mangueira Nascimento [2], Josean Fechine Tavares [2], Evandro Leite de Souza [3,*] and Hemerson Iury Ferreira Magalhães [1]

1 Laboratory of Toxicology, Department of Pharmaceutical Sciences, Health Sciences Center, Federal University of Paraíba, João Pessoa 58051-900, Brazil; paloma.oliveira05@hotmail.com (P.O.d.C.); clarissejmatos@hotmail.com (C.J.d.M.); hemersonufpb@gmail.com (H.I.F.M.)

2 Unity for Characterization and Analysis, Institute for Research in Pharmaceuticals and Medications, Federal University of Paraíba, João Pessoa 58051-900, Brazil; yurimangueira@ltf.ufpb.br (Y.M.N.); josean@ltf.ufpb.br (J.F.T.)

3 Laboratory of Food Microbiology, Department of Nutrition, Health Sciences Center, Federal University of Paraíba, João Pessoa 58051-900, Brazil

* Correspondence: evandroleitesouza@ccs.ufpb.br

Abstract: This study evaluated the efficacy of potentially probiotic fruit-derived *Lactobacillus* isolates, namely, *L. paracasei* 108, *L. plantarum* 49, and *L. fermentum* 111, to remove aflatoxin M_1 (AFM_1) from a phosphate buffer solution (PBS; spiked with 0.15 μg/mL AFM_1). The efficacy of examined isolates (approximately 10^9 cfu/mL) as viable and non-viable cells (heat-killed; 100 °C, 1 h) to remove AFM_1 was measured after 1 and 24 h at 37 °C. The recovery of AFM_1 bound to bacterial cells after washing with PBS was also evaluated. Levels of AFM_1 in PBS were measured with high-performance liquid chromatography. Viable and non-viable cells of all examined isolates were capable of removing AFM_1 in PBS with removal percentage values in the range of 73.9–80.0% and 72.9–78.7%, respectively. Viable and non-viable cells of all examined *Lactobacillus* isolates had similar abilities to remove AFM_1. Only *L. paracasei* 108 showed higher values of AFM_1 removal after 24 h for both viable and non-viable cells. Percentage values of recovered AFM_1 from viable and non-viable cells after washing were in the range of 13.4–60.6% and 10.9–47.9%, respectively. *L. plantarum* 49 showed the highest AFM_1 retention capacity after washing. *L. paracasei* 108, *L. plantarum* 49, and *L. fermentum* 111 could have potential application to reduce AFM_1 to safe levels in foods and feeds. The cell viability of examined isolates was not a pre-requisite for their capacity to remove and retain AFM_1.

Keywords: aflatoxin M_1; detoxification; *Lactobacillus*; probiotics; binding

Key Contribution: Viable and non-viable cells of all examined *Lactobacillus* isolates removed AFM_1; viable and heat-killed cells had a similar AFM_1 removal capability; AFM_1 retention efficacy of test isolates increased when contact time increased.

check for updates

Citation: Cruz, P.O.d.; Matos, C.J.D.; Nascimento, Y.M.; Tavares, J.F.; Souza, E.L.d.; Magalhães, H.I.F. Efficacy of Potentially Probiotic Fruit-Derived *Lactobacillus fermentum*, *L. paracasei* and *L. plantarum* to Remove Aflatoxin M_1 In Vitro. *Toxins* **2020**, *13*, 4. https://dx.doi.org/10.3390/toxins13010004

Received: 23 September 2020
Accepted: 18 November 2020
Published: 23 December 2020

1. Introduction

Aflatoxins are fungal secondary metabolites toxic to humans and animals, causing carcinogenic, mutagenic, teratogenic, and immunosuppressive effects [1]. Aflatoxins are produced by toxigenic *Aspergillus flavus*, *A. parasiticus*, and *A. nomius* isolates growing in a variety of food and feed commodities [2]. These metabolites are very stable to autoclaving, pasteurization, and other food processing procedures [3].

Aflatoxin M_1 (AFM_1) is a 4-hydroxy derivative of aflatoxin B_1 (AFB_1), which, although approximately ten-fold less toxigenic than aflatoxin B_1, exerts cytotoxic, genotoxic, and carcinogenic effects in a variety of species [2], being classified as belonging to group 1 (i.e., carcinogenic to humans) by the International Agency for Cancer Research [4]. AFM_1 is formed in the liver and excreted through the milk of lactating animals that have consumed feed contaminated with AFB_1. Approximately 0.3–6.2% of AFB_1 ingested by livestock is converted to AFM_1 in milk [5]. In Brazil and the USA, the maximum allowable limit of AFM_1 in raw milk is 0.5 μg/L [6,7]. The European Union has set a maximum limit of AFM_1 of 0.05 μg/L for raw milk, heat-treated milk, and milk used in dairy products formulation [8].

Control of aflatoxin in food and feed can be primarily achieved by a prevention of mold contamination and growth with the adoption of improved agricultural practices and control of storage conditions, as well as by the detoxification of contaminated products through chemical (e.g., ammonia, hydrogen peroxide, alkalis, and acids) or physical methods (e.g., heat, radiations, ultraviolet, and microwave) [9]. Some methods used for aflatoxins decontamination, although they have been shown to be effective to a certain extent, may have some drawbacks, such as negative impacts on nutritional and sensory characteristics of foods, production of potentially toxic by-products, or non-suitability for use in solid foods [2,9].

Use of lactic acid bacteria (LAB) has been considered a safe and environmentally friendly biological method for the detoxification of aflatoxins in foods and feeds [10,11]. Studies have found a variable capability among probiotic *Lactobacillus* species or isolates to bind aflatoxins [12–14]. These studies have mostly used commercial *Lactobacillus* cultures or isolates from dairy origin. Although a number of *Lactobacillus* isolates recovered from fruit, vegetables, or their processing by-products have shown good performance in in vitro tests for the selection of probiotics [15–17], none of these isolates have been examined for their capacity to remove aflatoxins. The use of select probiotic *Lactobacillus* isolates has been considered a promising biological tool for removing aflatoxins from foods through adsorption when compared to chemical and physical treatments. Furthermore, although still the fastest method for retaining high detoxification efficacy [18,19], many chemical agents are nonedible materials and need to be eliminated after aflatoxin decontamination [20,21], while *Lactobacillus* species have been usually considered safe for use in foods [16,17].

Considering the available evidence, it was expected that fruit-derived *L. fermentum*, *L. paracasei*, and *L. plantarum* isolates with aptitudes to be used as probiotics would be able to remove AFM_1 in a prospective view for application in food and feed detoxification. To test this hypothesis, this study evaluated the efficacy of these isolates as viable and non-viable (heat-killed) cells, in the removal of AFM_1 in vitro, as well as the recovery of the AFM_1 bound to bacterial cells.

2. Results and Discussion

Chromatograms for the quantification of AFM_1 in positive control, negative control, as well as in samples with viable cells of *L. paracasei* 108, *L. plantarum* 49, and *L. fermentum* 111 are shown in Figure 1. Chromatograms for the quantification of AFM_1 in assays evaluating the recovery of AFM_1 from cells after 1 h of incubation are shown in Figure 2.

Results of the capability of viable and heat-killed (non-viable) cells of *L. paracasei* 108, *L. plantarum* 49, and *L. fermentum* 111 for removing AFM_1 in PBS are presented in Table 1. Viable and heat-killed cells of all examined *Lactobacillus* isolates were able to remove AFM_1 in PBS, with removal percentage values in the range of 73.0 ± 1.2–80.0 ± 1.7% and 72.9 ± 1.1–78.7 ± 1.2%, respectively. Viable and heat-killed cells of the three examined isolates had similar values ($p > 0.05$) of AFM_1 removal. Only *L. paracasei* 108 had higher values ($p \leq 0.05$) of AFM_1 removal after 24 h for both viable and heat-killed cells compared to 1 h. Higher values of AFM_1 removal ($p \leq 0.05$) after 1 h were found for *L. plantarum* 49 and *L. fermentum* 111, but the three examined isolates had similar values of AFM_1 removal ($p > 0.05$) after 24 h.

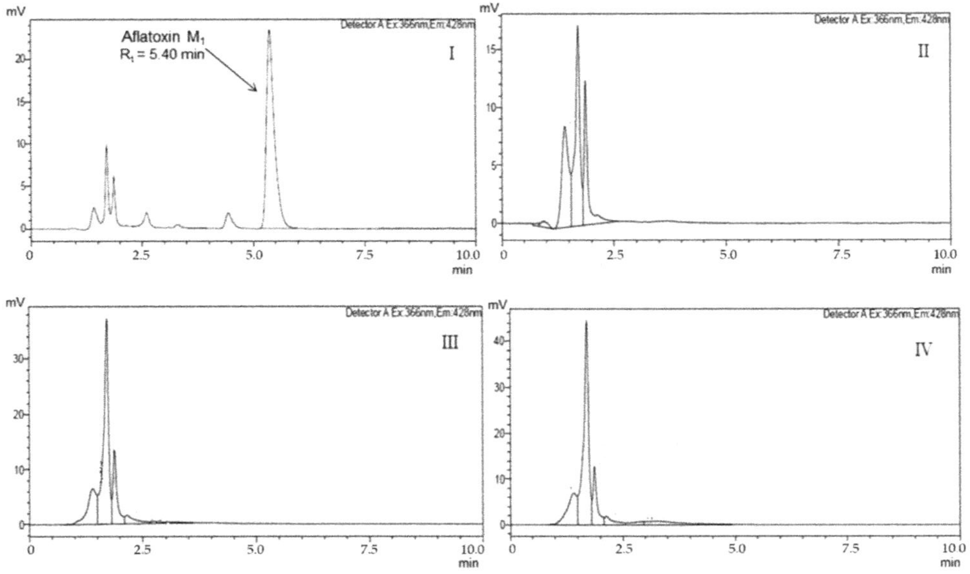

Figure 1. Chromatograms of aflatoxin M_1 (AFM_1) quantification in positive and negative control. (**I**) Positive control: phosphate buffer solution (PBS) with AFM_1. R_t = Retention time of AFM_1 in phosphate buffer solution; chromatographic peak area corresponding to AFM_1; (**II**) Negative control after 1 h of incubation: PBS + *L. paracasei* 108; (**III**) Negative control after 1 h of incubation: PBS + *L. plantarum* 49; (**IV**) Negative control after 1 h of incubation: PBS + *L. fermentum* 111.

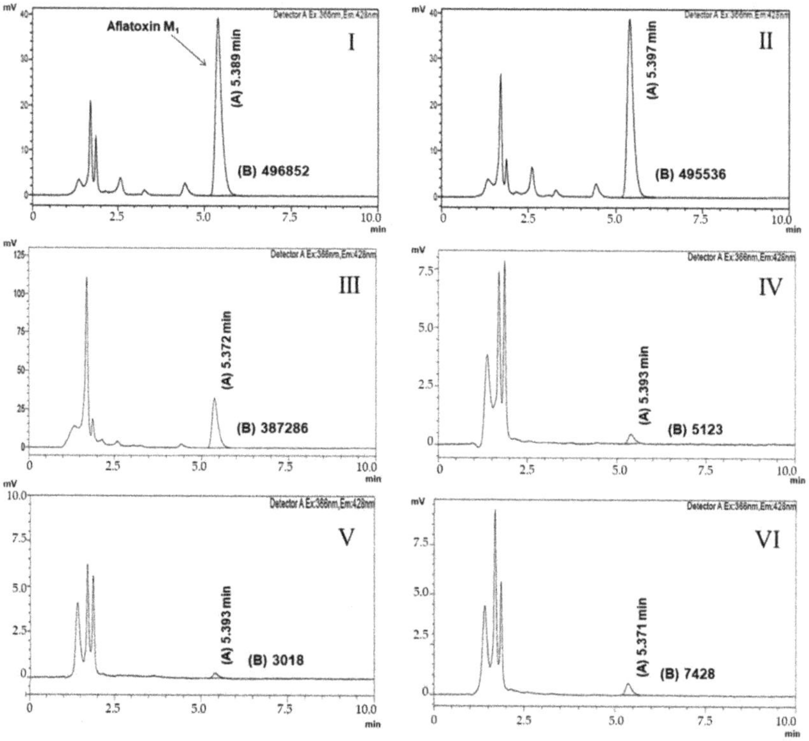

Figure 2. Chromatograms of aflatoxin M_1 (AFM_1) quantification in PBS. (**I**) Chromatogram of assays after 1 h of incubation: PBS + AFM_1 + *L. paracasei* 108; (**II**) Chromatogram of assays after 1 h of incubation: PBS + AFM_1 + *L. plantarum* 49; (**III**) Chromatogram of assays after 1 h of incubation: PBS + AFM_1 + *L. fermentum* 111; (**IV**) AFM_1 recovery chromatogram of *L. paracasei* 108 and AFM_1 complex after 1 h of incubation; (**V**) AFM_1 recovery chromatogram of *L. plantarum* 49 and AFM_1 complex after 1 h of incubation; (**VI**) AFM_1 recovery chromatogram of *L. fermentum* 111 and AFM_1 complex after 1 h of incubation. (**A**) Retention time (min) of aflatoxin M_1 in phosphate buffer solution; (**B**) chromatographic peak area corresponding to aflatoxin M_1.

Table 1. Percentage (average values ± standard deviation) of aflatoxin M_1 (AFM_1) removal in phosphate buffer solution by *L. paracasei* 108, *L. plantarum* 49, and *L. fermentum* 111.

Isolates	AFM_1 Removal (%)			
	1 h-Incubation		24 h-Incubation	
	Viable Cells	Heat-Killed Cells	Viable Cells	Heat-Killed Cells
L. paracasei 108	73.0 ± 1.2 ^{b,B}	72.9 ± 1.1 ^{b,B}	78.9 ± 0.5 ^{a,A}	78.7 ± 1.2 ^{a,A}
L. plantarum 49	78.1 ± 1.6 ^{a,A}	75.8 ± 1.0 ^{a,A,B}	77.0 ± 2.7 ^{a,A}	76.6 ± 1.5 ^{a,A}
L. fermentum 111	78.6 ± 2.1 ^{a,A}	78.4 ± 0.65 ^{a,A}	80.0 ± 1.7 ^{a,A}	78.3 ± 2.5 ^{a,A}

Different small letters in the same row (a,b) denote a significant difference ($p \leq 0.05$) among values, based on Tukey's test; different capital letters in the same column (A,B) denote a significant difference among values ($p \leq 0.05$), based on Tukey's test.

Previous studies have also verified that the capacity of LAB—either as viable or non-viable cells, of binding aflatoxins (e.g., aflatoxin B1, ochratoxin, trichothecene, and AFM_1) in PBS, laboratory media, or dairy matrices (e.g., milk and yoghurt)—varies in an isolate-dependent manner [2,11,22,23]. Aflatoxins bind to the surface components of LAB cells and variations in aflatoxin's binding capacities among LAB species or isolates could be associated with differences in the bacterial cell wall and cell envelope structures [7]. Early investigations have found lower capacity of AFM_1 removal by viable and/or heat-killed cells of different LAB (e.g., *L. plantarum*, *L. acidophilus*, *L. reuteri*, *L. johnsonii*, *L. rhamnosus*, *L. bulgaricus*, and *Streptococcus thermophilus*) [2,22,23], including probiotic *L. casei* [10], compared to *L. paracasei* 108, *L. plantarum* 49, and *L. fermentum* 111. The efficacy of AFM_1 removal from PBS as high (>60%) as those found for *Lactobacillus* isolates examined in this study was reported to *L. plantarum* MON03 and *L. rhamnosus* GAF01 after 6 or 24 h of incubation [24].

Results of the AFM_1 retention capacity of the viable and heat-killed cells of *L. paracasei* 108, *L. plantarum* 49, and *L. fermentum* 111 after washing with PBS are presented in Table 2. Percentage values of recovered AFM_1 from viable and heat-killed cells were in the range of 13.4 ± 1.5–60.6 ± 1.6% and 10.9 ± 1.2%–47.9 ± 1.5%, respectively. The highest values of recovered AFM_1 after 1 and 24 h were found for *L. fermentum* 111 and *L. paracasei* 108, respectively, for both viable and heat-killed cells. Only for *L. fermentum* 111 did the values of recovered AFM_1 decrease after 24 h for viable and heat-killed cells; for *L. paracasei* 108 and *L. plantarum* 49, these values varied with the viability/non-viability of cells and incubation time period. Overall, *L. plantarum* 49 had the higher AFM_1 retention capacity after washing. Variations in aflatoxin release have been linked to the differences in binding sites in different LAB isolates, or even in these binding sites being very similar. They could have minimal differences depending on each isolate [13,25,26].

Table 2. Percentage (average values ± standard deviation) of recovered aflatoxin M_1 (AFM_1) in solution after washing with phosphate buffer solution.

Isolates	AFM_1 Recovery, %			
	1 h-Incubation		24 h-Incubation	
	Viable Cells	Heat-Killed Cells	Viable Cells	Heat-Killed Cells
L. paracasei 108	34.6 ± 1.1 ^{b,B}	28.5 ± 1.7 ^{d,C}	31.7 ± 1.2 ^{c,A}	40.3 ± 1.6 ^{a,A}
L. plantarum 49	13.4 ± 1.5 ^{c,C}	43.8 ± 1.5 ^{a,B}	18.8 ± 1.0 ^{b,B}	10.9 ± 1.2 ^{d,C}
L. fermentum 111	60.6 ± 1.6 ^{a,A}	47.9 ± 1.5 ^{b,A}	14.1 ± 1.4 ^{c,C}	14.9 ± 1.6 ^{c,B}

Different small letters in the same row (a–c) denote a significant difference ($p \leq 0.05$) among values, based on Tukey's test; different capital letters in the same column (A,B) denote a significant difference among values ($p \leq 0.05$), based on Tukey's test.

For all examined isolates, the values of recovered AFM_1 decreased after 24 h of incubation, indicating that AFM_1 retention capacity increased when the length of the contact time increased. There was no clear association between the capability of removing AFM_1, initially, and of retaining AFM_1 after washing among examined isolates. Interestingly, a study with different *Lactobacillus* species found lower AFM_1 removal values than those found in this study, although the recovery of AFM_1 from bacterial cells was lower in the former [11].

Heat treatment positively affected the capability of retaining AFM_1 in *L. paracasei* 108 after 1 h of incubation, as well as of *L. plantarum* 49 and *L. fermentum* 111 after 24 h of incubation. Heating could increase the interaction capacity of bacterial cells/aflatoxin complexes by causing an increased exposure of the cell wall components, primarily polysaccharides and peptidoglycans, which act as binding sites to aflatoxin [14]. However, the destruction of specific components of the bacterial cell wall by heating, causing the denaturation of proteins and increased cell surface hydrophobicity, has been cited to result in a decreased capability of LAB cells of binding AFM_1 [7]. An increased capability of removing aflatoxin B1 was also found in *L. rhamnosus* after heating [27].

The recovery of the AFM_1 bound to the cells of examined *Lactobacillus* isolates after washing indicates that the binding was not strong and could not involve a non-covalent weak bond, but probably a physical association of AFM_1 with hydrophobic sites in the bacterial cell wall [13,20,25]. The lower AFM_1 recovery values found for the examined isolates could be linked to the interaction of AFM_1 molecules retained in the bacterial cell wall with other AFM_1 molecules retained in adjacent cells, forming a type of cross-linked matrix that avoids aflatoxin release during washing [10]. Probably, the efficacy of this type of cross-linked matrix decreased over time for *L. paracasei* 108 and *L. plantarum* 49. Although some authors have reported that a part of non-recovered AFM_1 might be degraded or biotransformed by a *Lactobacillus* metabolism [2,7], most of the available literature has indicated that aflatoxins are not removed by the metabolism of LAB, but because of a physical bound to the molecular components of bacterial cells, primarily peptidoglycans from the cell wall [19,21,25].

In agreement with available literature, the results of this study showed that the cell viability of the examined isolates is not a prerequisite for the removal and retaining of AFM_1 [13,28]. Cell concentration as high as 10^8–10^9 CFU/mL of viable or non-viable LAB is typically needed to reach a level of aflatoxins removal of $\geq$ 50% [22,28].

3. Conclusions

Results showed that potentially probiotic *L. fermentum* 111, *L. paracasei* 108, and *L. plantarum* 49 isolated from fruit processing by-products are capable of binding AFM_1 in vitro when assayed as either viable or non-viable cells. The recovery of AFM_1 from bacterial cell complexes varied with the examined isolate and contact time. Non-viable cells had a higher capability for retaining AFM_1 after 1 or 24 h of incubation. These results indicate that *Lactobacillus* isolates recovered from fruit with performance compatible to use as probiotics could have a satisfactory aflatoxin binding capacity, which could be exploited as a biological tool for the detoxification of foods and feeds, particularly, for the removal and restoration of AFM_1 to safe levels. Further studies are needed to investigate the mechanisms involved in removal of AFM_1 by these isolates and possible factors affecting the stability of formed complexes, including when exposed to conditions mimicking the human gastrointestinal tract.

4. Materials and Methods

4.1. Chemicals, Bacterial Isolates, and Inoculum Preparation

The AFM_1 standard was obtained from Sigma Aldrich (St. Louis, MO, USA). High-performance liquid chromatography (HPLC) grade solvents were obtained from Merck (Darmstadt, Germany).

The isolates *Lactobacillus plantarum* 49, *L. fermentum* 111, and *L. paracasei* 108 were examined separately for the removal of AFM_1. These isolates were recovered from fruit processing by-products, identified with a partial 16S rRNA gene sequence analysis and characterized as potential candidates for use as probiotics [17]. Stocks were stored at −20 °C in de Man, Rogosa, and Sharpe (MRS) broth (HiMedia, Mumbai, India) with glycerol (20 mL/100 mL; Sigma-Aldrich, St. Louis, MO, USA). Working cultures were maintained aerobically on MRS agar (HiMedia, Mumbai, India) at 4 °C and transferred to a new media monthly. Prior to use in assays, each isolate was cultivated anaerobically (Anaerobic System Anaerogen, Oxoid, Hampshire, UK) in MRS broth at 37 °C for 20–24 h (to reach the stationary growth phase), harvested by centrifugation (4500× *g*, 15 min, 4 °C), washed twice, and resuspended in phosphate buffer solution (PBS; 50 mM K_2HPO_4/KH_2PO_4; pH 6.9) to obtain cell suspensions with an optical density reading at 660 nm (OD_{660}) of 0.5. This suspension had viable counts of approximately 1.1×10^9 CFU/mL for each isolate when plated in MRS agar.

4.2. Evaluation of AFM_1 Removal and Recovery of AFM_1 from Bacterial Cells

The capability of examined *Lactobacillus* isolates to remove AFM_1 in PBS was assessed with viable and non-viable bacterial cell suspensions. To obtain non-viable bacterial cells, *Lactobacillus* cell suspensions were inactivated by boiling at 100 °C for 1 h. No visible colonies were found when heat-treated cell suspensions (named heat-killed cells) were plated onto MRS agar and followed by anaerobic incubation (using Anaerobic System Anaerogen, Oxoid, Hampshire, UK) for 48 h. For testing the AFM_1 removal capability, 1 mL of test isolate suspension (pure culture of viable and heat-killed cells) was mixed with 1.5 mL of PBS, previously spiked with 0.15 μg/mL AFM_1, and incubated aerobically at 37 °C [28]. After 1 and 24 h of incubation, the mixture was centrifuged (1500× *g*, 15 min, 4 °C) and the AFM_1 content in the supernatant was determined by HPLC, as detailed in Section 4.3.

Cell pellets collected from each monitored incubation period (contact time) were evaluated for the recovery of AFM_1 from cell complexes. Obtained pellets were washed with 1.5 mL of fresh PBS, the cells were re-pelleted (1500× *g*, 15 min, 4 °C), and supernatant was collected for the quantification of released AFM_1 [18]. For each isolate, a positive control consisting of free cells suspended in PBS with 0.15 μg/mL AFM_1, and a negative control, consisting of bacterial cells (viable or heat-killed), suspended in PBS were used.

4.3. Quantification of AFM_1

The quantification of AFM_1 in supernatants was done with high-performance liquid chromatography (HPLC) using a Shimadzu (Prominense, Tokyo, Japan) HPLC system, equipped with an auto sampler SIL 20A HT (Prominense, Shimadzu, Tokyo, Japan), fluorescence detector RF-20A (Prominense, Shimadzu, Tokyo, Japan), an LC-20AT pump (Prominense, Shimadzu, Tokyo, Japan), oven CTO-20A (Prominense, Shimadzu, Tóquio, Japão), a CBM-20A controller (Prominense, Shimadzu, Tokyo, Japan), a CLC-ODS (M) reverse phase column (4.6 × 150 mm; Shim-Pack, Prominense, Shimadzu, Tokyo, Japan) and pre-column G-ODS-4 (1.0 × 4.0 mm; Shim-Pack, Prominense, Shimadzu, Tokyo, Japan).

Chromatographic conditions were the same as those described in a previous study [7]. Excitation and emission wavelengths were 366 and 428 nm, and the injection volume was 20 μL. The mobile phase was water:methanol:acetonitrile (6:2:2) and the flow rate was 1 mL/min. The calibration curve was constructed using six concentrations of AFM_1 standard diluted in acetonitrile (20–60 ng/mL), performed in triplicate. From this analysis, the equation $y = 2E{+}07x + 873{,}267$ ($r^2 > 0.99$) was obtained. The limit of detection (LOD) and limit of quantification (LOQ) were estimated based on Resolution n° 899 of the Brazilian Agency for Health Surveillance [29]. The LOD and LOQ of AFM_1 were 0.20 and 0.67 ng/mL, respectively.

The percentage of AFM_1 removed by each isolate was determined with the Equation (1) [22,27,30]:

$$100 \times [1 - (\text{peak area of chromatographic peak of sample})/\text{area of positive control chromatographic peak})]. \quad (1)$$

4.4. Statistical Analysis

Assays were done in triplicate in three independent experiments (repetitions). A Kolmogorov–Smirnov normality test was run to assess whether obtained results had normal distribution. Results (average data ± standard deviation) were submitted to a one-way analysis of variance (ANOVA), followed by Tukey's test, considering a p value of ≤ 0.05 for significance. Statistical analyses were done with IBM SPSS Statistics 20 (Armonk, NY, USA).

Author Contributions: Conceptualization, P.O.d.C., H.I.F.M., E.L.d.S.; methodology, P.O.d.C., H.I.F.M., E.L.d.S., C.J.d.M., Y.M.N., J.F.T.; validation, P.O.d.C., H.I.F.M., C.J.d.M., Y.M.N., J.F.T.; investigation, P.O.d.C., C.J.d.M., Y.M.N.; writing—original draft preparation, P.O.d.C., H.I.F.M., E.L.d.S.; writing—review and editing; supervision, H.I.F.M.; funding acquisition, H.I.F.M., E.L.d.S., J.F.T. All authors have read and agreed to the published version of the manuscript.

Funding: This research was partially funded by CAPES (Brazil), finance code 001.

Acknowledgments: Authors thank the Coordenação de Aperfeiçoamento de Pessoal de Nível Superior (CAPES, Brazil) for partial funding of this research.

Conflicts of Interest: The authors declare no conflict of interest.

References

1. Bhat, R.; Rai, R.V.; Karim, A.A. Mycotoxins in food and feed: Present status and future concerns. *Compr. Rev. Food Sci. Food Saf.* **2010**, *59*, 57–81. [CrossRef]
2. Elsanhoty, R.M.; Salam, S.A.; Ramadan, M.F.; Badr, F.H. Detoxification of aflatoxin M1 in yoghurt using probiotics and lactic acid bacteria. *Food Cont.* **2014**, *43*, 129–134. [CrossRef]
3. Koppen, R.; Koch, M.; Slegel, D. Determination of mycotoxins in foods: Current state of analytical methods and limitations. *Appl. Microbiol. Biotechnol.* **2010**, *86*, 1595–1612. [CrossRef] [PubMed]
4. International Agency for Research on Cancer. Some traditional herbal medicine, some mycotoxins and styrene. In *Monographs on the Evaluation of Carginogenic Risks to Humans*; International Agency for Research on Cancer: Lyon, France, 2002.
5. Ayar, A.; Sert, D.; Lon, A.H. A study on the occurrence of aflatoxin in raw milk due to feeds. *J. Food Saf.* **2007**, *27*, 199–207. [CrossRef]
6. Ministry of Health; National Agency for Health Surveillance; Brazilian Legislation. *On the Maximum Tolerated Limit (MTL) for Mycotoxins in Foods*; Resolution No. 7 of 18 February 2011; National Agency for Health Surveillance: Brasilia, Brazil, 2011.
7. Corassin, C.H.; Bovo, F.; Rossim, R.E.; Oliveira, C.A.F. Efficiency of *Saccharomyces cerevisiae* and lactic acid bacteria strains to bind aflatoxin M1 in UHT skim milk. *Food Cont.* **2013**, *31*, 80–83. [CrossRef]
8. European Commission. Commission Regulation (EC) No 401/2006 of 23 February 2006 laying down the methods of sampling and analysis for the official control of the levels of mycotoxins in foodstuffs. *Off. J. Eur. Union* **2006**, *70*, 12–34.
9. Wang, B.; Mahoney, N.E.; Pan, Z.; Khir, R.; Wu, B.; Ma, H.; Zhao, L. Effectiveness of pulsed light treatment for degradation and detoxification of aflatoxin B1 and B2 in rough rice and rice bran. *Food Cont.* **2016**, *59*, 461–467. [CrossRef]
10. Hernandez-Mendoza, A.; Garcia, H.S.; Steele, J.L. Screening of *Lactobacillus casei* strains for their ability to bind aflatoxin B1. *Food Chem. Toxicol.* **2009**, *47*, 1064–1068. [CrossRef] [PubMed]
11. Serrano-Niño, J.C.; Cavazos-Garduño, A.; Hernandez-Mendoza, A.; Applegate, B.; Ferruzzi, M.C.; Martin-González, M.F.S.; García, H.S. Assessment of probiotic strains ability to reduce the bioaccessibility of aflatoxin M1 in artificially contaminated milk using an in vitro digestive model. *Food Cont.* **2013**, *31*, 202–207. [CrossRef]
12. Onilude, A.A.; Fagade, O.E.; Bello, M.M.; Fadahunsi, I.F. Inhibition of aflatoxin-producing aspergilli by lactic acid bacteria isolates from indigenously fermented cereal gruels. *Afr. J. Biotechnol.* **2005**, *4*, 1404–1408.
13. Azeem, N.; Nawaz, M.; Anjum, A.A.; Saeed, S.; Sana, S.; Mustafa, A.; Yousuf, M.R. Activity and anti-aflatoxigenic effect of indigenously characterized probiotic lactobacilli against *Aspergillus flavus*—A common poultry feed contaminant. *Animals* **2019**, *15*, 166. [CrossRef] [PubMed]
14. Elsanhoty, R.M.; Ramadan, M.F.; El-Gohery, S.S.; Abol-Ela, M.A.A. Ability of selected microorganisms for removing aflatoxins in vitro and fate of aflatoxins in contaminated wheat during baladi bread baking. *Food Cont.* **2013**, *33*, 287–292. [CrossRef]
15. Naeem, M.; Ilyas, M.; Haider, S.; Baig, S.; Saleem, M. Isolation characterization and identification of lactic acid bacteria from fruit juices and their efficacy against antibiotics. *Pak. J. Bot.* **2012**, *44*, 323–328.
16. Ilha, E.C.; Silva, T.; Lorenz, J.G.; De Oliveira Rocha, G.; Sant'Anna, E.S. *Lactobacillus paracasei* isolated from grape sourdough: Acid, bile, salt, and heat tolerance after spray drying with skim milk and cheese whey. *Eur. Food Res. Technol.* **2015**, *240*, 977–984. [CrossRef]
17. Garcia, E.F.; Luciano, W.A.; Xavier, D.E.; Da Costa, W.C.; De Sousa Oliveira, K.; Franco, O.L.; De Morais, M.A.J.; Lucena, B.T.; Picão, R.C.; Magnani, M.; et al. Identification of lactic acid bacteria in fruit pulp processing byproducts and potential probiotic properties of selected *Lactobacillus* strains. *Front. Microbiol.* **2016**, *7*, 1371. [CrossRef]
18. Ahlberg, S.H.; Joutsjoki, V.; Korhonen, H.J. Potential of lactic acid bacteria in aflatoxin risk mitigation. *Int. J. Food Microbiol.* **2015**, *207*, 87–102. [CrossRef]
19. Khanian, M.; Karimi-Torshizi, M.A.; Allameh, A. Alleviation of aflatoxin-related oxidative damage to liver and improvement of growth performance in broiler chickens consumed *Lactobacillus plantarum* 299v for entire growth period. *Toxicon* **2019**, *158*, 57–62. [CrossRef]
20. Assaf, J.C.; Nahle, S.; Chokr, A.; Louka, N.; Atoui, A.; El Khoury, A. Assorted methods for decontamination of aflatoxin m1 in milk using microbial adsorbents. *Toxins* **2019**, *11*, 304. [CrossRef]
21. Kim, S.; Lee, H.; Lee, S.; Lee, J.; Ha, J.; Choi, Y.; Yoon, Y.; Choi, K.H. Microbe-mediated aflatoxin decontamination of dairy products and feeds. *J. Dairy Sci.* **2017**, *100*, 871–880. [CrossRef]
22. El-Nezami, H.; Kankaanpää, P.; Salminen, S.; Ahokas, J. Physicochemical alterations enhance the ability of dairy strains of lactic acid bacteria to remove aflatoxin from contaminated media. *J. Food Prot.* **1998**, *61*, 466–468. [CrossRef]
23. Pierides, H.; El-Nezami, K.; Peltonem, S.; Salminem, J.; Ahokas, J.T. Ability of dairy strains of lactic acid bacteria to bind aflatoxin M1 in a food model. *J. Food Prot.* **2000**, *63*, 645–650. [CrossRef] [PubMed]
24. Jebali, R.; Abbes, S.; Salah-Abbès, J.B.; Younes, R.B.; Haous, Z.; Oueslati, R. Ability of *Lactobacillus plantarum* MON03 to mitigate aflatoxins (B1 and M1) immunotoxicities in mice. *J. Immunotoxicol.* **2014**, *12*, 290–299. [CrossRef] [PubMed]
25. Panwar, R.; Kumar, N.; Kashyap, V.; Ram, C.; Kapila, R. Aflatoxin M_1 detoxification ability of probiotic lactobacilli of Indian origin in in vitro digestion model. *Prob. Antimicrob. Proteins* **2019**, *11*, 460–469. [CrossRef] [PubMed]

26. Risa, A.; Divinyi, D.M.; Baka, E.; Krifaton, C. Aflatoxin B1 detoxification by cell-free extracts of *Rhodococcus* strains. *Acta Microbiol. et Immunol. Hung.* **2017**, *64*, 423–438. [CrossRef]
27. Abbès, S.; Salah-Abbès, J.B.; Sharafi, H.; Jebali, R.; Noghabi, K.A.; Oueslati, R. Ability of *Lactobacillus rhamnosus* GAF01 to remove AFM1 in vitro and to counteract AFM1 immunotoxicity in vivo. *J. Immunotoxicol.* **2013**, *10*, 279–286. [CrossRef]
28. Bovo, F.; Corassin, C.H.; Rosim, R.E.; De Oliveira, C.A. Efficiency of lactic acid bacteria strains for decontamination of aflatoxin M1 in phosphate buffer saline solution and in skim milk. *Food Bioproc. Technol.* **2012**, *5*, 1–5.
29. Brazilian Legislation, Ministry of Health, National Agency for Health Surveillance. *Guide for Validation of Analytical and Bioanalytical Methods. National Agency for Health Surveillance. Resolution n°899;* National Agency for Health Surveillance: Brasilia, Brazil, 2003.
30. Haskard, C.A.; El-Nezami, H.S.; Kankaanpää, P.E.; Salminen, S.; Ahokas, J.T. Surface binding of aflatoxin B1 by lactic acid bacteria. *Appl. Environ. Microbiol.* **2001**, *67*, 3086–3091. [CrossRef]

toxins

Article

Efficient and Simultaneous Chitosan-Mediated Removal of 11 Mycotoxins from Palm Kernel Cake

Atena Abbasi Pirouz [1,2], Jinap Selamat [1,3*], Shahzad Zafar Iqbal [4] and Nik Iskandar Putra Samsudin [1,3]

1 Laboratory of Food Safety and Food Integrity, Institute of Tropical Agriculture and Food Security, Universiti Putra Malaysia, 43400 UPM Serdang, Selangor, Malaysia; atenapirouz.upm@gmail.com (A.A.P.); nikiskandar@upm.edu.my (N.I.P.S.)
2 Faculty of Science, Institute of Biological Science, University of Malaya, 50603 UM Kuala Lumpur, Malaysia
3 Department of Food Science, Faculty of Food Science and Technology, Universiti Putra Malaysia, 43400 UPM Serdang, Selangor, Malaysia
4 Department Applied Chemistry, Faculty of Physical Science, Government College University Faisalabad, 38000 Punjab, Pakistan; shahzad@gcuf.edu.pk
* Correspondence: sjinap@gmail.com; Tel.: +603-9769-1043

Received: 19 September 2019; Accepted: 29 October 2019; Published: 12 February 2020

Abstract: Mycotoxins are an important class of pollutants that are toxic and hazardous to animal and human health. Consequently, various methods have been explored to abate their effects, among which adsorbent has found prominent application. Liquid chromatography tandem mass spectrometry (LC–MS/MS) has recently been applied for the concurrent evaluation of multiple mycotoxins. This study investigated the optimization of the simultaneous removal of mycotoxins in palm kernel cake (PKC) using chitosan. The removal of 11 mycotoxins such as aflatoxins (AFB_1, AFB_2, AFG_1 and AFG_2), ochratoxin A (OTA), zearalenone (ZEA), fumonisins (FB1 and FB2) and trichothecenes (deoxynivalenol (DON), HT-2 and T-2 toxin) from palm kernel cake (PKC) was studied. The effects of operating parameters such as pH (3–6), temperature (30–50 °C) and time (4–8 h) on the removal of the mycotoxins were investigated using response surface methodology (RSM). Response surface models obtained with R^2 values ranging from 0.89–0.98 fitted well with the experimental data, except for the trichothecenes. The optimum point was obtained at pH 4, 8 h and 35 °C. The maximum removal achieved with chitosan for AFB_1, AFB_2, AFG_1, AFG_2, OTA, ZEA, FB_1 and FB_2 under the optimized conditions were 94.35, 45.90, 82.11, 84.29, 90.03, 51.30, 90.53 and 90.18%, respectively.

Keywords: chitosan; mycotoxins; detoxification; LC-MS/MS; optimization

Key Contribution: This study presents for first time the removal of 11 mycotoxins simultaneously by using chitosan as adsorbent. Chitosan could efficiently adsorb eight mycotoxins simultaneously.

1. Introduction

Mycotoxins constitute a large number of naturally-occurring fungal secondary metabolites with considerable toxic impacts in plant and animal products, especially in developing countries [1]. These fungi usually attack cereals and other crops on the field or in storage, thereby causing significant economic losses and affecting trade globally. Furthermore, the presence of mycotoxins in feed and food commodities is a major health concern as the toxic effects cause serious problems to the health of animals, and ultimately humans. The major toxins of concern include aflatoxins (AFB_1, AFB_2, AFG_1, AFG_2), ochratoxinA OTA, fumonisins (FB_1, FB_2) and trichothecenes (ZEA, HT-2, T-2, and DON), which are placed in group 1, group 2 and group 3, respectively. According to the International Agency of Research on Cancer (IARC), AFB1 has been recognized as a class 1 carcinogen for animals and humans [2]. Animals often show symptoms of mycotoxicosis even when these mycotoxins are present below permitted levels. This is probably a result of the negative effects of the synergistic interactions between various mycotoxins when they occur simultaneously in the same feed [3].

Although palm kernel cake (PKC) has been commonly used in ruminant feed, its use in poultry, swine, and fish diets is limited due to its high fiber content [4]. While PKC is a valuable source of protein and energy, it is susceptible to infection with mycotoxin-producing fungi. It is abundantly produced in mainly in the equatorial tropics, including South East Asia, Africa and South America. The incidence and severity of the growing number of reports concerning the presence of mycotoxins in feed and food highlights the heightened need for practical detoxification procedures [3,5,6]. Numerous strategies involving physical, chemical and biological methods have been explored in order to detoxify mycotoxin-contaminated food and feed materials [7]. The successful removal of mycotoxins from contaminated agricultural commodities using biological and chemical methods is hindered by several issues [8]. Some of these include safety issues, failure to effectively inactivate different mycotoxins simultaneously, limited efficacy, potential loss of nutritional quality and unfavorable cost implications. Adsorption is one of the most effective and attractive physical processes for mycotoxin removal. Its major advantage is that it has minimal to no detrimental effects on the animal and this often does not outweigh the benefits gained from the high removal efficiency. The efficacy of adsorption appears to depend on the chemical structure and interactions between the solvent, adsorbate and adsorbent [9]. Several studies have reported the applicability of some inorganic and organic adsorbents such as activated charcoal, clay, yeast cell wall, hydrated sodium calcium aluminosilicates (HSCAS) and polymers for the binding and removal of mycotoxins [6,10–13]. In these cases, single adsorbents have been shown to be effective against one or two specific mycotoxins while few adsorbents may be used for various mycotoxins. However, none of them has been effective against all toxins [3,10,14,15]. Amongst numerous adsorbents, chitosan (CTS) is an effective, eco-friendly polymer and low-cost adsorbent which is used for the removal of pollutant effluents even at low concentrations because of its excellent adsorption capability [16].

Chitosan is a polyaminosaccharide that is derived through the deacetylation of chitin and it is predominantly comprised of unbranched chains of β-(1, 4)-linked 2-deoxy-2-amino-D-glucopyranose units. Chitin and CTS are the second most abundant bio- polymers after cellulose. They can be isolated from shells of crustaceans such as crabs, krills, shrimps and cell walls of some fungi [17]. Chitosan appears to be more attractive for use as adsorbent because of its beneficial properties such as hydrophilicity, biodegradability, non-toxic nature and anti-bacterial property. Likewise, CTS is a good scavenger for pollutants binding owing to the presence of amine ($-NH_2$) and hydroxyl ($-OH$) functional groups in its structure; these function as coordination and reaction sites [18]. In addition, CTS sorbents are conventionally used for adsorption of anionic pollutants from aqueous solutions because of their polycationic nature.

Chitin has very poor solubility in most organic solvents while CTS dissolves readily in dilute acidic solutions [19]. Aqueous acid solutions with pH below 6.0 have been found to be the best solvents for CTS. Such acids include acetic acid, hydrochloric acid, nitric acid and formic acid. However, sulfuric and phosphoric acids are not suitable solvents for CTS as it is insoluble in them [17]. Numerous articles have reviewed the application of chitosan and its derivatives in removing contaminants from water samples, wastewaters, dye compounds and heavy metals [20–24]. However, to date, there is limited number of literature on the successful simultaneous removal of mycotoxin with CTS as adsorbent [9,25,26].

To the best our knowledge, this is the first study on the simultaneous removal of 11 toxic mycotoxins in PKC using CTS.

2. Results and Discussion

Data Analysis

Table 1 shows the experimental treatments in the CCD design of RSM applied in optimizing the removal of mycotoxins from PKC using chitosan in Table 2, the estimated regression coefficients and the corresponding R^2 values, p-value and model lack of fit are presented. Each response was evaluated as a function of main (linear), quadratic and interaction effects of pH (x_1), time (x_2) and temperature (x_3). As revealed by ANOVA, the coefficients of multiple determination (R^2) for the responses ranged between 0.89 and 0.98, thus illustrating that the quadratic polynomial models obtained adequately represented the experimental data (Table 2). The models sufficiently related the studied independent variables to the simultaneous removal of eight mycotoxins by CTS, indicating a perfect fit ($p < 0.05$) with the second-order response surface equations. A good model fit is indicated by the R^2 values being at least 0.80 [27] Apparently, chitosan showed poor adsorption for DON, HT-2 and T-2 as the R^2 values for these responses were all less than 0.80 (i.e., 0.62, 0.55 and 0.71 respectively) and their p-values were likewise not significant ($p > 0.05$). These low R^2 values indicate that the predicted responses differed considerably from the experimental values and the models were not adequate. This observation may be due to the fact that trichothecenes, being non-ionizable molecules having a bulky epoxy group, have poor adsorption with plane surfaces. As a consequence, they adsorb on very few adsorbent agents [28].

Table 1. Experimental design (coded) of the central composite design (CCD).

Std Order	Block	Run Order	Pt Type	pH	Time (h)	Temperature (°C)
20	1	0	3	4.5	6	40
16	2	−1	3	4.5	8	40
17	3	−1	3	4.5	6	30
18	4	−1	3	4.5	6	50
19	5	0	3	4.5	6	40
13	6	−1	3	3.0	6	40
14	7	−1	3	6.0	6	40
15	8	−1	3	4.5	4	40
10	9	1	2	6.0	8	50
9	10	1	2	3.0	4	50
11	11	0	2	4.5	6	40
12	12	0	2	4.5	6	40
8	13	1	2	3.0	8	30
7	14	1	2	6.0	4	30
2	15	1	1	6.0	8	30
4	16	1	1	3.0	8	50
5	17	0	1	4.5	6	40
1	18	1	1	3.0	4	30
6	19	0	1	4.5	6	40
3	20	1	1	6.0	4	50

Table 2. Regression coefficient, R^2, *p*-value and lack of fit test for the reduced response surface models.

Regression Coefficient	DON	AFB_1	AFB_2	AFG_1	AFG_2	OTA	ZEA	HT-2	T-2	FB_1	FB_2
b_0	-	93.4	50.7	67.0	76.4	86.68	50.37	−53.0	-	72.2	81.8
b_1	-	−6.6	1.1	−3.9	−3.3	−0.20	−0.25	12.4	-	7.2	2.9
b_2	-	−2.5	0.88	22.1	2.7	1.9	3.3	-		15.8	3.5
b_3	-	−0.5	3.9	2.07	−7.0	0.23	−1.1	-	-	3.1	−6.7
b_{12}	-	−6.8	8.00	-	−21.8	−1.7	1.9	−31.9	-	2.2	-
b_{22}	-	−1.4	−5.8	-	5.3	1.6	−4.3	-	–	-	-
b_{32}	-	−6.72	-	-	−12.2	3.14	-	-	-		-
b_{12}	-	−9.5	−11.2	−11.9	-	−0.7	-	-	-	-	-
b_{13}	-	−8.3	-	15.7	3.3	1.4	-	-	-	5.5	-
b_{23}	0.9	−9.2	-	-	-	-	−3.9	-	-	−10.5	−5.0
R^2	0.72	0.98	0.97	0.96	0.98	0.98	0.89	0.61	0.71	0.98	0.92
R^2 (adj.)	0.53	0.96	0.95	0.94	0.97	0.96	0.82	0.47	0.38	0.97	0.89
Regression (*p*-value)	0.10 *	0.00	0.00	0.00	0.01	0.00	0.00	0.1 *	0.3 *	0.00	0.00
Lack of fit (*F*-value)	1.78	5.52	5.51	27.84	3.46	0.79	6.05	1.57	0.02	6.08	0.7
Lack of fit (*p*-value)	0.33 *	0.09 *	0.09 *	0.1 *	0.16 *	0.63 *	0.08 *	0.39 *	1.0 *	0.08 *	0.60 *

* Non-Significant ($p > 0.05$).

Judging from the *F* and *p* values for the main, quadratic and interaction effects of each independent variable (pH, time and temperature) as seen in Table 3, most of them showed significant effects ($p < 0.05$) for the removal of mycotoxins. Compared to the quadratic and interaction effects, the main linear effects were more significant ($p < 0.05$) for mycotoxin removal. As all factors had significant ($p < 0.05$) effects on the mycotoxin removal (Table 3), they should therefore be retained as critical parameters in the final reduced model for fitting with the experimental data. Furthermore, the interaction effects of all the independent variables were significant ($p > 0.05$) only in the removal of AFB_1. Except in the case of ZEA, the interaction effects of pH with the other two factors was significant ($p < 0.05$) in the removal of the mycotoxins. The reason may be due to the structure and the differences in the solubility of ZEA, owing to its polarity. The resorcinol moiety of ZEA is fused to a 14-atom macrocyclic lactone ring, with a double bond in the trans isomeric form with ketone and methyl groups [29], and its deprotonated form (ZEN) exists at pH > 7.62 [30,31]. Therefore, at acidic pH, the main binding mechanism will likely be hydrophobic interactions. Therefore, the removal of ZEA depended on temperature during equilibrium time. On the other hand, the results showed that the interaction of pH and temperature was significant ($p < 0.05$) for response variables, such as AFB_1, AFG_1, AFG_2, OTA and FB_1, with the effect being most significant for AFB_1 and OTA reduction as their *F* values were 97.42 and 70.21 respectively. The interaction effect of pH and time was significant ($p < 0.05$) for removal of AFB_1, AFB_2, AFG_1 and OTA (Table 3). Likewise, the interaction of pH and time had the highest influence on the removal of AFB_1 due to its rather high *F*-value of 127.30. Therefore, it can be observed that pH was more influential for mycotoxin removal than the other variables studied. An acidic pH causes the release of more H^+ ions that may react with the adsorbent or adsorbate, thereby affecting results. Being a polycationic polymer, the surface of chitosan would become strongly positively charged under more acidic conditions, due to protonation of amino groups. This would cause increased electrostatic reactions between it and the negatively-charged mycotoxin molecules, leading to better adsorption. However, with gradual increase in pH, the adsorbent (chitosan) surface carries more negative charges, causing repulsion between it and the mycotoxin molecules. This eventually results in reduced adsorption capacity [20].

Table 3. Significant Probability (p-value and F-value) of the independent variable effects in the reduced response surface models.

Variables	p and F Value	Linear Effects			Quadratic Effects			Interaction Effects		
		x_1	x_2	x_3	x_{12}	x_{22}	x_{32}	x_1x_2	x_1x_3	x_2x_3
AFB1(y_1)	p-value	0.00	0.009	0.011	0.002	0.002	-	0.00	0.000	0.00
	F-value	79.66	11.21	0.82	19.44	18.47	-	127.30	97.42	120.34
AFB2(y_2)	p-value	0.08a	0.15a	0.00	0.000	0.00	-	0.000	-	-
	F-value	3.72	2.40	46.57	59.37	59.84	-	304.58	-	-
AFG1(y_3)	p-value	0.001	0.000	0.26a	-	-	-	0.00	0.00	-
	F-value	25.90	203.65	1.94	-	-	-	45.96	74.78	-
AFG2(y_4)	p-value	0.001	0.004	0.00	0.00	0.00	0.00	-	0.002	-
	F-value	−3.33	2.72	−7.00	−21.94	5.09	−12.38	-	14.60	-
OTA(y_5)	p-value	0.21a	0.00	0.15a	0.00	0.00	0.00	0.002	0.00	-
	F-value	1.90a	180.22	2.44a	33.64	32.26	119.93	18.84	79.21	-
ZEA(y_6)	p-value	0.66a	0.00	0.06	0.03	0.001	-	-	-	0.003
	F-value	0.2	34.04	4.10	6.20	19.61	-	-	-	33.46
FB1(y_7)	p-value	0.00	0.00	0.001	-	-	-	-	0.00	0.00
	F-value	98.15	483.12	19.42	-	-	-	-	45.99	171.58
FB2(y_8)	p-value	0.000	0.005	0.007	-	-	-	-	-	0.00
	F-value	13.69	20.69	74.65	-	-	-	-	-	40.01

[a] Non-Significant ($p > 0.05$).

The interaction effects of the processing variables on mycotoxin removal, shown to be significant from ANOVA results (Table 3), are explained visually with three-dimensional (3-D) response surface plots in Figure 1a–m. It can be seen from Figure 1a–c that the removal of AFB1 was significantly affected ($p > 0.05$) by the interaction of all the independent variables. The interaction effect x_1x_3 was also significant ($p < 0.05$) for almost all the target mycotoxins except ZEA, AFB_2 and FB_2, thus indicating an overall positive effect on mycotoxin reduction. Maximum removal of AFB_1 and AFG_2 were seen in the middle of pH (x_1) with two other factors (x_2, x_3) for AFB_1 (Figure 1a–c) and pH (x_1) and temperature (x_3) for AFG_2 (Figure 1g). Likewise, maximum removal of ZEA was illustrated in the middle of x_2 and x_3 in Figure 1j.

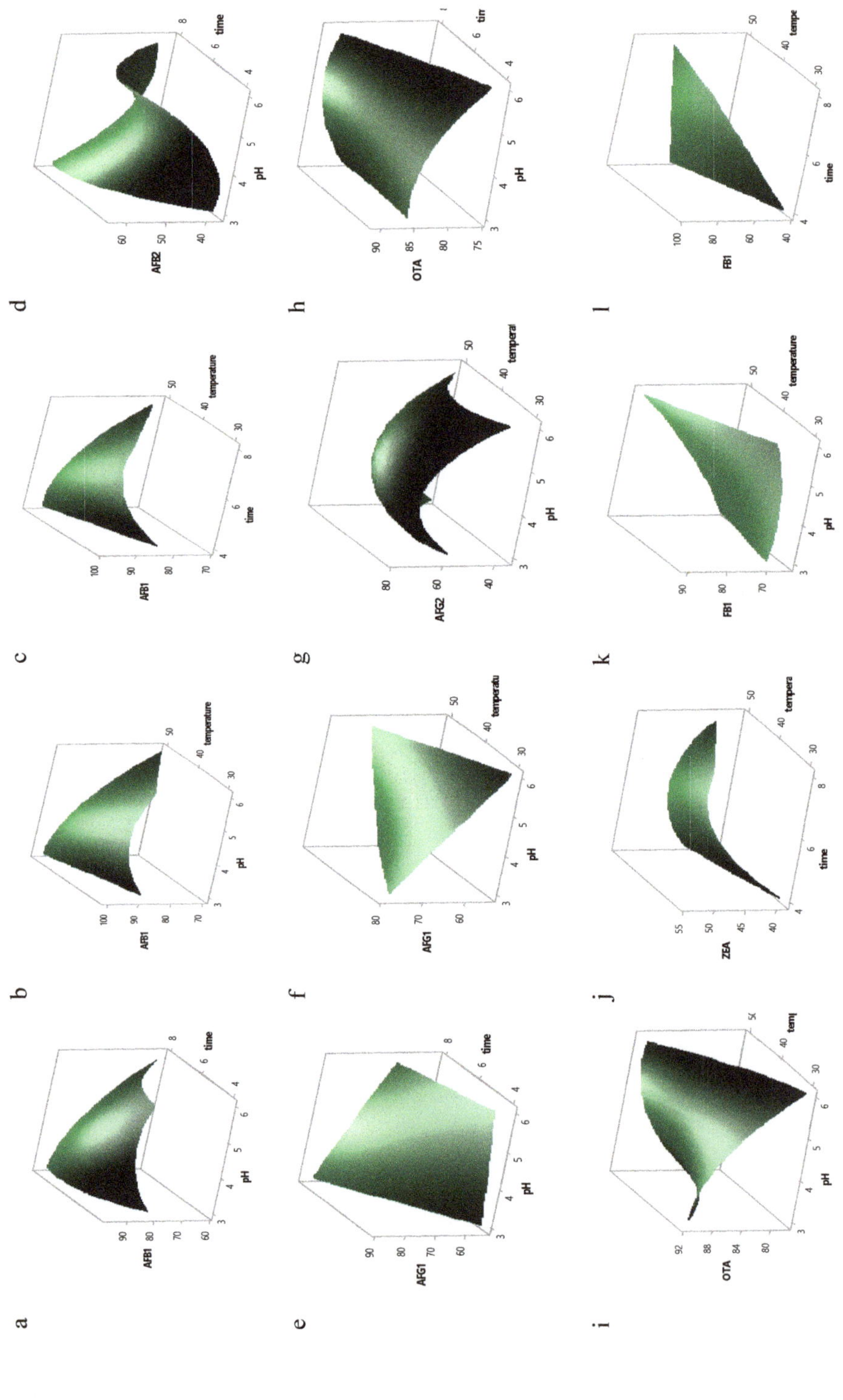

Figure 1. *Cont.*

m

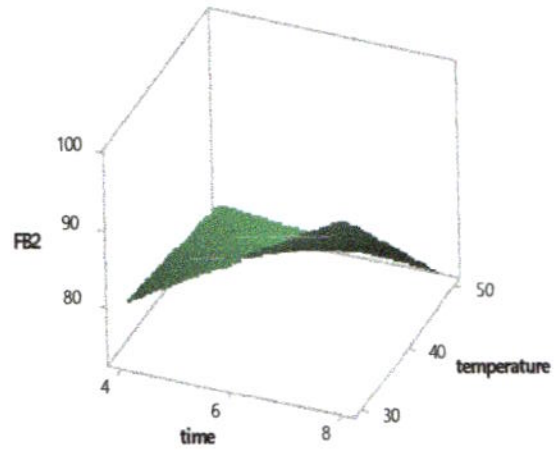

Figure 1. Response surface plots showing the interaction effect of independent variables on the reduction of 8 mycotoxins (**a–c**) AFB_1, (**d**) AFB_2, (**e–f**) AFG_1, (**g**) AFG_2, (**h–i**) OTA), (**j**) ZEA), (**k–l**) FB_1, (**m**) FB_2.

3. Statistical Design

Three independent variables, i.e., pH (x_1), equilibrium time (x_2) and temperature (x_3), were evaluated for their effect on the response variables y_1–y_{11}, denoting the removal of DON, AB_1, AB_2, AG_1, AG_2, OTA, ZEA, HT-2, T-2 toxin, FB1 and FB2 respectively. These variables were selected for the study based on findings from literature and preliminary studies. A composite central design (CCD) with 20 experimental runs was employed to study the main and interaction effects of the variables on the mycotoxin removal. The range of values applied on the independent variable ranges studied were: pH 3–6, equilibrium time of 3–8 h and 30–50 °C temperature, all set at three levels for each variable, as illustrated in Table 4. The center point was replicated six times reproducibility [32].

Table 4. Levels of experimental variables established in accordance with central composite design (CCD).

Independent Variable	Independent Variable Level		
	Low	Center	High
pH	3	5	6
Time (h)	4	5	8
Temperature (°C)	30	40	50

4. Statistical Analysis

Regression analysis as well as analysis of variance (ANOVA) was applied to establish the nature of the relationship between the responses and the three independent variables. To fit the regression models to the experimental data with the objective of achieving the overall optimal region for all response variables studied [33]. For all tests the *p*-value adopted was less than 0.05. The generalized polynomial model proposed for relating the response to independent variables is given below:

$$y_i = b_0+b_1x_1+b_2x_2+b_3x_3+b_{12}x_1x_2+b_{13}x_1x_3+b_{23}x_2x_3+b_{11}x_{12}+b_{22}x_{22}+b_{33}x_{32} \quad (1)$$

where y_i represents the predicted dependent variables; b_0 is the offset term (constant); b_1, b_2 and b_3 are the linear effects; b_{11}, b_{22} and b_{33} are quadratic effects; and b_{12}, b_{13}, b_{23}, b_{31} and b_{32} are the interaction effects. The terms x_ix_j and x_i^2 (i = 1, 2 or 3) denote the interaction and quadratic terms respectively [34,35]. The adequacy of the model was tested using model analysis, lack of fit test and coefficient of determination (R^2) analysis.

5. Optimization and Validation Procedure

The final reduced models in optimization can be presented as 3-D response surface plots. These can reveal the significant interactive effects of the independent variables on the response [36]. Here, the relationship of each response to the independent variables was expressed with 3-D plots by fixing two variables at the centre point while varying the third within the chosen experimental range. The levels of the independent variables for achieving the optimum goal of the individual and overall responses were determined with the aid of the response optimizer.

The response optimizer allows the attainment of a fair balance in the optimization of several response variables by identifying the best combination of input variable settings that favour maximum value of response(s) [37]. It was thus applied in the current study in order to simultaneously reduce the 11 target mycotoxins. The final reduced models were verified by conducting five replicate experimental runs at the optimal settings and comparing the observed results with the predicted responses. Significant difference between the predicted and experimental results were further confirmed by one sample *t*-test Experimental design, model generation, prediction and other statistical analysis were done using a statistical package (Minitab 17 software, State College, PA, USA).

6. Adsorption Studies

About 2 kg of fresh representative PKC samples were kept at 4 °C ahead of sample extraction and subsequent analysis. Three different concentrations (5.0, 25.0 and 100.0 ng/g) of AFB_1, AFB_2, AFG_1, AFG_2, OTA, ZEA, DON, HT-2, T-2, FB1 and FB2 standards were mixed with approximately 5 g of PKC, each in triplicate solvent evaporation was allowed to occur in the spiked samples by storing them overnight in the dark. Preliminary studies conducted within the range of 0.005 to 0.04 g of CTS revealed that decrease in mycotoxins was not observed beyond 0.035 g. Therefore, this amount was utilized in the adsorption experiments. In the sorption experiments, 350 mg of CTS adsorbent was added to 5 g of mycotoxin-contaminated PKC samples in 50 mL flasks. A 20 mL volume of solvent (acetonitrile/water/formic acid at 70:29:1, *v*/*v*/*v*) was added to the flask and the pH (3–6) was adjusted as needed using 0.01 M HCl. Adsorption was then carried out at controlled temperatures (30–50 °C) and at desired equilibrium times (4–8 h) under constant shaking (300 rpm). The mixture of solution was centrifuged at 3000 rpm for 10 min and 1 mL of the final solution was mixed with 3 mL of water for dilution [38]. The purpose of sample dilution during the sample preparation procedure was to reduce the possible matrix effect [39]. The extract obtained was then filtered with nylon syringe filter (0.22 μm). At the end of this process, residual mycotoxins present were measured using LC/MS-MS [40]. Adsorption was estimated based on the initial and final amounts of mycotoxins present in the aqueous, as presented in the following Equation (2) [41]:

$$E = (C0 - Ce)/C0/100$$

In Equation (2), C0 is the concentration (ng/mL) of the mycotoxin in the blank control and Ce is its concentration (ng/mL) in the supernatant.

7. Optimization for Maximum Mycotoxin Removal

To identify the optimum settings of the independent variables for the desired goal of mycotoxin removal, multiple response optimizations (numerical and visual) were conducted. Two stages may be considered in optimization: (a) visualize the significant interaction effects of independent variables on the response variables and (b) the actual optimization, where the factors are further examined in order to determine the best applicable conditions. Presented in Figure 2 are the respective response plots for simultaneous removal of eight mycotoxins obtained with different settings of the studied variables. Maximum removal of all mycotoxins was predicted to occur at the optimal condition of pH 4, time 8 h and temperature 35 °C (Figure 2).

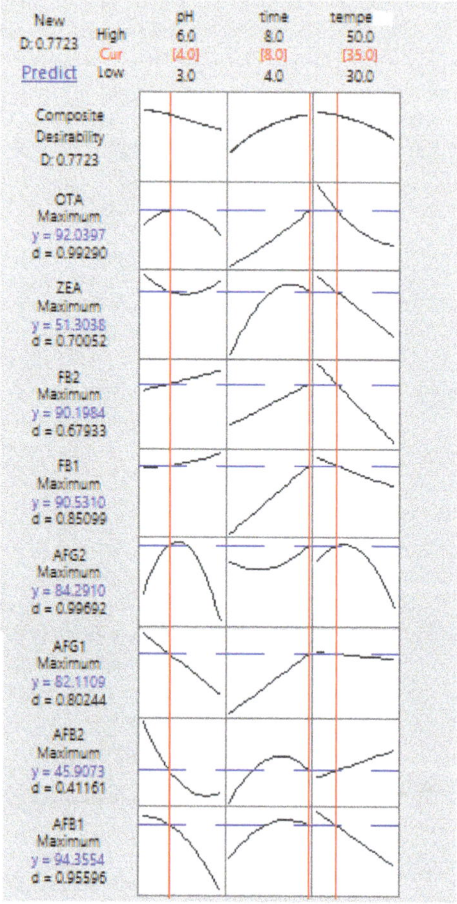

Figure 2. Response optimization, parameters, predicted response (y) and desirability of multi-mycotoxin by CTS.

8. Reduced Response Model Validation

Adequacy of the response-regression equations was evaluated using t-test. The corresponding experimental responses were compared with predicted values and the results are presented in Table 5. In the validation process, there must be no significant difference ($p > 0.05$) between the predicted and actual experimental values; this implies good agreement between the two values. This observation verifies adequate fitness of the response equations by RSM. Applying the optimum conditions predicted by the reduced models in this study, reduction for AFB_1, AFB_2, AFG_1, AFG_2, OTA, ZEA, FB_1 and FB_2 were 94.35, 45.90, 82.11, 84.29, 90.03, 51.30, 90.53 and 90.18% respectively. The total desirability was 0.77 as shown in Table 5. Hence, the final reduced models fitted by RSM were adequate.

Table 5. Comparison between predicted and experimental values based on the final reduced model.

Response	pH	Time	Temperature	y_0	y_i	y_0–y_i	Desirability
AFB_1	4	8	35	94.35 ± 1.94	92.95 ± 2.1	1.4	0.95
AFB_2	4	8	35	45.90 ± 0.003	46.58 ± 0.05	−0.68	0.41
AFG_1	4	8	35	82.11 ± 0.84	79.48 ± 0.08	−2.63	0.81
AFG_2	4	8	35	84.29 ± 0.31	83.11 ± 0.43	−1.18	0.99
OTA	4	8	35	90.03 ± 0.5	87.96 ± 0.27	−2.07	0.99
ZEA	4	8	35	51.30 ± 0.21	52.61 ± 0.05	2.31	0.70
FB_1	4	8	35	90.53 ± 0.43	89.85 ± 0.52	−0.68	0.85
FB_2	4	8	35	90.18 ± 2.3	88.73 ± 0.12	−1.45	0.68

y_0: predicted value, y_i: experimental value, y_0–y_i: residue.

Results of the recovery all the experimental response values showed that this method is acceptable to be used for mycotoxin removal with chitosan in PKC. Recovery values ranged from 81% to 112% for all mycotoxins as reported [38,42].

Results from this study have shown that CTS is promising as an adsorbent for removal of various types of mycotoxins. Its application for the removal of OTA in contaminated drinks has been previously demonstrated [9,43]. Dietary supplementation in poultry for removal of AFB1 and ZEA [44], demonstrated the effectiveness of CTS in reducing the levels of one or two mycotoxins. In this study, CTS showed a moderate to high adsorbent capacity against eight of the eleven mycotoxins evaluated simultaneously, though it showed poor adsorption against HT2, T-2 and DON. These findings indicate better performance against a wider range of mycotoxins than was achieved in a similar study [45] and with cross-linked chitosan [30]. This study further suggests that CTS can remarkably bind all eight of the mycotoxins assessed simultaneously.

9. Conclusions

We report for the first time, the simultaneous CTS adsorption of 11 mycotoxins in PKC as an ingredient of animal feed. Statistical optimization using RSM (CCD) was a valuable tool for maximizing the effects and interactions of pH, time and temperature for removal of mycotoxins. The optimum condition for the removal of mycotoxins was at pH 4 for 8 h and at temperature of 35 °C, with high overall desirability (D 0.77). The overall coefficient of determination values for the regression models were high ($0.89 < R^2 < 0.98$), as revealed by ANOVA. Results from the current study revealed the removal of eight target mycotoxins using Chitosan. Mycotoxin removal efficiency was 45.90% and 94.35% for AFB2 and AFB1 respectively. In increasing order, removal efficiency generally followed this trend: AFB_1 > FB_1 > FB_2 > OTA > AFG_2 > AFG_1 > ZEA and AFB_2. The present method offers clear advantages in terms of simplicity, speed, cost-effectiveness and ensuring low concentration of adverse mycotoxins in the sample. This finding is important as the mycotoxins were diminished to a greater extent than was reported using other adsorbents. The results clearly showed that pH is an important primary factor to be considered in the removal of mycotoxins with CTS. Lastly, CTS is relatively inexpensive and is thus a good candidate for practical applications involving simultaneous removal of mycotoxins in animal feed.

10. Materials and Methods

Palm kernel cake (PKC) samples were collected from local mills across different regions in Malaysia (Shah Alam and Kelantan in Selangor and Kelantan state respectively). Representative samples of the PKC were prepared as described previously [46]. Analytical pure standards of the aflatoxins (AFB_1, AFB_2, AFG_1, and AFG_2), ochratoxin A (OTA) zearalenone (ZEA), trichothecenes (deoxynivalenol (DON), HT-2 and T-2 toxin) and fumonisins (FB_1-FB_2), were purchased from VICAM (Watertown, MA, USA). Chitosan (CTS > 85% deacetylation) was sourced from Sigma-Aldrich (St. Louis, MO, USA). Deionized water was prepared with a water purifier (Elga Classic UV MK2; Elga, Marlow,

UK). HPLC-grade solvents (acetonitrile, methanol and formic acid) were from Merck (Darmstadt, Germany). Filtration of all eluents was done using 0.22-μm Whatman membrane filters (Whatman, 110 Maidstone, UK).

Mycotoxins Analysis by LC–MS/MS

The mass spectrometer used for the analyses was an Agilent 1290 Infinity UHPLC module LC/MS-MS with a Triple Quad LC/MS (Agilent 6410, Agilent technologies, Palo Alto, CA, USA). This system consisted of an auto sampler, a degasser and column oven. Separation was performed using a Zorbax Eclipse plus C18 column (2 × 150 mm, 3 μm) at column temperature of 30 °C manufactured by Agilent Technologies (Palo Alto, CA, USA). The analysis was operated in positive and negative modes with electrospray interface (ESI±) with the following parameters: capillary voltage of 4 kV, nitrogen as spray gas and desolvation temperature 40 °C. Mycotoxins were analyzed in multi reaction monitoring (MRM) mode while matrix-matched standard calibration was used for quantification. As shown in Table 6, the mobile phase consisted of a gradient of 2 solvents: mobile phase A (methanol) slightly acidified with mobile phase B (0.1% formic acid in water), at a flow-rate of 0.2 mL/min. Validation of the LC-MS/MS method was carried out by investigating the basic performance characteristics included linearity, limit of detection, limit of quantification and recovery in accordance with the European Commission regulation for the performance of analytical methods (EC 657/2002).

Table 6. Gradient elution program of the LC/MS-MS.

Step	Time (min)	Solvent A%	Solvent B%	Flow Rate (mL/min)
1	0–8	10	90	0.4
2	8–10	90	10	0.4
3	10–17	0	100	0.4
4	17–20	90	10	0.4

Author Contributions: A.A.P. carried out the entire experiments and wrote the manuscripts with support from J.S., A.A.P., J.S., S.Z.I. and N.I.P.S. designed the experiments. J.S. supervised the project. A.A.P., J.S., N.I.P.S. and S.Z.I. discussed the results and contributed to the final manuscript. All authors approved the final manuscripts. All authors have read and agreed to the published version of the manuscript.

Funding: This research was funded by Ministry of Education Malaysia [grant number 6369114] and HICOE environment set at the Institute of Tropical Agriculture and Food Security.

Acknowledgments: The authors would like to acknowledge the contribution of the Ministry of Education Malaysia [grant number 6369114] and HICOE environment set at the Institute of Tropical Agriculture and Food Security.

Conflicts of Interest: The authors declare no conflict of interest.

References

1. Signorini, M.; Gaggiotti, M.; Molineri, A.; Chiericatti, C.; de Basílico, M.Z.; Basilico, J.; Pisani, M. Exposure assessment of mycotoxins in cow's milk in Argentina. *Food Chem. Toxicol.* **2012**, *50*, 250–257. [CrossRef] [PubMed]
2. da Rocha, M.E.B.; Freire, F.D.C.O.; Maia, F.E.F.; Guedes, M.I.F.; Rondina, D.J.F.C. Mycotoxins and their effects on human and animal health. *Food Control* **2014**, *36*, 159–165. [CrossRef]
3. Vila-Donat, P.; Marin, S.; Sanchis, V.; Ramos, A. A review of the mycotoxin adsorbing agents, with an emphasis on their multi-binding capacity, for animal feed decontamination. *Food Chem. Toxicol.* **2018**, *114*, 246–259. [CrossRef] [PubMed]
4. Sharmila, A.; Alimon, A.; Azhar, K.; Noor, H.; Samsudin, A. Improving nutritional values of Palm Kernel Cake (PKC) as poultry feeds: A review. *Malays. J. Anim. Sci.* **2014**, *17*, 1–18.
5. Peng, W.-X.; Marchal, J.; van der Poel, A. Strategies to prevent and reduce mycotoxins for compound feed manufacturing. *Anim. Feed Sci. Technol.* **2018**, *237*, 129–153. [CrossRef]

6. Jard, G.; Liboz, T.; Mathieu, F.; Guyonvarc'h, A.; Lebrihi, A. Review of mycotoxin reduction in food and feed: from prevention in the field to detoxification by adsorption or transformation. *Food Addit. Contam.* **2011**, *28*, 1590–1609. [CrossRef]
7. Jans, D.; Pedrosa, K.; Schatzmayr, D.; Bertin, G.; Grenier, B. Mycotoxin Reduction in Animal Diets. In *Mycotoxin Reduction in Grain Chains*; Wiley: Hoboken, NJ, USA, 2014; Chapter 8; pp. 101–110.
8. Smith, T.; Girish, C. Prevention and control of animal feed contamination by mycotoxins and reduction of their adverse effects in livestock. In *Animal Feed Contamination*; Elsevier: Guelph, ON, Canada, 2012; pp. 326–351.
9. Mine Kurtbay, H.; Bekçi, Z.; Merdivan, M.; Yurdakoç, K. Reduction of ochratoxin A levels in red wine by bentonite, modified bentonites, and chitosan. *J. Agric. Food Chem.* **2008**, *56*, 2541–2545. [CrossRef]
10. Avantaggiato, G.; Havenaar, R.; Visconti, A. Assessment of the multi-mycotoxin-binding efficacy of a carbon/aluminosilicate-based product in an in vitro gastrointestinal model. *J. Agric. Food Chem.* **2007**, *55*, 4810–4819. [CrossRef]
11. Phillips, T.; Afriyie-Gyawu, E.; Williams, J.; Huebner, H.; Ankrah, N.-A.; Ofori-Adjei, D.; Jolly, P.; Johnson, N.; Taylor, J. Marroquin-Cardona, A. Reducing human exposure to aflatoxin through the use of clay: A review. *Food Addit. Contam.* **2008**, *25*, 134–145. [CrossRef]
12. Kong, C.; Shin, S.Y.; Kim, B.G. Evaluation of mycotoxin sequestering agents for aflatoxin and deoxynivalenol: An in vitro approach. *SpringerPlus* **2014**, *3*, 346. [CrossRef]
13. Wielogórska, E.; MacDonald, S.; Elliott, C. A review of the efficacy of mycotoxin detoxifying agents used in feed in light of changing global environment and legislation. *World Mycotoxin J.* **2016**, *9*, 419–433. [CrossRef]
14. Kabak, B. Prevention and management of mycotoxins in food and feed. In *Mycotoxins in Food, Feed and Bioweapons*; Springer: Corum, Turkey, 2009; pp. 201–227.
15. Di Gregorio, M.C.; Neeff, D.V.D.; Jager, A.V.; Corassin, C.H.; Carão, Á.C.D.P.; Albuquerque, R.D.; Azevedo, A.C.D.; Oliveira, C.A.F. Mineral adsorbents for prevention of mycotoxins in animal feeds. *Toxin Rev.* **2014**, *33*, 125–135. [CrossRef]
16. Azlan, K.; Saime, W.N.W.; Liew, L. Chitosan and chemically modified chitosan beads for acid dyes sorption. *J. Environ. Sci.* **2009**, *21*, 296–302. [CrossRef]
17. Yeul, V.S.; Rayalu, S.S. Unprecedented chitin and chitosan: A chemical overview. *J. Polym. Environ.* **2013**, *21*, 606–614. [CrossRef]
18. Yen, M.-T.; Yang, J.-H.; Mau, J.-L. Antioxidant properties of chitosan from crab shells. *Carbohydr. Polym.* **2008**, *74*, 840–844. [CrossRef]
19. Pillai, C.; Paul, W.; Sharma, C.P. Chitin and chitosan polymers: Chemistry, solubility and fiber formation. *Prog. Polym. Sci.* **2009**, *34*, 641–678. [CrossRef]
20. Ngah, W.W.; Teong, L.; Hanafiah, M.A.K.M. Adsorption of dyes and heavy metal ions by chitosan composites: A review. *Carbohydr. Polym.* **2011**, *83*, 1446–1456. [CrossRef]
21. Chatterjee, S.; Chatterjee, T.; Lim, S.R.; Woo, S.H. Adsorption of a cationic dye, methylene blue, on to chitosan hydrogel beads generated by anionic surfactant gelation. *Environ. Technol.* **2011**, *32*, 1503–1514. [CrossRef]
22. Chatterjee, S.; Lee, M.W.; Woo, S.H. Adsorption of congo red by chitosan hydrogel beads impregnated with carbon nanotubes. *Bioresour. Technol.* **2010**, *101*, 1800–1806. [CrossRef]
23. Kyzas, G.Z.; Lazaridis, N.K.; Kostoglou, M. Adsorption/desorption of a dye by a chitosan derivative: Experiments and phenomenological modeling. *Chem. Eng. J.* **2014**, *248*, 327–336. [CrossRef]
24. Ren, Y.; Abbood, H.A.; He, F.; Peng, H.; Huang, K. Magnetic EDTA-modified chitosan/SiO_2/Fe_3O_4 adsorbent: Preparation, characterization, and application in heavy metal adsorption. *Chem. Eng. J.* **2013**, *226*, 300–311. [CrossRef]
25. Peng, X.; Liu, B.; Chen, W.; Li, X.; Wang, Q.; Meng, X.; Wang, D. Effective biosorption of patulin from apple juice by cross-linked xanthated chitosan resin. *Food Control* **2016**, *63*, 140–146. [CrossRef]
26. Kaushik, A.; Solanki, P.R.; Ansari, A.A.; Ahmad, S.; Malhotra, B.D. Chitosan–iron oxide nanobiocomposite based immunosensor for ochratoxin-A. *Electrochem. Commun.* **2008**, *10*, 1364–1368. [CrossRef]
27. Pirouz, A.; Selamat, J.; Iqbal, S.; Mirhosseini, H.; Karjiban, R.A.; Bakar, F.A. The use of innovative and efficient nanocomposite (magnetic graphene oxide) for the reduction on of Fusarium mycotoxins in palm kernel cake. *Sci. Rep.* **2017**, *7*, 12453. [CrossRef] [PubMed]
28. Afsah-Hejri, L.; Jinap, S.; Arzandeh, S.; Mirhosseini, H. Optimization of HPLC conditions for quantitative analysis of aflatoxins in contaminated peanut. *Food Control* **2011**, *22*, 381–388. [CrossRef]

29. Ko, W.-C.; Chang, C.-K.; Wang, H.-J.; Wang, S.-J.; Hsieh, C.-W. Process optimization of microencapsulation of curcumin in γ-polyglutamic acid using response surface methodology. *Food Chem.* **2015**, *172*, 497–503. [CrossRef]
30. Liu, D.; Xu, H.; Tian, B.; Yuan, K.; Pan, H.; Ma, S.; Yang, X.; Pan, W. Fabrication of carvedilol nanosuspensions through the anti-solvent precipitation–ultrasonication method for the improvement of dissolution rate and oral bioavailability. *Aaps Pharmscitech* **2012**, *13*, 295–304. [CrossRef]
31. Huang, Y.; Yuan, Y.; Zhou, Z.; Liang, J.; Chen, Z.; Li, G. Optimization and evaluation of chelerythrine nanoparticles composed of magnetic multiwalled carbon nanotubes by response surface methodology. *Appl. Surf. Sci.* **2014**, *292*, 378–386. [CrossRef]
32. Mirhosseini, H.; Tan, C.P.; Taherian, A.R.; Boo, H.C. Modeling the physicochemical properties of orange beverage emulsion as function of main emulsion components using response surface methodology. *Carbohydr. Polym.* **2009**, *75*, 512–520. [CrossRef]
33. Mehrnoush, A.; Tan, C.P.; Hamed, M.; Aziz, N.A.; Ling, T.C. Optimisation of freeze drying conditions for purified serine protease from mango (Mangifera indicaCv. Chokanan) peel. *Food Chem.* **2011**, *128*, 158–164. [CrossRef]
34. Yibadatihan, S.; Jinap, S.; Mahyudin, N.J.F.A. Simultaneous determination of multi-mycotoxins in palm kernel cake (PKC) using liquid chromatography-tandem mass spectrometry (LC-MS/MS). *Food Addit. Contam. Part A* **2014**, *31*, 2071–2079. [CrossRef] [PubMed]
35. Patel, D.; Sciences, B. Matrix effect in a view of LC-MS/MS: An overview. *Int. J. Pharma Biol. Sci.* **2011**, *2*, 559–564.
36. Rubert, J.; Soler, C.; Mañes, J.J.F.C. Application of an HPLC–MS/MS method for mycotoxin analysis in commercial baby foods. *Food Chem.* **2012**, *133*, 176–183. [CrossRef]
37. Fan, L.; Luo, C.; Sun, M.; Li, X.; Lu, F.; Qiu, H. Preparation of novel magnetic chitosan/graphene oxide composite as effective adsorbents toward methylene blue. *Bioresour. Technol.* **2012**, *114*, 703–706. [CrossRef] [PubMed]
38. Kathiravan, T.; Nadanasabapathi, S.; Kumar, R. Pigments and antioxidant activity of optimized Ready-to-Drink (RTD) Beetroot (*Beta vulgaris* L.)-passion fruit (*Passiflora edulis* var. flavicarpa) juice blend. *Croat. J. Food Sci. Technol.* **2015**, *7*, 9–21. [CrossRef]
39. Boudergue, C.; Burel, C.; Dragacci, S.; Favrot, M.-C.; Fremy, J.-M.; Massimi, C.; Pringent, P.; Debongnie, P.; Pussemier, L.; Boudra, H. Review of mycotoxin-detoxifying agents used as feed additives: Mode of action, efficacy and feed/food safety. *EFSA Support. Publ.* **2009**, *6*, 22E. [CrossRef]
40. Gromadzka, K.; Waskiewicz, A.; Chelkowski, J.; Golinski, P. Zearalenone and its metabolites: Occurrence, detection, toxicity and guidelines. *World Mycotoxin J.* **2008**, *1*, 209–220. [CrossRef]
41. Zhao, Z.; Liu, N.; Yang, L.; Wang, J.; Song, S.; Nie, D.; Yang, X.; Hou, J.; Wu, A. Cross-linked chitosan polymers as generic adsorbents for simultaneous adsorption of multiple mycotoxins. *Food Control* **2015**, *57*, 362–369. [CrossRef]
42. Faucet-Marquis, V.; Joannis-Cassan, C.; Hadjeba-Medjdoub, K.; Ballet, N.; Pfohl-Leszkowicz, A. Development of an in vitro method for the prediction of mycotoxin binding on yeast-based products: Case of aflatoxin B 1, zearalenone and ochratoxin A. *Appl. Microbiol. Biotechnol.* **2014**, *98*, 7583–7596. [CrossRef]
43. Soleimany, F.; Jinap, S.; Abas, F.J.F.C. Determination of mycotoxins in cereals by liquid chromatography tandem mass spectrometry. *Food Chem.* **2012**, *130*, 1055–1060. [CrossRef]
44. Bornet, A.; Teissedre, P. Chitosan, chitin-glucan and chitin effects on minerals (iron, lead, cadmium) and organic (ochratoxin A) contaminants in wines. *Eur. Food Res. Technol.* **2008**, *226*, 681–689. [CrossRef]
45. Khajarern, J.; Khajarern, S.; Moon, T.; Lee, J. Effects of dietary supplementation of fermented chitin-chitosan (fermkit) on toxicity of mycotoxin in ducks. *Asian-Australas. J. Anim. Sci.* **2003**, *16*, 706–713. [CrossRef]
46. Solís-Cruz, B.; Hernández-Patlán, D.; Beyssac, E.; Latorre, J.; Hernandez-Velasco, X.; Merino-Guzman, R.; Tellez, G.; López-Arellano, R. Evaluation of chitosan and cellulosic polymers as binding adsorbent materials to prevent aflatoxin B1, fumonisin B1, ochratoxin, trichothecene, deoxynivalenol, and zearalenone mycotoxicoses through an in vitro gastrointestinal model for poultry. *Polymers* **2017**, *9*, 529. [CrossRef] [PubMed]

toxins

MDPI

Article

Effect of Ozone and Electron Beam Irradiation on Degradation of Zearalenone and Ochratoxin A

Kai Yang [1], Ke Li [1], Lihong Pan [1], Xiaohu Luo [1,2,3,4,*], Jiali Xing [5], Jing Wang [2], Li Wang [1], Ren Wang [1], Yuheng Zhai [1] and Zhengxing Chen [1,*]

1 National Engineering Laboratory for Cereal Fermentation Technology, Jiangnan University, Wuxi 214122, China; yangkai164@outlook.com (K.Y.); 6160112134@vip.jiangnan.edu.cn (K.L.); yelanplh@outlook.com (L.P.); legend0318@hotmail.com (L.W.); nedved_wr@jiangnan.edu.cn (R.W.); 6190112167@stu.jiangnan.edu.cn (Y.Z.)
2 Beijing Advanced Innovation Center for Food Nutrition and Human Health, Beijing Technology and Business University (BTBU), Beijing 100048, China; jwang010@126.com
3 College of Food and Pharmaceutical Science, Ningbo University, Ningbo 315000, China
4 Research Institute of Gang Yagou Healthy Food and Biotechnology, Ningbo 315205, China
5 Ningbo Institute for Food Control, Ningbo 315048, China; hellojiali77@gmail.com
* Correspondence: xh06326@gmail.com (X.L.); zxchen2007@foxmail.com (Z.C.)

Received: 16 January 2020; Accepted: 21 February 2020; Published: 24 February 2020

Abstract: Zearalenone (ZEN) and ochratoxin A (OTA) are key concerns of the food industry because of their toxicity and pollution scope. This study investigated the effects of ozone and electron beam irradiation (EBI) on the degradation of ZEN and OTA. Results demonstrated that 2 mL of 50 μg/mL ZEN was completely degraded after 10 s of treatment by 2.0 mg/L ozone. The degradation rate of 1 μg/mL ZEN by 16 kGy EBI was 92.76%. Methanol was superior to acetonitrile in terms of degrading ZEN when the irradiation dose was higher than 6 kGy. The degradation rate of 2 mL of 5 μg/mL OTA by 50 mg/L ozone at 180 s was 34%, and that of 1 μg/mL OTA by 16 kGy EBI exceeded 90%. Moreover, OTA degraded more rapidly in acetonitrile. Ozone performed better in the degradation of ZEN, whereas EBI was better for OTA. The conclusions provide theoretical and practical bases for the degradation of different fungal toxins.

Keywords: ozone; electron beam irradiation; degradation; zearalenone; ochratoxin A

Key Contribution: (1) ZEN and OTA in methanol and acetonitrile can be efficiently degraded by electron beam irradiation (EBI). (2) ZEN in standard solution can be efficiently degraded by ozone; OTA required a higher ozone concentration and longer treatment time than ZEN. (3). EBI induces reactions involving acetonitrile and between acetonitrile and ZEN and OTA.

---

1. Introduction

Crop pollution by fungal toxins is a global issue that causes massive annual economic losses. Large territorial areas of China are located in temperate and subtropical zones, offering favorable climatic conditions for the growth and reproduction of toxic fungi [1]. Zearalenone (ZEN) of *Fusarium* [2] and ochratoxin A (OTA) of *Aspergillus* and *Penicillium* [3] exhibited the most extensive distribution and strongest toxicity among the more than 400 toxic fungi discovered thus far [4]. Numerous studies have reported on the reproduction, genetic, and immune toxicities of ZEN, which causes nausea, vomiting, and diarrhea in humans and animals [5]. Animal toxicological experiments and clinical studies have demonstrated the strong nephrotoxicity, immunotoxicity, and carcinogenicity of OTA [6,7].

Ozone, as a strong oxidant, can attack the double bond in organic compounds through molecules and free radicals in a liquid system [8–10]. In addition, ozone exhibits acceptable permeability and can automatically decompose into oxygen without generating toxic residues [11]. Hence, ozonation is a fungal toxin degradation technology with promising potential, and has been the focus of numerous studies in recent decades. Xu et al. discussed the reduction of ZEN in corn flour by ozone treatment, and four ozonation products were identified by a method involving the use of ultra-performance liquid chromatography-tandem mass spectrometry [12]. Inan et al. degraded aflatoxin B_1 (AFB_1) in sliced and ground pimiento by 33 and 66 mg/L ozone and obtained degradation rates of 80% and 93%, respectively [13]. Zorlugenc et al. treated AFB_1 in dry figs by ozone gas and ozonated water for 180 min, and the degradation rates of AFB_1 were 95.21% and 88.62%, respectively [14]. These studies proved the strong degradation capability of ozonated gas and ozone water for fungal toxins.

Electron beam irradiation (EBI) is the process of irradiating products by using the electron beam generated by an electron accelerator. This technology is characterized by high energy utilization, simple operation, and safe use. EBI is a safe and effective green-processing technology. Researchers have explored the application of EBI in agricultural products and food storage, crop breeding, radiation sterilization, radiation pest control, and other emerging fields such as radiation chemical and radiation material engineering [15,16]. The degradation of fungal toxins in foods based on EBI has recently been discussed. Stepanik et al. investigated the degradation of deoxynivalenol (DON) in three production intermediates in distillers dried grain and solubles by using a dose of EBI treatment [17]. Wang et al. discussed the degradation of AFB_1 by EBI and found that 8.6 kGy of EBI was adequate to completely degrade 5 ng/g AFB_1 [18]. The mechanism of action was similar to that of γ-ray [19]. Water molecules were activated and ionized after EBI, generating hydroxyl radicals and hydration molecules. Hydroxyl radicals further destroy the molecular structure of the toxin.

Few studies on the degradation of ZEN and OTA by ozone and EBI are available presently, although numerous studies have focused on the degradation of AFB_1 [20]. The effects of ozone and EBI on the degradation of ZEN and OTA cannot be easily understood due to the different structures of ZEN and OTA from AFB_1, thereby limiting the applications of ozone and EBI in ZEN- and OTA-contaminated foods. The influences of ozone concentration, sample concentration, treatment time, and radiation dose in acetonitrile and methanol systems on the degradation rates of ZEN and OTA were discussed on the basis of previous studies on DON [21] and AFB_1 [22] degradation by ozone and EBI. The present study provides theoretical and practical bases for OTA and ZEN degradation in food by ozone and EBI in the future.

2. Results

2.1. *Standard Curves of Zearalenone (ZEN) and Ochratoxin A (OTA)*

The linear correlation between the peak area and concentration (0.5–5.0 and 0.1–1.0 μg/mL) was clarified on the basis of the standard curves of ZEN and OTA (Figure 1). The regression equations of the ZEN and OTA standard curves are marked in Figure 1. R^2 represents the square of the correlation coefficient, and the determination coefficient R^2 is a relative index of goodness of fit between the regression line and the observed value of the sample, reflecting the proportion of the fluctuations of the dependent variable that can be explained by the independent variable. The closer R^2 is to 1, the better the goodness of fit. R^2 of the regression equations in the ZEN and OTA standard curves were 0.9999 and 0.9998, respectively, indicating a high degree of linear regression.

2.2. *Degradation Rates of ZEN and OTA by Ozone*

The degradation rates of 2 mL of 50 μg/mL ZEN standard working solution (a) and 2 mL of 5 μg/mL OTA standard working solution (b) by ozone under different treatment time periods are shown in Figure 2. The degradation rate of ZEN at 1 s was higher than 50%. The degradation of ZEN slowed down with the increase in treatment time. No ZEN was detected in the solution at 10 s. The degradation curve of OTA from 0–180 s was a reverse S-shaped curve. The degradation rate of

OTA increased during the first 30 s and decreased between 30–60 s, but it increased gradually between 60–180 s and reached the peak (34%) at 180 s.

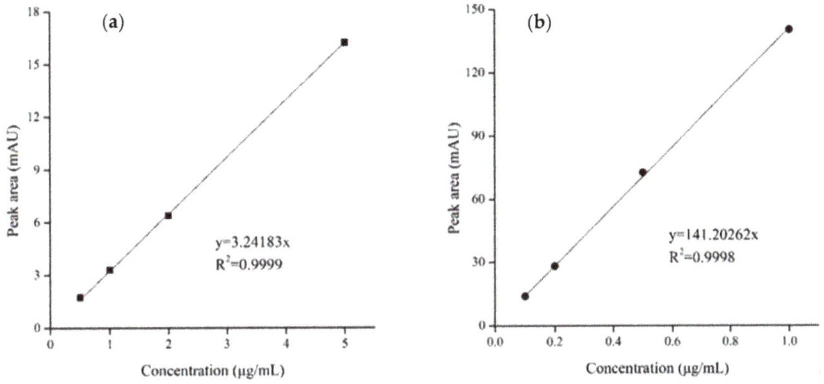

Figure 1. High-performance liquid chromatography (HPLC) standard curves of zearalenone (ZEN) (**a**) and ochratoxin A (OTA) (**b**).

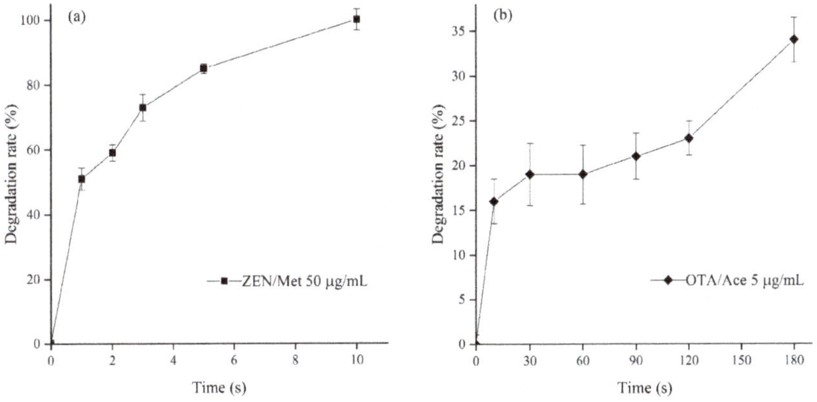

Figure 2. Degradation curves of ZEN (**a**) and OTA (**b**) by ozone at different treatment time periods.

2.3. Degradation of ZEN and OTA by Electron Beam Irradiation (EBI)

2.3.1. Degradation of ZEN by EBI

The degradation curves of 1.0 μg/mL ZEN in methanol and acetonitrile solution under different EBI doses (i.e., 0, 2, 4, 6, 8, 10, 12, 14, and 16 kGy) are shown in Figure 3. The degradation rate of ZEN in the acetonitrile solution was higher than that in the methanol solution under 0–6 kGy. However, the degradation rate of ZEN in acetonitrile decreased gradually with the increase in dose, higher than that in acetonitrile at an irradiation dose exceeding 6 kGy. The degradation of ZEN slowed down in methanol with the increase in irradiation dose. The degradation rates of ZEN in methanol and acetonitrile were 92.76% and 72.29%, respectively, at 16 kGy. Methanol was conducive to the degradation of ZEN by EBI at high irradiation doses. According to the literature, EBI possesses unique advantages in degrading fungal toxins, and considerable development of this approach has been complicated. Liu et al. processed AFB_1 in sewage by EBI [23]. The 1 and 5 μg/mL toxin samples were degraded completely at 8 kGy. Peng et al. irradiated OTA in different solvent systems by electron beams and disclosed the degradation rates of OTA under the same concentration as follows:

water > acetonitrile > methanol–water (60:40, v/v) [24]. Therefore, EBI can also degrade ZEN in a methanol solution.

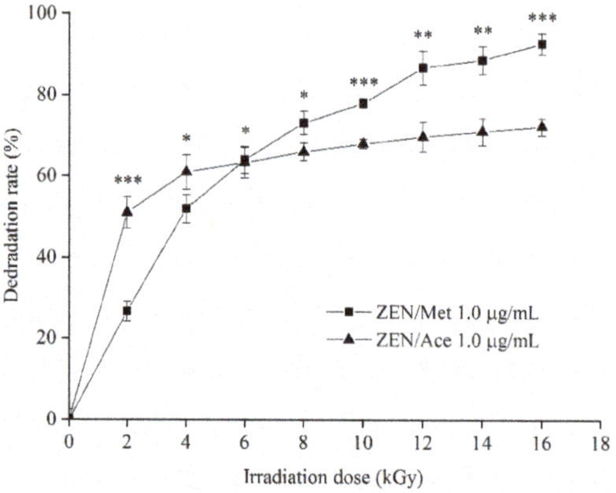

Figure 3. Degradation curve of ZEN in methanol (Met) and acetonitrile (Ace) at different electron beam irradiation (EBI) doses. Data are presented as means ± standard deviation (SD). *** $p < 0.01$, ** $0.01 < p < 0.05$, and * $p > 0.05$.

2.3.2. Degradation of OTA by EBI

The degradation of 1 μg/mL OTA in methanol and acetonitrile solution at different EBI doses (i.e., 0, 2, 4, 6, 8, 10, 12, 14, and 16 kGy) is shown in Figure 4 with S-shaped curves, indicating that the contents of the active substances (such as free radicals and active oxygen), which can react with OTA in the solvent system, initially increased and then decreased. In the irradiation dose range of 0–6 kGy, the degradation rate of OTA in the two solvent systems gradually increased and slowly degraded at 6 kGy. The degradation rates of OTA in methanol and acetonitrile at 16 kGy reached the maximum values of 84.16% and 91.56%, respectively.

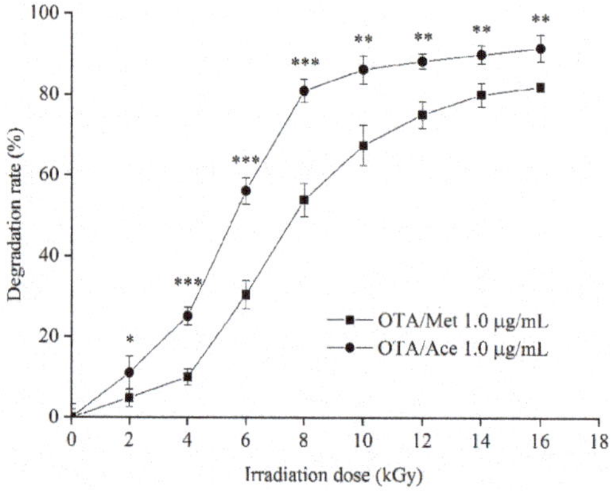

Figure 4. Degradation curve of OTA in Met and Ace at different EBI doses. Data are presented as means ± SD. *** $p < 0.01$, ** $0.01 < p < 0.05$, and * $p > 0.05$.

2.3.3. Effects of Solvents on Degradation of ZEN and OTA by EBI

Methanol is a common protic solvent and ·OH and e_{aq}^{-} quencher [25]. Acetonitrile is a common aprotic polar solvent. Both are widely used as solvents of fungal toxins. The acetonitrile solutions of ZEN and OTA after EBI application turned yellow, with its color deepening as the radiation dose increased. In contrast, the methanol solution remained transparent. The acetonitrile solutions of ZEN and OTA after EBI (i.e., 0, 4.0, 8.0, 12.0, and 16.0 kGy) are shown in the order from left to right in Figure 5a,b, respectively. Kameneva et al. irradiated acetonitrile molecules in a solid inert gas matrix by x-ray [26]. The Fourier infrared spectrum detection showed that acetonitrile molecules generated CH_3NC, CH_2CNH, and CH_2NCH molecular polymers and free radicals such as CH_2CN and CH_2NC.

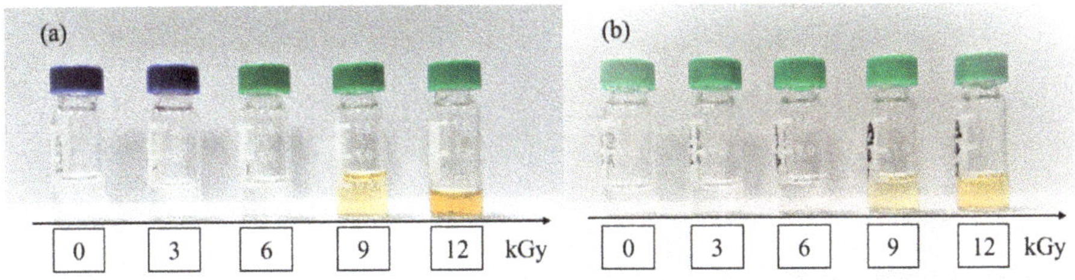

Figure 5. Degradation samples of ZEN (**a**) and OTA (**b**) treated with EBI in Ace.

3. Discussion

High degradation velocities of OTA in the early reaction stage may be related to the active materials in the reaction system in the reaction of degrading OTA by using ozone. Active substances were consumed completely as the reaction continued, thus resulting in the decelerated degradation. Ozone molecules degraded OTA and generated free radicals at the end of the reaction, resulting in the gradual increase in degradation speeds. This finding confirmed the research conclusions of Qi et al. [20].

The degradation rate of ZEN/Ace samples in the reaction of degrading ZEN/Met and ZEN/Ace by EBI was observably higher than that of ZEN/Met samples within 0–6 kGy. Schmelling et al. reported that organic solvents (i.e., acetonitrile and methanol solutions) treated with EBI produced less free radicals, and free radicals were in the dynamic process of generation and annihilation [27]. Guo et al. proved that methanol is a free radical scavenger [25]. In 0–6 kGy, free radicals generated by EBI in acetonitrile can be used for ZEN degradation, whereas free radicals in methanol were eliminated by methanol molecules once generated, so the degradation rate of ZEN in methanol was low. At 6–16 kGy, the degradation rate of both ZEN samples slowed down, and the degradation rate of the ZEN/Met samples was higher than that of the ZEN/Ace samples. A possible reason for this trend was that at 6–16 kGy, the degradation of ZEN in acetonitrile resulted in a sharp decline in its concentration. Acetonitrile generated a large amount of free radicals by irradiation that slowed down the degradation rate of ZEN/Ace. In the methanol system, the free radical-scavenging effect of methanol was limited and relatively more free radicals were present in the solution. Thus, the degradation rate of ZEN/Met was still higher than that of ZEN/Ace.

Within the irradiation dose range of 0–16 kGy, the degradation rate of OTA in the acetonitrile solution exceeded that in the methanol solution, contradicting the results of Peng et al. [24]. This result may be due to different processing conditions such as volume, container, and handling operations. This study demonstrated that EBI can effectively degrade OTA in methanol and acetonitrile with a higher degradation rate in acetonitrile. On one hand, the free radicals of degrading OTA were reduced because of the free radical-scavenging effect of methanol. On the other hand, the molecular structure of OTA contained more free radical-charged sites, and acetonitrile free radicals produced by EBI were still relatively more in the degrading process, thus the phenomenon of a ZEN/Ace degradation rate lower than that in ZEN/Met at 6–16 kGy was not observed.

Moreover, different substrates can considerably affect the reaction. High-performance liquid chromatography (HPLC) chromatograms of ZEN and OTA degradation by a 3 kGy EBI dose in acetonitrile solution were compared with those in methanol (Figure 6). Within the retention time range of 1.5–5 min, the HPLC chromatograms of ZEN and OTA in acetonitrile exhibited numerous absorption peaks, whereas no absorption peaks were observed in the methanol solution and the blank group. The degradation curves of ZEN and OTA were remarkably different under the same conditions, indicating the considerable difference of their reaction mechanisms. This difference can be used to interpret the reaction results of ZEN and OTA in different solvents. In addition, this difference may be partially attributed to the different molecular structures of ZEN and OTA.

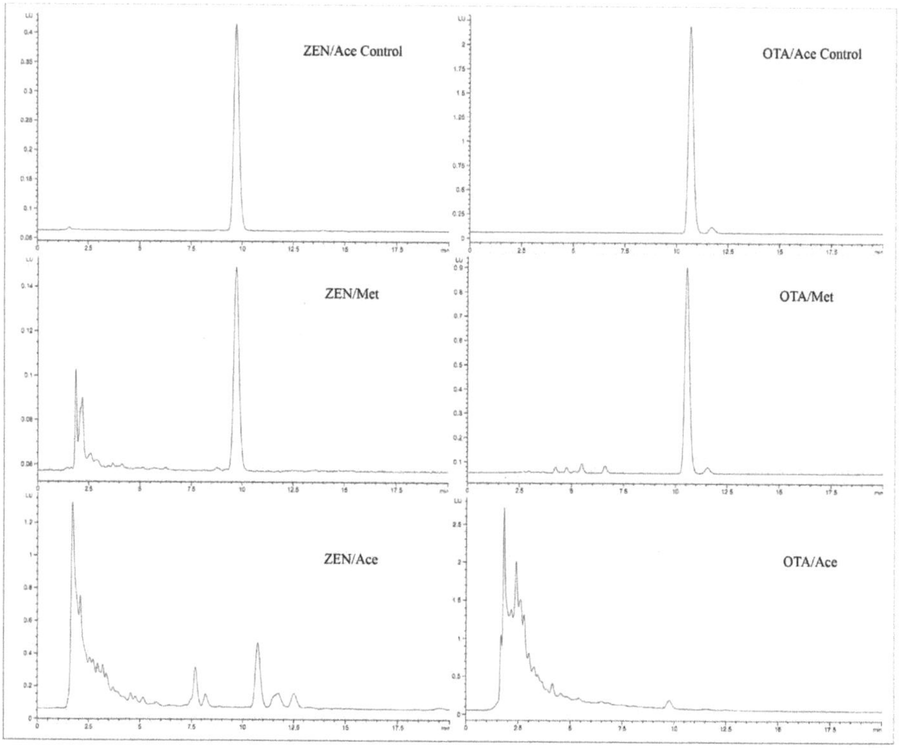

Figure 6. HPLC chromatograms of ZEN and OTA treated with 3 kGy EBI dose in Met and Ace.

4. Conclusions

Ozone and EBI were proven to be a safe, efficient, and environmentally friendly processing method in degrading ZEN and OTA. In this study, the degradation rate of the ZEN and OTA standard working solutions increased with the extension of ozone treatment time. ZEN was completely degraded within 10 s at 2 mg/L of ozone concentration, and the degradation rate of OTA was 34% at 180 s by ozone treatment, suggesting that ZEN was more sensitive to ozone. The degradation rate of ZEN and OTA solutions by EBI increased with the irradiation dose. At high radiation dose, methanol was beneficial to the degradation of ZEN by EBI and acetonitrile was more beneficial to the degradation of OTA by EBI. EBI can induce the reaction among acetonitrile molecules and between acetonitrile and toxin molecules by comparing the degradation rates of ZEN and OTA in different solutions using HPLC chromatograms. However, the high cost of equipment limits the wide application of ozone treatment and EBI. In addition, a high EBI dose on grain will affect the color of the product, which is not conducive to the subsequent processing and utilization. Further research needs to be done to investigate the mechanism of degradation of mycotoxin by ozone and EBI and discuss the different process conditions and instrument parameters in degrading mycotoxins in cereals and cereal-derived food products.

5. Materials and Methods

5.1. Materials and Instruments

5.1.1. Materials and Reagent

Standard ZEN and OTA products (purity ≥ 99.8%) and acetic acid (HPLC grade) were obtained from J&K Scientific Ltd. (Shanghai, China). HPLC-grade methanol (Met) and acetonitrile (Ace) were purchased from Fisher Scientific Company (Waltham, MA, USA). Milli-Q quality water (resistance ≥ 18.2 MΩ/cm) was prepared by a Millipore-QSP ultrapure water instrument (Millipore, Bedford, MA, USA). Nitrogen (purity ≥ 99.8%) and oxygen (purity ≥ 99.8%) were obtained from Wuxi Xinnan Chemical Gas Co., Ltd., Wuxi, China. The other analytical pure reagents were purchased from China Pharmaceutical Chemical Reagent Co., Ltd., Shanghai, China.

5.1.2. Major Apparatus

HPLC (HPLC 1260) with a fluorescence detector and ZORBAX SB-C18 column was purchased from Agilent Technologies (Palo Alto, CA, USA). The AB5.0 electron beam accelerator was obtained from Wuxi EL PONT Radiation Technology Co., Ltd. (Wuxi, China) and the CFG-3-20 g-type ozone generator was purchased from Qingdao Guolin Industrial Co., Ltd. (Qingdao, China). An Ideal 2000 Ozone concentration analysis recorder was obtained from Zibo ADEL Measurement Control Co., Ltd. (Zibo, China) and the MD200-1 pressure-blowing instrument was purchased from Hangzhou Allsheng Instrument Co., Ltd. (Hangzhou, China).

5.2. Experimental Methods

5.2.1. Preparation of Standard Stock and Working Solutions of ZEN and OTA

ZEN was dissolved in a methanol solution, and OTA was dissolved in an acetonitrile solution to prepare 100 and 10 μg/mL standard stock solutions, respectively. The solutions were stored at −20 °C. A certain amount of ZEN standard stock solution was collected and dried using nitrogen. Then, methanol and acetonitrile were added for secondary dissolution to prepare 1.0 μg/mL ZEN/Met and ZEN/Ace standard working solutions, respectively. The solutions were stored at 4 °C for EBI. A certain amount of ZEN standard stock solution and methanol was used to prepare 50 μg/mL of standard working solution and stored at 4 °C for subsequent ozone treatment. A certain amount of OTA standard stock solution was obtained and dried by nitrogen. Then, methanol and acetonitrile were added for secondary dissolution to prepare 1.0 μg/mL OTA/Met and OTA/Ace standard working solutions, respectively. The solutions were stored at 4 °C for EBI. A portion of OTA standard stock solution and acetonitrile was used to prepare a 5 μg/mL working solution and stored at 4 °C for subsequent ozone treatment.

5.2.2. Measurement of ZEN and OTA Contents

An Agilent 1260 HPLC with a G1321B fluorescence detector was employed. The chromatographic column was a ZORBAX SB-C18 column (4.6 mm × 150 mm). The filling diameter and column temperature were 5 μm and 35 °C, respectively. The injection volume was 20 μL. The flow phase of ZEN was methanol/water (60/40, v/v) with the flow rate set at 1.0 mL/min. The detection wavelength was 274 and 440 nm for the excitation and emission wavelengths, respectively. The flow phase of OTA was water/acetonitrile/acetic acid (56/43/1, v/v/v), and the flow rate was 0.9 mL/min. The detection wavelength consisted of 333 and 477 nm for the excitation and emission wavelengths, respectively.

5.2.3. Drawing of Standard ZEN and OTA Curves

Several ZEN and OTA standard stock solutions were selected. ZEN (i.e., 0.5, 1.0, 2.0, and 5.0 μg/mL) and OTA standard working solutions (i.e., 0.1, 0.2, 0.5, and 1.0 μg/mL) were prepared by the flow phase.

The relation curves between the absorption peak area in the liquid chromatograph and concentration of solutions were drawn and the standard curves of ZEN and OTA were drawn according to these relation curves.

5.2.4. Degradation of ZEN and OTA by Ozone

Ozone was generated by a high-pressure discharger from an ozone generator connected with an external oxygen source. Ozone concentration was adjusted by controlling the current of the ozone generator, and changes in ozone concentration were monitored online by ozone concentration detectors. The excess ozone was eliminated by the decomposition of the ozone destroyer.

A total of 2 mL ZEN (50 μg/mL) and OTA (5 μg/mL) working solutions were dissolved in a piece of 10 mL polyethylene centrifuge tube, which was supplied with ozone. The ozone treatment conditions for ZEN were as follows: concentration = 2.0 mg/L, flow rate = 1.0 L/min, and treatment time = 0, 1, 2, 3, 5, and 10 s. The ozone treatment conditions for OTA were as follows: concentration = 50.0 mg/L, flow rate = 1.0 L/min, and treatment time = 0, 10, 30, 60, 90, 120, and 180 s. After the ozone treatment, nitrogen was supplied for 3 min, and then the reaction was terminated. Subsequently, 1 mL flow phase was used for secondary dissolution.

5.2.5. Degradation of ZEN and OTA by EBIs

A total of 2 mL ZEN and 2 mL OTA working solutions were placed in a 5 mL polyethylene centrifuge tube. Irradiation doses were 0, 2, 4, 6, 8, 10, 12, 14, and 16 kGy. The accelerated electron energy was 5 MeV, and the electron beam current was 20 mA with a 1000 mm scan width. The dose rate was 2 kGy/s. The samples were dried by nitrogen after irradiation, and a 1 mL flow phase was used for secondary dissolution.

5.2.6. Data Processing

Sample processing and detection were repeated at least three times. One-way analysis of variance was performed by the Statistical Package for the Social Sciences version 17.0. $p < 0.05$ was considered to be statistically significant. $p > 0.05$ was not statistically significant.

Author Contributions: Conceptualization, K.Y. and K.L.; Data curation, K.Y. and L.P.; Formal analysis, K.L.; Funding acquisition, K.Y.; Investigation, L.P. and X.L.; Methodology, K.Y. and L.P.; Project administration, X.L.; Resources, K.Y. and X.L.; Software, K.L., J.X., Y.Z. and Z.C.; Supervision, J.X. and L.W.; Validation, K.L. and J.W.; Visualization, L.W.; Writing—original draft, K.Y.; Writing—review & editing, K.Y., R.W. and Z.C. All authors have read and agreed to the published version of the manuscript.

Funding: This research was financially supported by the National Key Research and Development Program of China (2017YFC1600904), the Jiangsu Agriculture Science and Technology Innovation Fund CX(17)1003, the China Agriculture Research System (CARS-02-32), the Open Foundation of Beijing Advanced Innovation Center for Food Nutrition and Human Health (20182014), the National Natural Science Foundation of China (31771898), and the National Top Youth for Grain Industry (LQ2018302).

Conflicts of Interest: The authors declare no conflict of interest.

References

1. Abramson, D.; Richter, W.; Rintelen, J.; Sinha, R.N.; Schuster, M. Ochratoxin-A Production in Bavarian Cereal-Grains Stored at 15-Percent and 19-Percent Moisture-Content. *Arch. Environ. Contam. Toxicol.* **1992**, *23*, 259–265. [CrossRef] [PubMed]
2. Bennett, J.W.; Klich, M. Mycotoxins. *Clin. Microbiol. Rev.* **2003**, *16*, 497–516. [CrossRef] [PubMed]
3. Janati, S.S.F.; Beheshti, H.R.; Asadi, M.; Mihanparast, S.; Feizy, J. Preliminary Survey of Aflatoxins and Ochratoxin A in Dried Fruits from Iran. *Bull. Environ. Contam. Toxicol.* **2012**, *88*, 391–395. [CrossRef] [PubMed]
4. Hussein, H.S.; Brasel, J.M. Toxicity, metabolism, and impact of mycotoxins on humans and animals. *Toxicology* **2001**, *167*, 101–134. [CrossRef]

5. World Health Organization; International Agency for Research on Cancer. *Some Naturally Occurring Substances: Food Items and Constituents, Heterocyclic Aromatic Amines and Mycotoxins*; World Health Organization: Geneva, Switzerland, 1993.
6. Castegnaro, M.; Canadas, D.; Vrabcheva, T.; Petkova-Bocharova, T.; Chernozemsky, I.N.; Pfohl-Leszkowicz, A. Balkan endemic nephropathy: Role of ochratoxins A through biomarkers. *Mol. Nutr. Food Res.* **2006**, *50*, 519–529. [CrossRef] [PubMed]
7. Heller, M.; Rosner, H.; Burkert, B.; Moller, U.; Hinsching, A.; Rohrmann, B.; Thierbach, S.; Kohler, H. In vitro studies into the influence of ochratoxin A on the production of tumor necrosis factor alpha by the human monocytic cell line THP-1. *Dtsch. Tierarztl. Wochenschr.* **2002**, *109*, 200–205.
8. Hoigné, J.; Bader, H.J.W.R. Rate constants of reactions of ozone with organic and inorganic compounds in water—I: Non-dissociating organic compounds. *Water Res.* **1983**, *17*, 173–183. [CrossRef]
9. Kleiser, G.; Frimmel, F.H. Removal of precursors for disinfection by-products (DBPs)—Differences between ozone- and OH-radical-induced oxidation. *Sci. Total Environ.* **2000**, *256*, 1–9. [CrossRef]
10. Staehelin, J.; Hoigne, J. Decomposition of ozone in water in the presence of organic solutes acting as promoters and inhibitors of radical chain reactions. *Environ. Sci. Technol.* **1985**, *19*, 1206–1213. [CrossRef]
11. Luo, X.; Wang, R.; Wang, L.; Li, Y.; Zheng, R.; Sun, X.; Wang, Y.; Chen, Z.; Tao, G. Analyses by UPLC Q-TOF MS of products of aflatoxin B-1 after ozone treatment. *Food Addit. Contam. Part A* **2014**, *31*, 105–110. [CrossRef]
12. Xu, Y.; Wang, Y.F.; Ji, J.; Wu, H.; Pi, F.W.; Zhang, Y.Z.; Sun, X.L. Chemical and toxicological alterations of zearalenone under ozone treatment. *Food Addit. Contam. Part A* **2019**, *36*, 163–174. [CrossRef] [PubMed]
13. Inan, F.; Pala, M.; Doymaz, I. Use of ozone in detoxification of aflatoxin B-1 in red pepper. *J. Stored Product. Res.* **2007**, *43*, 425–429. [CrossRef]
14. Zorlugenc, B.; Zorlugenc, F.K.; Oztekin, S.; Evliya, I.B. The influence of gaseous ozone and ozonated water on microbial flora and degradation of aflatoxin B-1 in dried figs. *Food Chem. Toxicol.* **2008**, *46*, 3593–3597. [CrossRef] [PubMed]
15. Manaila, E.; Stelescu, M.D.; Craciun, G.; Ighigeanu, D. Wood Sawdust/Natural Rubber Ecocomposites Cross-Linked by Electron Beam Irradiation. *Materials* **2016**, *9*, 503. [CrossRef] [PubMed]
16. Stelescu, M.; Manaila, E.; Craciun, G.; Ighigeanu, D. Electron beam processing of ethylene-propylene-terpolymer-based rubber mixtures. *Int. Sch. Sci. Res. Innov.* **2018**, *12*, 258–262.
17. Stepanik, T.; Kost, D.; Nowicki, T.; Gabay, D. Effects of electron beam irradiation on deoxynivalenol levels in distillers dried grain and solubles and in production intermediates. *Food Addit. Contam.* **2007**, *24*, 1001–1006. [CrossRef] [PubMed]
18. Wang, R.Q.; Liu, R.J.; Chang, M.; Jin, Q.Z.; Huang, J.H.; Liu, Y.F.; Wang, X.G. Ultra-performance Liquid Chromatography Quadrupole Time-of-Flight MS for Identification of Electron Beam from Accelerator Degradation Products of Aflatoxin B-1. *Appl. Biochem. Biotechnol.* **2015**, *175*, 1548–1556. [CrossRef]
19. Getoff, N. Radiation-induced degradation of water pollutants—State of the art. *Radiat. Phys. Chem.* **1996**, *47*, 581–593. [CrossRef]
20. Qi, L.J.; Li, Y.L.; Luo, X.H.; Wang, R.; Zheng, R.H.; Wang, L.; Li, Y.F.; Yang, D.; Fang, W.M.; Chen, Z.X. Detoxification of zearalenone and ochratoxin A by ozone and quality evaluation of ozonised corn. *Food Addit. Contam. Part A* **2016**, *33*, 1700–1710. [CrossRef]
21. Wang, L.; Luo, Y.P.; Luo, X.H.; Wang, R.; Li, Y.F.; Li, Y.N.; Shao, H.L.; Chen, Z.X. Effect of deoxynivalenol detoxification by ozone treatment in wheat grains. *Food Control* **2016**, *66*, 137–144. [CrossRef]
22. Luo, X.H.; Qi, L.J.; Liu, Y.T.; Wang, R.; Yang, D.; Li, K.; Wang, L.; Li, Y.N.; Zhang, Y.W.; Chen, Z.X. Effects of Electron Beam Irradiation on Zearalenone and Ochratoxin A in Naturally Contaminated Corn and Corn Quality Parameters. *Toxins* **2017**, *9*, 84. [CrossRef] [PubMed]
23. Liu, R.; Wang, R.; Lu, J.; Chang, M.; Jin, Q.; Du, Z.; Wang, S.; Li, Q.; Wang, X. Degradation of AFB(1) in aqueous medium by electron beam irradiation: Kinetics, pathway and toxicology. *Food Control* **2016**, *66*, 151–157. [CrossRef]
24. Peng, C.H.; Ding, Y.; An, F.P.; Wang, L.; Li, S.Y.; Nie, Y.; Zhou, L.Y.; Li, Y.R.; Wang, C.G.; Li, S.R. Degradation of ochratoxin A in aqueous solutions by electron beam irradiation. *J. Radioanal. Nucl. Chem.* **2015**, *306*, 39–46. [CrossRef]
25. Guo, Z.B.; Zhou, F.; Zhao, Y.F.; Zhang, C.Z.; Liu, F.L.; Bao, C.X.; Lin, M.Y. Gamma irradiation-induced sulfadiazine degradation and its removal mechanisms. *Chem. Eng. J.* **2012**, *191*, 256–262. [CrossRef]

26. Kameneva, S.V.; Volosatova, A.D.; Feldman, V.I. Radiation-induced transformations of isolated CH3CN molecules in noble gas matrices. *Radiat. Phys. Chem.* **2017**, *141*, 363–368. [CrossRef]
27. Schmelling, D.; Poster, D.; Chaychian, M.; Neta, P.; McLaughlin, W.; Silverman, J.; Al-Sheikhly, M. Applications of ionizing radiation to the remediation of materials contaminated with heavy metals and polychlorinated biphenyls. *Radiat. Phys. Chem.* **1998**, *52*, 371–377. [CrossRef]

toxins

MDPI

Article

Acetamiprid Affects Destruxins Production but Its Accumulation in *Metarhizium* sp. Spores Increases Infection Ability of Fungi

Monika Nowak [1], Przemysław Bernat [1], Julia Mrozińska [2] and Sylwia Różalska [1,*]

1 Department of Industrial Microbiology and Biotechnology, Faculty of Biology and Environmental Protection, University of Łódź, 90–237 Łódź, Poland; monika.nowak@unilodz.eu (M.N.); przemyslaw.bernat@biol.uni.lodz.pl (P.B.)
2 Scientific Students Group "SKN Bio-Mik", Faculty of Biology and Environmental Protection, University of Łódź, 90–237 Łódź, Poland; julia.mrozia@gmail.com
* Correspondence: sylwia.rozalska@biol.uni.lodz.pl

Received: 10 August 2020; Accepted: 5 September 2020; Published: 11 September 2020

Abstract: *Metarhizium* sp. are entomopathogenic fungi that inhabit the soil environment. Together, they act as natural pest control factors. In the natural environment, they come into contact with various anthropogenic pollutants, and sometimes, they are used together and interchangeably with chemical insecticides (e.g., neonicotinoids) for pest control. In most cases, the compatibility of entomopathogens with insecticides has been determined; however, the influence of these compounds on the metabolism of entomopathogenic fungi has not yet been studied. Secondary metabolites are very important factors that influence the fitness of the producers, playing important roles in the ability of these pathogens to successfully parasitize insects. In this study, for the first time, we focus on whether the insecticide present in the fungal growth environment affects secondary metabolism in fungi. The research revealed that acetamiprid at concentrations from 5 to 50 mg L^{-1} did not inhibit the growth of all tested *Metarhizium* sp.; however, it reduced the level of 19 produced destruxins in direct proportion to the dosage used. Furthermore, it was shown that acetamiprid accumulates not only in plant or animal tissues, but also in fungal cells. Despite the negative impact of acetamiprid on secondary metabolism, it was proofed to accumulate in *Metarhizium* spores, which appeared to have a stronger infectious potential against mealworm *Tenebrio molitor*, in comparison to the insecticide or the biological agent alone.

Keywords: entomopathogens; mycoinsecticides; secondary metabolites; insect pathogenesis; acetamiprid accumulation

Key Contribution: Acetamiprid represses destruxins production by *Metarhizium* sp.; Spores of *M. brunneum* with accumulated acetamiprid have increased infectivity against *T. molitor*.

1. Introduction

Synthetic insecticides are important pesticides for both agricultural and domestic pest control. Among them, neonicotinoids (e.g., acetamiprid, imidacloprid, thiacloprid) are the most extensively used worldwide because of their high effectiveness in controlling crop and domestic pests [1]. They account for more than 25% of the global insecticide market and are now being considered as a replacement for many existing conventional insecticide classes [2]. Neonicotinoids' popularity is largely due to their physicochemical properties, high effectiveness, low resistance, and the fact that they are less harmful to mammals compared to other insecticides. For example, to protect fruit plants against pests, up to 3 g per 100 m^2 of a popular pest control product (e.g., Mospilan 20 SP) is used with acetamiprid as the active substance are used and, as a consequence, acetamiprid penetrates the soil and bioaccumulates. According to data from the European Food Safety Authority (EFSA), ^{14}C-acetamiprid was identified as the major constituent of the radioactive residues in all plant parts (the study included eggplants, apples, carrots and cabbage) in an amount of 30–90% within 14–90 days after the last application [3]. The ability of neonicotinoids to accumulate in plants is known to increase the probability of environmental contamination and exposure to nontarget organisms [3–5]. In addition, despite the lack of recognition of acetamiprid as a compound persisting in soil, its degradation in environmental conditions has been found to last up to 43 days [3].

Among all methods of insect control, biological methods deserve special attention. *Metarhizium* sp., the common insect pathogens in wildlife, are very efficient bioinsecticides usually applied in practice [6]. Their effectiveness against insects depends mainly on their infective potential, i.e., the ability to produce extracellular lytic enzymes and secondary metabolites [7,8]. While the extracellular enzymes are well studied, equally important secondary metabolites, which play critical roles in the ability of *Metarhizium* to successfully parasitize their hosts and ultimately contribute to the success or failure of these fungi as biological control agents, are quite often neglected [9]. Entomopathogenic fungi produce a variety of bioactive metabolites including >40 cyclic hexadepsipeptides destruxins (dtxs) [8]. It is suggested that in attacked insects, dtxs induce paralysis and muscle contraction via muscle depolarization by the direct opening of Ca^{2+} channels in the membrane [10,11]. Besides their insecticidal activity, dtxs have also potential as pharmaceuticals showing antiviral, antitumor, cytotoxic, immunosuppressant or antiproliferative effects [12,13]. However, due to the endophytic properties of *Metarhizium* sp., the presence of dtxs can be found in, e.g., potatoes [14], maize and strawberries [15], causing dtxs to enter the food chain and pose a threat to human health.

The aim of this work was to determine the influence of acetamiprid on the growth and the secondary metabolism of *Metarhizium*, which is considered as a significant factor during the pest infection process. Furthermore, we checked whether acetamiprid could be accumulated by *Metarhizium*, how it affected the production of dtxs, and whether it affected the ability of fungi to infect insects. This study could help to understand the potential risks of a harmful influence of acetamiprid on soil-inhabiting fungi and their infectious potential, which plays an important role in maintaining the ecological balance.

2. Results

2.1. Fungal Biomass Yield of Metarhizium sp. in the Presence of Acetamiprid

Among the tested strains, *M. anisopliae* and *M. robertsii* IM2358 were the best growing species, while *M. brunneum* and *M. robertsii* ARSEF727 grew at a similar medium rate (biomass yield about 6 g L^{-1}). The slowest growing species was *M. globosum*. It turned out that acetamiprid did not inhibit growth in any of the tested strains, even at the highest concentration of 50 mg L^{-1} ($p > 0.05$) (Figure 1). Literature data also provides information that acetamiprid has no harmful effect on conidia germination and production or vegetative growth in *M. anisopliae*—strain E9 (ESALQ/USP) [16]. The lack of toxic effect was also confirmed in the presented study.

2.2. Quantitative Analyses of the Content of Acetamiprid in Metarhizium Fungal Cultures

In this study, the fungal ability to eliminate acetamiprid added to cultures at concentrations of 5, 25 and 50 mg L^{-1} was verified (Figure S1). None of the tested *Metarhizium* sp. showed the highly effective ability to remove acetamiprid from the Czapek Dox culture medium after seven days of incubation. At the concentration of 5 mg L^{-1}, a slight elimination capacity was demonstrated for *M. brunneum* and *M. robertsii* IM6519 (the average removal rate reached 29 and 24%, respectively). In a situation where five times more acetamiprid was added to the fungal culture, a loss was observed in the samples of all tested strains. *M. anisopliae*, *M. globosum* and *M. brunneum* removed respectively 31, 25 and 24% of acetamiprid from the culture medium. In the case of the other species, the substrate elimination was below 20%. In the fungal cultures, where the insecticide concentration was 50 mg L^{-1} there was no loss of more than 20% of the insecticide for any species. However, studies of the content of acetamiprid separately in the mycelium and culture medium showed that it was accumulated in the fungal cells.

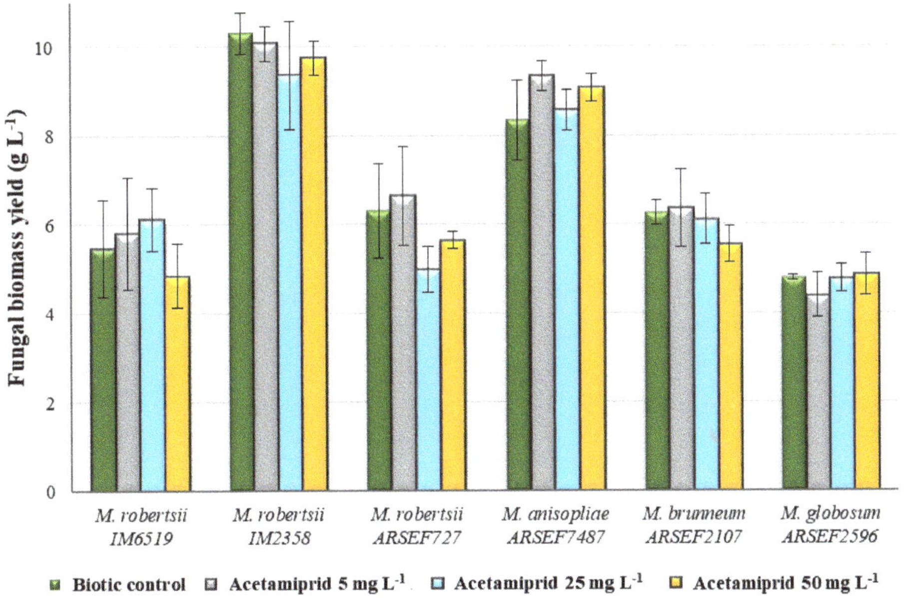

Figure 1. Influence of acetamiprid at concentrations of 5, 25 and 50 mg L^{-1} on fungal biomass yield of *Metarhizium* sp. One-way ANOVA was used for investigations of statistical significance. All differences are statistically insignificant ($p > 0.05$).

This insecticide has proved the ability to accumulate, inter alia, in the tissues of plants where, through translocation, it can even move from the roots to the shoots [17,18]. It was found that due to its good solubility in water, acetamiprid has a strong toxic effect on aquatic organisms where it bioaccumulates by sorption mechanisms characteristic for compounds with high polarity [19,20]. Although acetamiprid accumulation ability has been described for several different species, in this paper, we present for the first time that entomopathogens, which are often used interchangeably or alternatively with various insecticides in agriculture, can also accumulate this compound, without metabolizing it inside the cells (during seven days of incubation). Herein, the amount of acetamiprid on the mycelium dry weight (mg g^{-1}) was directly proportional to the increasing concentration ($p < 0.05$) (Figure 2). This trend was similar for each tested species while *M. brunneum* exhibited the highest accumulation potential. The rest of the strains showed statistically significant differences in the amounts of acetamiprid accumulated in the cells at the three concentrations used. At the concentration of 25 mg L^{-1} in *M. anisopliae* the highest amount of the accumulated insecticide (0.69 mg per g of dry weight) was observed ($p < 0.05$), but it is worth noting that this species had been previously found to have high biomass yield (Figure 1). *M. robertsii* IM6519, *M. robertsii* IM2358 and *M. globosum* accumulated in the cells' comparable amounts of acetamiprid (approximately 0.36–0.45 mg per g of dry weight, $p > 0.05$). By comparison, 0.12 mg per g of dry weight was found in *M. brunneum* ($p < 0.05$). The situation changed for the acetamiprid concentration of 50 mg L^{-1} in the fungal culture and the amount of the toxic substrate accumulated in the mycelium leveled out (Figure 2). The largest quantity was detected for *M. globosum* (1.05 mg per g of dry weight), which was different from the other species (except *M. anisopliae*, $p > 0.05$). In all *M. robertsii* strains and the *M. anisopliae* strain studied, the acetamiprid amounts determined per g of dry weight were comparable.

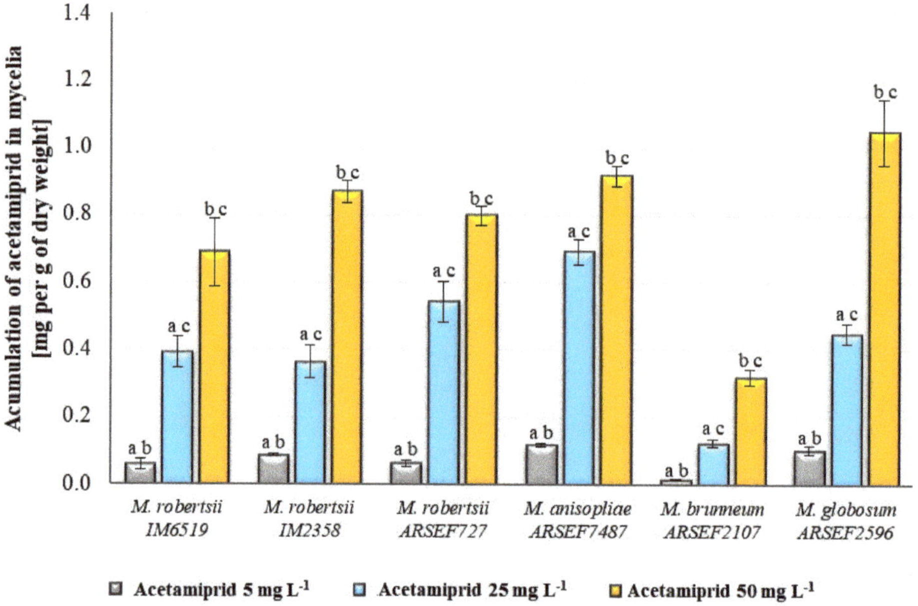

Figure 2. Accumulation of acetamiprid at concentrations of 5, 25 and 50 mg L^{-1} in the mycelium of *Metarhizium* sp. One-way ANOVA and Tukey's test were used for investigations of statistical significance. (**a–c**) $p < 0.05$. Statistically significant differences between samples at individual concentrations within the species. (**a**) Between samples with acetamiprid at concentrations of 5 and 25 mg L^{-1}; (**b**) between samples with acetamiprid at concentrations of 5 and 50 mg L^{-1}; (**c**) between samples with acetamiprid at concentrations of 25 and 50 mg L^{-1}.

2.3. *Analyses of Destruxins in Fungal Cultures of Metarhizium sp.*

According to literature data, *M. anisopliae*, *M. robertsii* and *M. brunneum* species have genes responsible for the production of dtxs [8]. Dtxs in *M. globosum* were also marked in this work, but their content was very low compared to the other species (in the order of 0.002 and 0.004 mg L^{-1} for dtx A and dtx B, respectively), so this species was excluded from further analyses. *M. robertsii* ARSEF727 had the lowest content of dtxs in the biotic control compared to the other species. The expression of genes responsible for the production of specific units making up the dtxs structure might not be as high as in the case of the other strains [8]. It cannot be said that the low concentrations of dtxs in *M. robertsii* ARSEF727 and *M. globosum* were caused by the poor growth of these fungi, because their growth rate was similar to that of *M. brunneum* and *M. robertsii* IM6519, which turned out to be the species with the highest content of dtxs in the biotic controls. Interestingly, *M. anisopliae*, in which the synthesis of dtxs has been accurately described, did not turn out to be the best producer [21]. *M. robertsii* IM2358 was also found to have higher levels of dtxs than *M. anisopliae*.

According to literature data, none of the fungal species has the capacity to produce all 39 types of dtxs, but *M. anisopliae* produces the majority of them [8]. In all tested strains, except *M. globosum*, 19 dtxs were determined. Due to the lack of chromatography standards, accurate quantitative analyses were performed only for dtx A and B. Therefore, the amounts of dtx A and B and the other types were described separately. It is worth noting that dtx A and dtx B are the main metabolites and occur in higher concentrations compared to other dtxs [22], which was also confirmed in this work.

It was checked whether, despite the lack of the influence of acetamiprid on the growth of the tested fungi, this insecticide affected the secondary metabolism. As mentioned above, three concentrations of acetamiprid (5, 25 and 50 mg L^{-1}) were examined. It turned out that the lowest concentration caused disturbances in the synthesis of the secondary metabolites of *Metarhizium* ($p < 0.05$). The use of higher doses of acetamiprid contributed to a gradual reduction in the amount of detected dtxs. Declines in the content of dtxs A and B were quite proportional (Figure 3). For *M. brunneum* there were no statistically significant differences between the amounts of dtx A at concentrations of 25 and 50 mg L^{-1}. The differences between all the concentrations used, which were determined for dtx B were statistically significant. The amounts of dtx A for *M. robertsii* IM2358 did not differ significantly between the concentrations of 5 and 25 mg L^{-1}, and for dtx B between the concentrations of 25 and 50 mg L^{-1}. No statistically significant differences between the concentrations of 25 and 50 mg L^{-1} for dtx A and B were found for *M. robertsii* ARSEF727.

The most harmful effect of acetamiprid on the production of dtxs was noted for *M. brunneum*, despite the fact that the growth rate and amounts of dtxs in the biotic sample were similar to those observed for *M. robertsii* IM6519. At the concentration of 5 mg L^{-1}, the contents of dtxs A and B were 56.43 and 41.93% lower than in the biotic controls, respectively. The highest dose of the insecticide resulted in a very large reduction in the contents of dtxs A and B to 11.99 and 14.58% of the biotic control, respectively. As mentioned above, *M. brunneum* accumulated in the mycelium the lowest quantities of acetamiprid per g of dry weight (Figure 2). It seems that *M. brunneum* defended itself against the presence of the insecticide in the mycelium. This could have been the reason why acetamiprid so heavily influenced the contents of dtxs in this strain. Dtxs production in *M. robertsii* ARSEF727 and *M. robertsii* IM6519 was also inhibited at the highest concentration of the insecticide and for dtx A the amounts were 90.99 and 72.09% lower than in the biotic control, and for dtx B 82.53 and 73.15%, respectively (Figure 3).

Comparable decreases in the contents of dtxs A and B were observed for *M. anisopliae* and *M. robertsii* IM2358 strains. With the increase in the acetamiprid concentration, the amounts of dtx A were lower by 10.04, 17.33 and 43.05% for *M. robertsii* IM2358 and by 13.10, 33.24 and 43.61% for *M. anisopliae*. It was noticed that the dose of 25 mg L^{-1} was more toxic to *M. anisopliae* than to *M. robertsii* IM2358. The concentration of dtx B for *M. anisopliae* decreased in a similar way to the content of dtx A (9.49, 33.05 and 40.03% less than in the biotic control, with the increase in the acetamiprid concentration). For *M. robertsii* IM2358 at the of concentrations 5 and 25 mg L^{-1} the decreases were similar to dtx A (7.94 and 19.68% less than in the biotic control, respectively), while at the concentration of 50 mg L^{-1}, the content of dtx B decreased by 24.21% (the reduction was almost two-fold smaller than for dtx A).

The levels of the other 17 dtxs, for which chromatographic standards are not available, were estimated based on the chromatographic peak areas. It turned out that the tested species differed in terms of the profile of dtxs, which was confirmed by the PCA (Figure 4). To the best of our knowledge, this kind of analysis had never been done before.

A similar dtxs profile was obtained for *M. anisopliae* and *M. robertsii* IM2358 (Figure 4). These strains differed from the others due to the high levels of dtx B1 and dtx Ed. A superior decrease in the levels of these dtxs and dtx D was observed for *M. robertsii* IM2358 with the acetamiprid concentration of 50 mg L^{-1}, hence in the PCA chart, this tested sample was distinguished and shown to migrate towards *M. robertsii* IM6519 (tested samples with acetamiprid at concentrations of 5 and 25 mg L^{-1}), in which the levels of these dtxs were also low (Figure 4). The level of dtx DesmA distinguished *M. anisopliae* from *M. robertsii* IM2358, as lower values were obtained for *M. anisopliae*. The level of synthesized dtx A1 was definitely a factor differentiating *M. anisopliae* from the other tested species, because for this strain, the highest level of dtx A1 was determined. Such close proximity of *M. anisopliae* and *M. robertsii* IM2358 on the PCA chart was in line with the presented previously. These species were characterized by a similar growth (Figure 1) and the effect of acetamiprid at concentrations of 5, 25 and 50 mg L^{-1} on the decrease in the amounts of dtxs A and B (Figure 3).

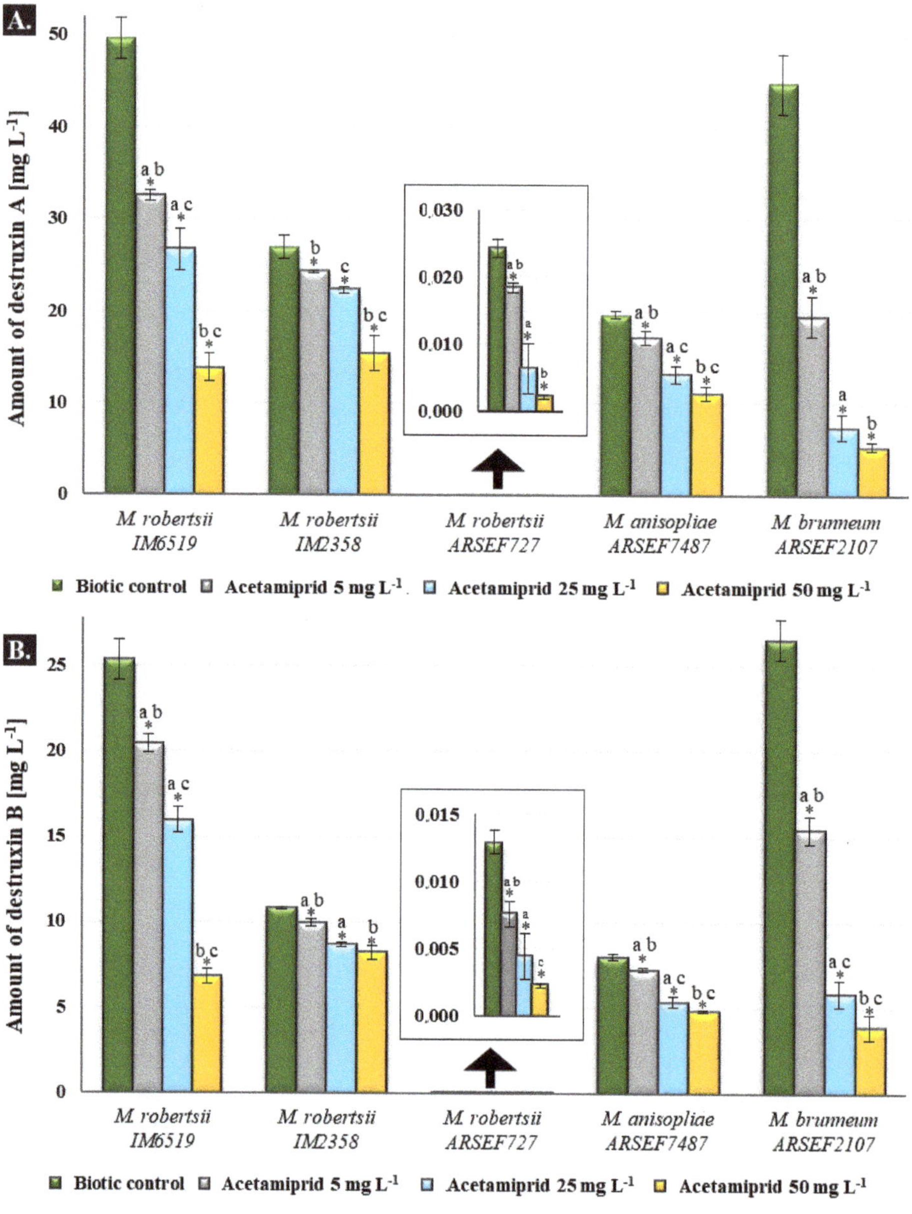

Figure 3. Effect of acetamiprid at concentrations of 5, 25 and 50 mg L^{-1} on the amounts of destruxins A (**A**) and B (**B**) produced by *Metarhizium* species. One-way ANOVA and Tukey's test were used for investigations of statistical significance. * $p < 0.05$. Statistically significant differences between samples with acetamiprid at concentrations of 5, 25 and 50 mg L^{-1} and their biotic controls within the species; (a–c) $p < 0.05$—statistically significant differences between samples at individual concentrations within the species. (a) Between samples with acetamiprid at concentrations of 5 and 25 mg L^{-1}; (b) between samples with acetamiprid at concentrations of 5 and 50 mg L^{-1}; (c) between samples with acetamiprid at concentrations of 25 and 50 mg L^{-1}.

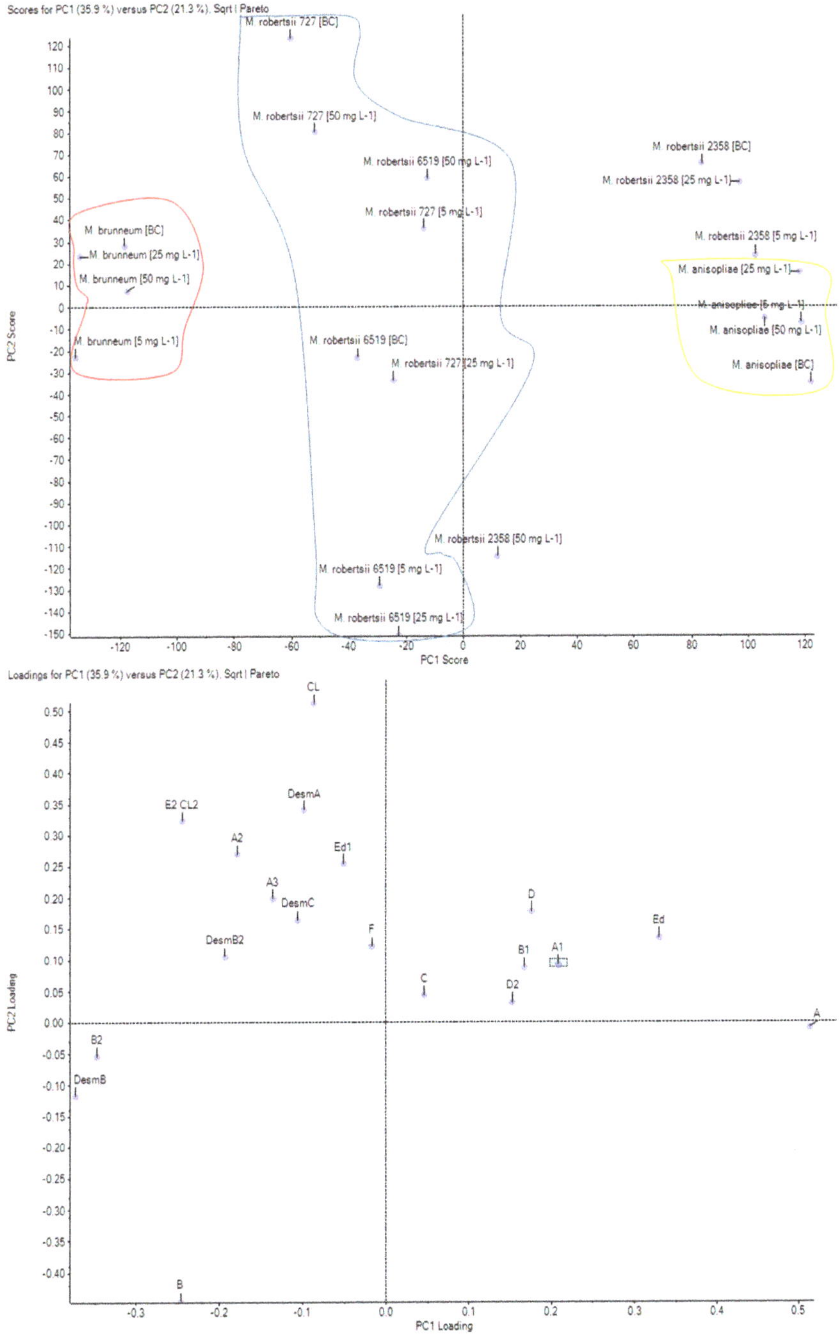

Figure 4. Results of principal component analysis (PCA) on the profile of destruxins of *Metarhizium* species in samples without the addition of acetamiprid and with acetamiprid at concentrations of 5, 25 and 50 mg L^{-1}. PC1 against PC2 scores chart (**top**); PC1 against PC2 loadings chart (**bottom**).

The above-mentioned results of the accumulation of acetamiprid in the mycelium showed that *M. brunneum* differed from the other species because of the lowest quantity of the insecticide bound in the fungal cells (Figure 2). It turned out that the dtxs profile of this strain also contributed to its differentiation, particularly to the high levels of dtxs DesmB, B2, DesmB2 and E2CL2 and the relatively low levels of dtxs Ed and D2.

Analysis of the PCA chart was more complicated for the strains *M. robertsii* ARSEF727 and *M. robertsii* IM6519. Their profiles were quite similar; however, it was possible to see differences in the contents of individual dtxs (Figure 4). The differentiating factor for *M. robertsii* ARSEF727 was the high level of dtx Ed1, particularly for the sample with acetamiprid at the concentration of 50 mg L^{-1}, where the addition of acetamiprid did not reduce the level of dtx Ed1 more than in the sample with the addition of acetamiprid at the concentration of 25 mg L^{-1}. The high level of dtx E2CL2 slightly differentiated from the biotic sample with *M. robertsii* ARSEF727 from the other samples of this species. Dtx CL was at a high level in *M. robertsii* IM6519, but in the sample with acetamiprid at a concentration of 50 mg L^{-1}, it definitely decreased. The close proximity of *M. robertsii* IM6519 (the biotic control and the sample with acetamiprid at a concentration of 50 mg L^{-1}) to *M. robertsii* ARSEF727 was due to the high level of dtx A3. However, the low level of this dtx in the tested sample with acetamiprid at a concentration of 25 mg L^{-1} in *M. robertsii* ARSEF727 made this strain more similar to *M. robertsii* IM6519 (samples with acetamiprid at concentrations of 5 and 25 mg L^{-1}).

2.4. Permeability of the Cell Membrane and the Content of Acetamiprid in Spores and Subcellular Fractions of the M. brunneum

M. brunneum was chosen to conduct an experiment on the effect of acetamiprid on the permeability of biological membranes, due to the greatest inhibition of dtxs production by this compound, even to 88% at the concentration of 50 mg L^{-1} (Figure 3). Dtxs are extracellular metabolites; however, their synthesis takes place in fungal cells [23]. The properties of the cell membrane, including permeability, potential and fluidity, have an influence on the cell secretion process [24]. Acetamiprid did not reduce the permeability of biological membranes at any of the used concentrations ($p > 0.05$). The reduced amount of dtxs determined in the samples with the addition of the toxic insecticide was not associated with a disorder of the membrane permeability system (Table S1).

Due to the high inhibition of dtxs production, it was checked whether acetamiprid accumulated in the spores of *M. brunneum*. Additionally, its amount in the cell wall and other subcellular structures of the fungus was determined. It turned out that acetamiprid accumulated in the spores (0.280 ± 0.05 µg per 10^6 of spores), while in cell fractions almost 6-fold more acetamiprid was detected in the cell wall (27.61 ± 3.75 µg per g of dry weight) than in the other subcellular structures (4.78 ± 0.65 µg per g of dry weight).

2.5. Influence of Acetamiprid, Spores of M. brunneum ARSEF2107 and the Combination of Spores and Acetamiprid on the Mortality of Tenebrio molitor (Mealworm)

Acetamiprid is used worldwide as an effective insect control agent. The dose of acetamiprid at used in these studies (5, 25 and 50 mg L^{-1}) caused mortality of *T. molitor* (Figure 5).

Additionally, the action of the neonicotinoid was compared to the killing properties of *M. brunneum* spores. The obtained results of acetamiprid accumulation in the fungal spores prompted us to determine what effect could be generated by the combination of *M. brunneum* spores with the accumulated acetamiprid and whether such a mixture could be an alternative to using the chemical insecticide alone. The results were surprising because a dose of 25 µg acetamiprid (50 mg L^{-1}) caused similar mealworm mortality resulting from a combination of spores with the insecticide accumulated in the amount of 140 ng, i.e., almost 180-fold less. The difference in LT_{50} was one day, and for the highest dose of acetamiprid this value was determined on the fifth day of testing, and for the combination of spores and insecticide on day six. Acetamiprid at the highest dose acted slightly faster, while at the end of the experiment it turned out that the highest mortality was achieved for the combined action of spores and acetamiprid. Similarly to chemical insecticides, entomopathogens do not kill insects immediately and their lethal effect is delayed even up to 14 days [13]. When a combination of spores and acetamiprid was used, an effect similar to that achieved by the insecticide applied alone was observed. This suggests that when using a combination of spores and acetamiprid, the mechanism of action of the insecticide is can be followed, but due to the accumulation of acetamiprid in the spores, the form of application of the toxic compound has been changed, and therefore, it could be used in a smaller amount than in a situation when it is applied as the only insect-killing agent.

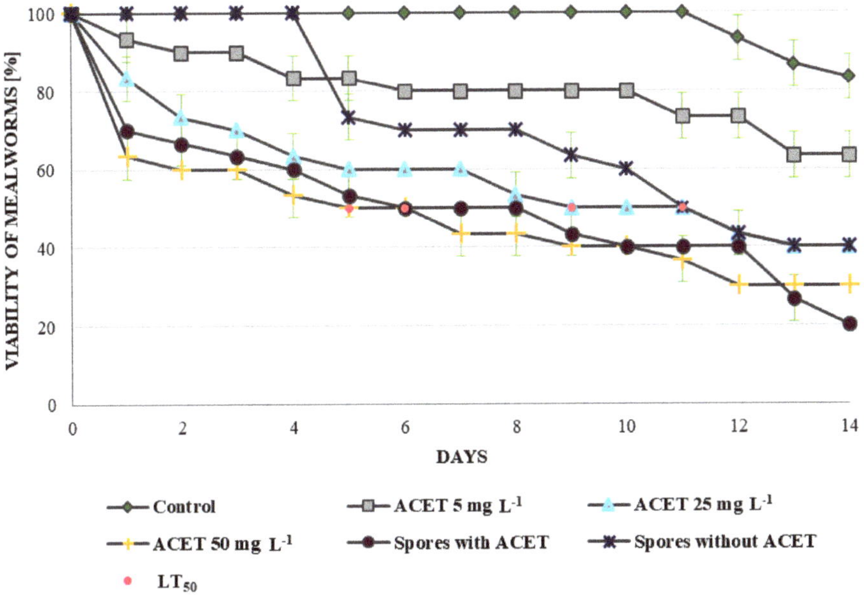

Figure 5. Viability of *Tenebrio molitor* mealworms treated with acetamiprid (ACET) at the concentrations of 5, 25 and 50 mg L^{-1}, with *Metarhizium brunneum* spores and a combination of spores and ACET. Statistical significance was assessed by standard deviations.

In the natural environment, acetamiprid can impair dtxs production, thereby affecting the functioning of *Metarhizium* sp. in their habitat and the fight for an ecological niche. Due to the increased infectivity of *Metarhizium* spores applied with acetamiprid, it is possible that not only pests, but also beneficial arthropod species may be exposed to this toxic action.

3. Conclusions

The study reveals that, although acetamiprid does not inhibit the growth of *Metarhizium* sp., it affects the metabolism of the fungus by decreasing its ability to produce dtxs. This phenomenon may have environmental implications because dtxs are produced not only during infection but can also be important for the survival of *Metarhizium* in soil. It has been proved for the first time that acetamiprid accumulates in fungi, not only in plant and animal tissues, which could have some ecological implications as well. However, in the case of *Metarhizium*, the most important finding is the fact that acetamiprid increases its infectivity as in the experiments the spores with the accumulated insecticide were shown to cause the highest mortality of the tested larvae. On the other hand, in the light of the results obtained, it cannot be conclusively stated that a decrease in the production of dtxs caused by acetamiprid does not disturb the infection process because acetamiprid is a strong insecticide whose combined action with *M. brunneum* was revealed to be the most effective in the mortality tests of *T. molitor*.

4. Materials and Methods

4.1. Chemicals and Reagents

All reagents and solvents were of analytical or liquid chromatography-mass spectrometry (LC–MS) grade and were purchased from Sigma-Aldrich (Steinheim, Germany) unless otherwise stated. Destruxin A (dtx A) from *M. anisopliae* and destruxin B (dtx B; Cayman Chemical, Ann Arbor, MI, USA) were used as chromatography standards. LC–MS grade water (Merck, Darmstadt, Germany) was used for chromatography. Fungi were cultivated on Czapek Dox broth (BD-Difco, Le Pont-de-Claix, France). Acetamiprid (99% purity) was added to the fungal cultures and was also used as a chromatography standard.

4.2. Microorganisms and Cultivation Conditions

Six fungal strains of the genus *Metarhizium* (*M. robertsii* IM6519, *M. robertsii* IM2358, *M. robertsii* ARSEF727, *M. anisopliae* ARSEF7487, *M. brunneum* ARSEF2107, *M. globosum* ARSEF2596) from the strains collection of the ARSEF (The Agricultural Research Service Collection of Entomopathogenic Fungal Cultures) and the Department of Industrial Microbiology and Biotechnology, University of Lodz (Poland), were used during the investigations. All strains were maintained on ZT agar slants(glucose (4 g L^{-1}); Difco yeast extract (4 g L^{-1}); agar (25 g L^{-1}); and malt extract (6 °Blg), up to 1 L; pH 7.0) as described previously [25–27]. Cultures for tests with *Metarhizium* spore suspension adjusted to 1×10^6 spores mL^{-1} were prepared on Czapek Dox liquid medium (total volume 40 mL in 100 mL Erlenmeyer flasks; BD-Difco, Le Pont-de-Claix, France). Acetamiprid stock dissolved in acetonitrile at the concentration of 50 mg mL^{-1} was added to fungal cultures to a final concentration of 5, 25 and 50 mg L^{-1}. Additionally, abiotic controls (without fungal biomass) and biotic controls (without acetamiprid) were prepared. All samples were incubated on a rotary shaker (120 rpm) at 28 °C for 7 days.

4.3. Destruxins Extraction by a Modified QuEChERS Method

After the incubation, the fungal cultures were filtrated through Whatman filter paper Number 1 (Sigma-Aldrich, Steinheim, Germany) to separate the culture media from the mycelia. The mycelia (for biomass estimation) were harvested and dried at 105 °C until a constant weight was obtained. The culture media were centrifuged for 5 min at 10,000 rpm, and subsequently, 20 mL was transferred to each 50 mL Falcon tube with 10 mL acetonitrile. After vigorous vortexing for 1 min, 3000 rpm, *QuEChERS* salts (4 g $MgSO_4$; 1 g NaCl; 1 g C_6H_5 $Na_3O_7{\cdot}2H_2O$; 0.5 g $C_6H_6Na_2O_7{\cdot}1.5\ H_2O$) were added and the tubes were again vortexed for 1 min. Afterwards, the tubes were centrifuged for 5 min at 8000 rpm. Eight milliliters of the upper layer was transferred to each 15 mL Falcon tube and evaporated to dryness under reduced pressure at 40 °C. After evaporation, the samples were dissolved in 5 mL LC–MS grade water (Merck, Darmstadt, Germany) and 4 mL of the extracts were cleaned on the Solid Phase Extraction Column with octadecyl sorbent C18. Subsequently, 5 mL of acetonitrile was added to rinse the metabolites bound on the sorbent, and next, 4 mL of the extract was transferred to each 15 mL Falcon tube and again evaporated to dryness as described above. After evaporation, the samples were dissolved in 2.5 mL of LC–MS grade water and 1 mL was subjected to LC–MS/MS.

4.4. Acetamiprid Extraction by a Modified QuEChERS Method

The mycelia were separated from Czapek Dox medium by filtration through Whatman filter paper Number 1 (Sigma-Aldrich, Steinheim, Germany). Then, 20 mL of deionized water and 10 mL of acetonitrile were added to each mycelium sample and ultrasonic extraction was done (2 min, Am 36%, pulse for 10 s). Then, 10 mL of acetonitrile was added to the culture medium in the volume 20 mL, and ultrasonic extraction was performed as mentioned above. The subsequent procedure was the same for both types of samples. The samples were transferred to each 50 mL Falcon tube and extracted with a Ball Mill (Retch MM400, Idar-Oberstein, Germany) for 5 min and at 25/s frequency.

After homogenization, *QuEChERS salts* were added and the tubes were vortexed 3000 rpm for 1 min. Subsequently, the extracts were centrifuged for 5 min at 5000 rpm. Then, 1 mL of the top layer was collected for the LC–MS/MS analysis.

4.5. Acetamiprid Extraction from M. brunneum Spores and Subcellular Fractions

To determine the acetamiprid concentration in spores, 7-day-old fungal cultures were filtered through the nylon net. The filtrates were centrifuged for 10 min at 10,000 rpm, and after supernatant removal, 20 mL of deionized water was added to the spores' pellet. The number of spores were counted in the Thoma cell counting chamber. Then, 10 mL of acetonitrile was added and the *QuEChERS* procedure was done as described above.

For acetamiprid presence in cell fractions, fungal cultures were centrifuged (10 min at 10,000 rpm), and after supernatant removal, the precipitate was washed twice with 20 mL of deionized water [28]. Then, the mycelium was suspended in 20 mL of deionized water and ultrasonic extraction was performed (2 min, Am 36%, pulse for 10 s). Mycelia disintegration was controlled by cell oscopic observations. After mycelia disruption, the samples were centrifuged for 10 min at 1200 rpm. The supernatant was separated from the precipitate with the cell wall fraction, then it was transferred into Eppendorf tubes and centrifuged for 20 min at 20,000 rpm at 4 °C. Obtained precipitates were suspended in 20 mL of deionized water, then 10 mL of acetonitrile was added and the *QuEChERS* extraction procedure was performed as described above. The cell wall fraction precipitate was washed twice in 20 mL of deionized water by centrifugation for 10 min at 1200 rpm. Then, it was suspended in 20 mL of deionized water, 10 mL of acetonitrile was added and the extraction procedure was followed as described above.

4.6. LC–MS/MS Quantitative and Qualitative Analyses of Destruxins

Quantitative and qualitative analyses of dtxs were carried out by using LC–MS/MS (LC Agilent 1200 coupled with a tandem mass spectrometer, AB Sciex QTRAP 4500, Framingham, MA, USA). The separation was performed with a Kinetex C18 column maintained at 40 °C. Water with 5 mM ammonium formate (AF, Solvent A) and methanol with 5 mM ammonium formate (Wolvent B) were used as mobile phases at a flow rate of 0.5 mL min^{-1}. The injection volume was 5 μL. The eluent gradient was conducted as follows: hold 90% A from 0 to 0.25 min, linear increase from 90% A to 90% B to 2 min, hold 90% B from 2 to 4 min, reverse to the initial conditions from 4 to 4.1 min, and maintained for column equilibration to 6.0 min.

The detection of dtxs was conducted using MS/MS with an electrospray ion source (ESI) in the positive ionization scheduled multiple reaction monitoring (sMRM) scan mode. The MRM detection window was set to 25 s. The optimized ESI parameters were as follows: CUR: 25; IS: 5000 V; TEMP: 500 °C; GS1: 50; GS2:50. MRM parameters of 19 dtxs are presented in Table S2 [29]. Dtxs were detected in the culture medium of each of the tested strains. The quantitative analyses of dtx A and dtx B were carried out using standard curves in the linearity range 2.5–100 ng mL^{-1} ($r = 0.9997$ and $r = 0.9999$, respectively). The levels of the other dtxs were determined based on chromatographic peak areas and compared between samples using principal component analysis (PCA).

4.7. LC–MS/MS Quantitative Analyses of Acetamiprid

Quantitative analyses of acetamiprid were carried out using LC–MS/MS (LC Agilent 1200 coupled with a tandem mass spectrometer, AB Sciex QTRAP 3200). The separation was performed with a Kinetex C18 column maintained at 40 °C. Water with 5 mM AF (solvent A) and acetonitrile with 5 mM AF and 0.1% formic acid (FA, Solvent B) were used as mobile phases at a flow rate of 0.5 mL min^{-1}. The injection volume was 10 μL. The eluent gradient was conducted as follows: hold 90% A from 0 to 0.25 min, linear increase from 90% A to 90% B to 0.5 min, hold 90% B from 0.5 to 4 min, reverse to initial conditions from 4 to 4.1 min, and maintained for column equilibration to 6.0 min.

The detection of acetamiprid was conducted using MS/MS with ESI in the positive ionization MRM scan mode (223.2/126.1 *m/z*; 223.2/73.0 *m/z*). The optimized ESI parameters were as follows: CUR: 25; IS: 5500 V; TEMP: 500 °C; GS1: 50; GS2:60. The quantitation curve of acetamiprid was accomplished in the quadratic regression in the range 25–1000 ng mL^{-1} and $r = 0.9999$.

4.8. Permeability of the Cell Membranes

The intention was to check whether acetamiprid simply interferes with the transport of dtxs from the fungal cell to the culture medium, or its action is connected with another mechanism. The procedure was performed according to the method described by Siewiera et al., 2015 [30] with some modifications. Briefly, 1 mL each of the control samples and the tested samples with acetamiprid concentrations of 5, 25 and 50 mg L^{-1} was transferred into Eppendorf tubes and then centrifuged for 10 min at 12,000 rpm. The supernatant was removed and 1 mL of Phosphate Buffered Saline (PBS) and 2 μL of propidium iodide (stock solution 0.1 mg mL^{-1}) were added to the precipitate and the mixture was vortexed for 30 s at 3000 rpm. After incubation in the dark for 5 min, the supernatant was removed. The mycelium was washed twice in PBS by centrifugation in the conditions described previously. Finally, the samples were suspended in 1 mL of PBS and propidium iodide fluorescence was measured at $\lambda_{ex} = 540$ and $\lambda_{em} = 630$ (FLUOstar Omega, BMG LABTECH, Ortenberg, Germany). The final results were presented as fluorescence intensity per mg of dry weight.

4.9. Mortality Test of Larvae of Tenebrio molitor (Mealworm)

Three concentrations of acetamiprid (5, 25 and 50 mg L^{-1}) and *Metarhizium* sp. spores (1×10^6 spores mL^{-1}) with and without accumulated acetamiprid were tested. Control samples without any stressful factors were also done. The effects of the individual variants were checked using 10 mealworms, kept in the dark in plastic boxes with holes in the lid, and the bottom was lined with tissue paper. Before starting the experiment, the larvae were fed with oat flakes, which eliminates the death of starvation. Insect vitality was assessed daily for 14 days.

4.10. Data Analysis

Fungal biomass estimation and quantitative analyses of acetamiprid were conducted in four repetitions, analyses of dtxs in six repetitions. Measurements of propidium iodide fluorescence were carried out in four repetitions. The mortality test of larvae of *T. molitor* was conducted in triplicates. Variabilities of samples were given as standard deviations (±SD). The one-way analysis of variance (ANOVA) and the posthoc Tukey test were used for investigations of statistical significance, using the concentrations of acetamiprid as a factor on transformed data. Scores at $p < 0.05$ were classified as significant. Statistica 13.1 (StatSoft, Tulsa, OK, USA) was used to analyze the data. The qualitative data of dtxs were submitted to PCA in orthogonal rotation and normalization using total area sums and Pareto scaling (Marker View Software 1.2.1., AB Sciex, Framingham, MA, USA).

5. Patents

Patent application No. P.434091 in the Patent Office of the Republic of Poland.

Supplementary Materials: The following are available online at http://www.mdpi.com/2072-6651/12/9/587/s1, Figure S1: Elimination of acetamiprid at the concentrations of 5 (A), 25 (B) and 50 mg L^{-1} (C) after 7 days of incubation by *Metarhizium* sp. considering the residual content in the culture medium and mycelium; Table S1: Effect of acetamiprid on the permeability of the *Metarhizium brunneum* ARSEF2107 fungal cell wall; Table S2: Multiple Reaction Monitoring (MRM) parameters for determining 19 types of destruxins.

Author Contributions: M.N.: Conceptualization, Investigation, Methodology, Writing—review and editing; J.M.: Investigation; P.B.: Methodology; S.R.: Investigation, Methodology, Funding acquisition, Writing—review and editing. All authors have read and agreed to the published version of the manuscript.

Funding: This work was supported by the National Science Center in Krakow (Poland), grant number UMO-2016/23/B/NZ9/00840.

Conflicts of Interest: The authors declare no conflict of interest.

References

1. Han, W.; Tian, Y.; Shen, X. Human exposure to neonicotinoid insecticides and the evaluation of their potential toxicity: An overview. *Chemosphere* **2018**, *192*, 59–65. [CrossRef]
2. Bass, C.; Denholm, I.; Williamson, M.S.; Nauen, R. The global status of insect resistance to neonicotinoid insecticides. *Pestic. Biochem. Physiol.* **2015**, *121*, 78–87. [CrossRef] [PubMed]
3. EFSA (European Food Safety Authority). Conclusion on the peer review of the pesticide risk assessment of the active substance acetamiprid. *EFSA J.* **2016**, *14*, 26. [CrossRef]
4. Xiong, J.; Wang, Z.; Ma, X.; Li, H.; You, J. Occurrence and risk of neonicotinoid insecticides in surface water in a rapidly developing region: Application of polar organic chemical integrative samplers. *Sci. Total Environ.* **2019**. [CrossRef] [PubMed]
5. Ihara, M. Neonicotinoids: Molecular mechanisms of action, insights into resistance and impact on pollinators. *Curr. Opin. Insect Sci.* **2018**, *30*, 86–92. [CrossRef] [PubMed]
6. Lovett, B.; St. Leger, R.J. Genetically engineering better fungal biopesticides. *Pest Manag. Sci.* **2018**, *74*, 781–789. [CrossRef]
7. Mondal, S.; Baksi, S.; Koris, A.; Vatai, G. Journey of enzymes in entomopathogenic fungi. *Pac. Sci. Rev. A Nat. Sci. Eng.* **2016**. [CrossRef]
8. Wang, B.; Kang, Q.; Lu, Y.; Bai, L.; Wang, C. Unveiling the biosynthetic puzzle of destruxins in Metarhizium species. *Proc. Natl. Acad. Sci. USA* **2012**, *109*, 1287–1292. [CrossRef]
9. Donzelli, B.G.G.; Krasnoff, S.B. Molecular Genetics of Secondary Chemistry in Metarhizium Fungi. *Adv. Genet.* **2016**. [CrossRef]
10. Pedras, M.S.C.; Irina Zaharia, L.I.; Ward, D.E. The destruxins: Synthesis, biosynthesis, biotransformation, and biological activity. *Phytochemistry* **2002**, *59*, 579–596. [CrossRef]
11. Wang, X.; Gong, X.; Li, P.; Lai, D.; Zhou, L.; Wang, X.; Gong, X.; Li, P.; Lai, D.; Zhou, L. Structural diversity and biological activities of cyclic depsipeptides from fungi. *Molecules* **2018**, *23*, 169. [CrossRef] [PubMed]
12. Liu, B.L.; Tzeng, Y.M. Development and applications of destruxins: A review. *Biotechnol. Adv.* **2012**, *30*, 1242–1254. [CrossRef] [PubMed]
13. Litwin, A.; Nowak, M.; Różalska, S. Entomopathogenic fungi: Unconventional applications. *Rev. Environ. Sci. Biotechnol.* **2020**, *19*, 23–42. [CrossRef]
14. Ríos-Moreno, A.; Garrido-Jurado, I.; Resquín-Romero, G.; Arroyo-Manzanares, N.; Arce, L.; Quesada-Moraga, E. Destruxin A production by *Metarhizium brunneum* strains during transient endophytic colonisation of *Solanum tuberosum*. *Biocontrol Sci. Technol.* **2016**, *26*, 1574–1585. [CrossRef]
15. Taibon, J.; Sturm, S.; Seger, C.; Strasser, H.; Stuppner, H. Quantitative assessment of destruxins from strawberry and maize in the lower parts per billion range: Combination of a QuEChERS-based extraction protocol with a fast and selective UHPLC-QTOF-MS assay. *J. Agric. Food Chem.* **2015**, *63*, 5707–5713. [CrossRef]
16. Neves, P.M.O.J.; Hirose, E.; Tchujo, P.T.; Moino, J.R.A. Compatibility of entomopathogenic fungi with neonicotinoid insecticides. *Neotrop. Entomol.* **2001**, *30*, 263–268. [CrossRef]
17. Li, Y.; Long, L.; Yan, H.; Ge, J.; Cheng, J.; Ren, L.; Yu, X. Comparison of uptake, translocation and accumulation of several neonicotinoids in komatsuna (*Brassica rapa* var. perviridis) from contaminated soils. *Chemosphere* **2018**, *200*, 603–611. [CrossRef] [PubMed]
18. De Laet, C.; Matringe, T.; Petit, E.; Grison, C. Eichhornia crassipes: A Powerful Bio-indicator for Water Pollution by Emerging Pollutants. *Sci. Rep.* **2019**, *9*, 7326. [CrossRef]
19. Barbieri, M.V.; Postigo, C.; Guillem-Argiles, N.; Monllor-Alcaraz, L.S.; Simionato, J.I.; Stella, E.; Barceló, D.; López de Alda, M. Analysis of 52 pesticides in fresh fish muscle by QuEChERS extraction followed by LC-MS/MS determination. *Sci. Total Environ.* **2019**, *653*, 958–967. [CrossRef]
20. Bartlett, A.J.; Hedges, A.M.; Intini, K.D.; Brown, L.R.; Maisonneuve, F.J.; Robinson, S.A.; Gillis, P.L.; de Solla, S.R. Acute and chronic toxicity of neonicotinoid and butenolide insecticides to the freshwater amphipod, Hyalella azteca. *Ecotoxicol. Environ. Saf.* **2019**, *175*, 215–223. [CrossRef]

21. Dong, T.; Zhang, B.; Weng, Q.; Hu, Q. The production relationship of destruxins and blastospores of Metarhizium anisopliae with virulence against Plutella xylostella. *J. Integr. Agric.* **2016**, *15*, 1313–1320. [CrossRef]
22. Ríos-Moreno, A.; Carpio, A.; Garrido-Jurado, I.; Arroyo-Manzanares, N.; Lozano-Tovar, M.D.; Arce, L.; Gámiz-Gracia, L.; García-Campaña, A.M.; Quesada-Moraga, E. Production of destruxins by *Metarhizium* strains under different stress conditions and their detection by using UHPLC-MS/MS. *Biocontrol Sci. Technol.* **2016**, *26*, 1298–1311. [CrossRef]
23. Ravindran, K.; Akutse, S.; Sivaramakrishnan, S.; Wang, L. Determination and characterization of destruxin production in Metarhizium anisopliae Tk6 and formulations for Aedes aegypti mosquitoes control at the field level. *Toxicon* **2016**. [CrossRef] [PubMed]
24. Bernat, P.; Nykiel-Szymańska, J.; Stolarek, P.; Słaba, M.; Szewczyk, R.; Ró, S. 2,4-dichlorophenoxyacetic acid-induced oxidative stress: Metabolome and membrane modifications in Umbelopsis isabellina, a herbicide degrader. *PLoS ONE* **2018**, *13*, e0199677. [CrossRef]
25. Różalska, S.; Pawłowska, J.; Wrzosek, M.; Tkaczuk, C.; Długoński, J. Utilization of 4-n-nonylphenol by Metarhizium sp. isolates. *Acta Biochim. Pol.* **2013**, *60*, 677–682. [CrossRef]
26. Rózalska, S.; Glińska, S.; Długoński, J. Metarhizium robertsii morphological flexibility during nonylphenol removal. *Int. Biodeterior. Biodegrad.* **2014**, *95*, 285–293. [CrossRef]
27. Nowak, M.; Soboń, A.; Litwin, A.; Różalska, S. 4-n-nonylphenol degradation by the genus Metarhizium with cytochrome P450 involvement. *Chemosphere* **2019**, *220*, 324–334. [CrossRef]
28. Słaba, M.; Szewczyk, R.; Bernat, P.; Długoński, J. Simultaneous toxic action of zinc and alachlor resulted in enhancement of zinc uptake by the filamentous fungus Paecilomyces marquandii. *Sci. Total Environ.* **2009**, *407*, 4127–4133. [CrossRef]
29. Arroyo-Manzanares, N.; Diana Di Mavungu, J.; Garrido-Jurado, I.; Arce, L.; Vanhaecke, L.; Quesada-Moraga, E.; De Saeger, S. Analytical strategy for determination of known and unknown destruxins using hybrid quadrupole-Orbitrap high-resolution mass spectrometry. *Anal. Bioanal. Chem.* **2017**, *409*, 3347–3357. [CrossRef]
30. Siewiera, P.; Bernat, P.; Rózalska, S.; Długoński, J. Estradiol improves tributyltin degradation by the filamentous fungus Metarhizium robertsii. *Int. Biodeterior. Biodegrad.* **2015**, *104*, 258–263. [CrossRef]

toxins

MDPI

Article

Interactions of Destruxin A with Silkworms' Arginine tRNA Synthetase and Lamin-C Proteins

Jingjing Wang, Qunfang Weng, Fei Yin and Qiongbo Hu *

Key Laboratory of Bio-Pesticide Innovation and Application of Guangdong Province; College of Agriculture, South China Agricultural University, Guangzhou 510642, China; wangjingjing@stu.scau.edu.cn (J.W.); wengweng@scau.edu.cn (Q.W.); yfei2020@stu.scau.edu.cn (F.Y.)

* Correspondence: hqbscau@scau.edu.cn

Received: 30 December 2019; Accepted: 21 February 2020; Published: 22 February 2020

Abstract: Destruxin A (DA), a cyclodepsipeptidic mycotoxin produced by entomopathogenic fungus *Metarhizium anisopliae*, has good insecticidal activity and potential to be a new pesticide. However, the mechanism of action is still obscure. Our previous experiments showed that DA was involved in regulation of transcription and protein synthesis and suggested that silkworms' arginine tRNA synthetase (BmArgRS), Lamin-C Proteins (BmLamin-C) and ATP-dependent RNA helicase PRP1 (BmPRP1) were candidates of DA-binding proteins. In this study, we employed bio-layer interferometry (BLI), circular dichroism (CD), cellular thermal shift assay (CETSA), and other technologies to verify the interaction of DA with above three proteins in vitro and in vivo. The results of BLI indicated that BmArgRS and BmLamin-C were binding-protein of DA with K_D value 5.53×10^{-5} and 8.64×10^{-5} M, but not BmPRP1. These interactions were also verified by CD and CETSA tests. In addition, docking model and mutants assay in vitro showed that BmArgRS interacts with DA at the pocket including Lys228, His231, Asp434 and Gln437 in its enzyme active catalysis region, while BmLamin-C binds to DA at His524 and Lys528 in the tail domain. This study might provide new insight and evidence in illustrating molecular mechanism of DA in breaking insect.

Keywords: Destruxins; *Bombyx mori*; BmArgRS; BmLamin-C; RNA helicase; binding protein

Key Contribution: BmArgRS and BmLamin-C are binding protein of Destruxin A in silkworm Bm12 cells. BmArgRS interacts with DA in its enzyme active catalysis region at Lys228, His231, Asp434 and Gln437. BmLamin-C binds to DA in its lamin tail domain at His524 and Lys528.

1. Introduction

Destruxin A (DA, Figure 1A) isolated from entomopathogenic fungus *Metarhizium anisopliae* is a cyclodepsipeptidic mycotoxin with insecticidal, antifeedant, and anti-immunity effects on host insects [1,2]. It is also reported that DA is a key pathogenic factor of *M. anisopliae* against insects [3]. DA is considered as a new potential pesticide to contract researchers interesting. For this, it is necessary to elucidate the targets of DA acting on insects. In the past decade, several studies indicated that DA changes the morphology of hemocytes and brings on equilibrium chaos of intra- and extra- cellular hydrogen and calcium ion in *Bombyx mori* [4,5], and regulates immune related gene expression [6,7]. Recently, a few DA binding-proteins in silkworm were found [8–10]. However, these results are not enough to explain the mechanisms of DA against insects.

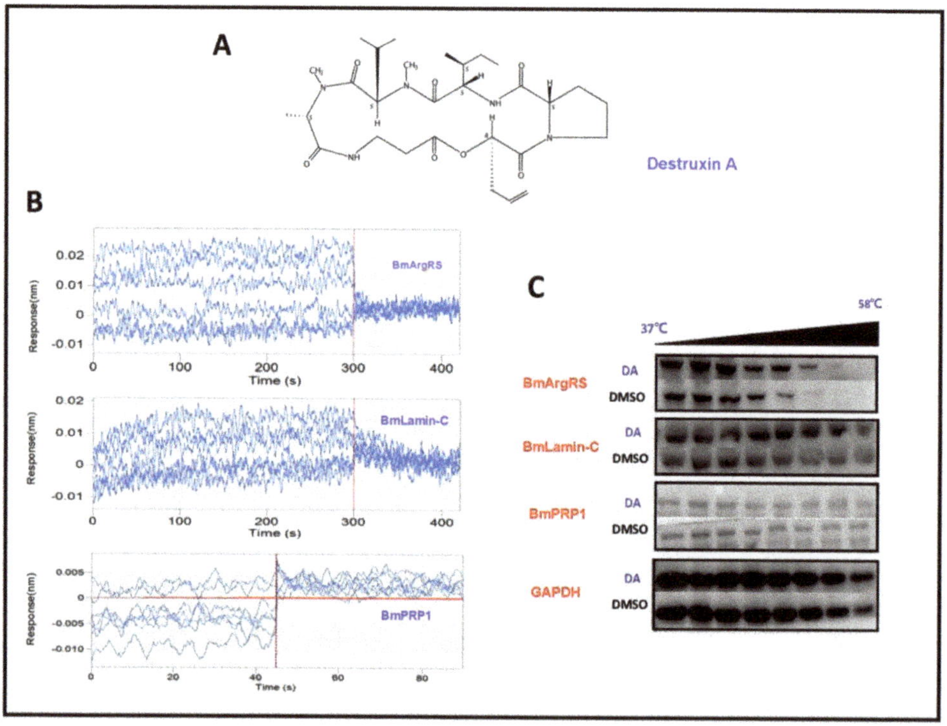

Figure 1. Profiles of interaction between Destruxin A (DA) with BmArgRS, BmLamin-C and BmPRP1 (**A**) The structure of Destruxin A. (**B**) BLI analysis showed the interactions of DA with BmArgRS and BmLamin-C but not BmPRP1 in vitro. (**C**) Cellular thermal shift assay (CETSA) results showed the interations of DA with BmArgRS and BmLamin-C in vivo.

To discover the DA target molecules, we conducted experiments based on drug affinity responsive target stability (DARTS) [11] in Bm12 cells; nuclear membranes protein Lamin-C (BmLamin-C), arginine tRNA synthetase (BmArgRS), and ATP-dependent RNA helicase PRP1 (BmPRP1) were detected. These three proteins have been studied thoroughly in human and model organisms to date. Summarily, Lamin-C belongs to nuclear intermediate filament proteins which provides mechanical stability, organizes chromatin and regulates transcription and other nuclear activities [12]. Moreover, recent studies have shown that Lamin-C plays role in development, tissue responsing to mechanical, reactive oxygen species, and thermal stresses [7]. ArgRS is significant in protein synthesis process, which provides arginine and maintaining fidelity in peptide chain extension [13,14]. While PRP1 has the functions of pre-mRNA-splicing and its fidelity of recognition [14,15]. However, these proteins have been rarely studied in *B. mori* and related biological pathways were never associated with DA target research before. In this study, we will validate the interaction of DA with these proteins in vivo and vitro. The results will provide new insights on better understanding for the DA-binding proteins.

2. Results

2.1. Interactions of Destruxin A with Three Proteins by BLI and CETSA Analysis

In order to evaluate whether BmLamin-C, BmArgRS and BmPRP1 proteins interact with DA, we conducted the experiments of bio-layer interferometry (BLI) in vitro and cellular thermal shift assay (CETSA) in vivo. In BLI assays, the results indicated that the responses of BmArgRS and BmLamin-C proteins were positively correlated with DA concentrations. There were affinity constant (K_D) values of

5.53×10^{-5} and 8.64×10^{-5} M respectively for DA with BmArgRS and BmLamin-C (Table 1, Figure 1B). However, the results showed that BmLamin-C is not a DA-binding protein, because a significant correlation between DA concentration and response of BmPRP1 was not detected. Meanwhile, the results of CETSA experiments exhibited that DA induced the thermal stability shift of BmArgRS and BmLamin-C but not BmPRP1 (Figure 1C), which suggested that the two proteins interact with DA in vivo. Obviously, both the BLI and CETSA experiments provided in vitro and in vivo evidences for that DA binds to BmArgRS and BmLamin-C but not BmPRP1.

Table 1. Detailed results of bio-layer interferometry (BLI) assay.

Proteins	DA Con. (μM)	Response (nm)	K_{on} (1/Ms) [1]	K_{dis} (1/s) [2]	K_D (M) [3]
BmArgRS	25	−0.0006	6.68×10^2	3.70×10^{-2}	5.53×10^{-5}
	200	0.0093			
	300	0.0192			
BmLamin-C	25	−0.0015	3.61×10^2	3.12×10^{-2}	8.64×10^{-5}
	200	0.008			
	300	0.0148			
BmPRP1	15.6	0.0107	/	/	/
	62.5	−0.0047			
	125	−0.0119			
	500	−0.0422			

[1] K_{on}: association rate constant; [2] K_{dis}: dissociation rate constant; [3] K_D: affinity constant.

2.2. Key Sites of Interaction of DA with BmArgRS and BmLamin-C

In the circular dichroism (CD) tests, the scanning results in 190–260 nm ultraviolet region indicated the CD shifts of DA-treated BmArgRS and BmLamin-C, which suggest that DA damages the α-helixes of the two proteins (Figure 2A). Meanwhile, in the 250–340 nm ultraviolet scanning, the protein CD changes caused by DA were found, which indicated that DA brings on the transformation of disulfide bonds and some side chains of BmArgRS and BmLamin-C (Figure 2A). These data provide the evidences for the interactions of DA with BmArgRS and BmLamin-C.

Furthermore, in analysis of homologue modeling (Figure 2B,C), DA interacts with BmArgRS and BmLamin-C with the scores −9.71 and −8.08 kcal/mol, respectively. The molecular docking predicted that there are many hydrogen bonds between DA and BmArgRS, which provide a pocket consisted of Lys228, His231, Gln437, Lys475, Val468, and Asp434 to DA binding (Figure 2D). However, there is only a hydrogen bond between DA and Lys528 in BmLamin-C (Figure 2E), although a pocket formed by His524, Thr526, Lys528, Glu530, Ser535, Ile552, and Met554 was predicted.

Based on the analysis above, each of amino acids of comprising hydrogen bond was mutated to alanine and the interactions of all mutant proteins with DA were investigated through BLI assay. Interestingly, in BmArgRS, 4 mutants, His231Ala, Lys228Ala, Asp434Ala, and Gln437Ala, displayed no interaction with DA (Figure 3). However, the interactions were still found in the mutants Val468Ala and Lys475Ala with DA, because the K_D values of 5.3×10^{-5} and 5.71×10^{-6} were respectively recorded, which were at same level compared with wild type (Figure 3). Those illustrated that DA binds to BmArgRS in the pocket including Lys228, His231, Asp434, and Gln437. Strikingly, the interaction site is just located in the conserved enzyme active catalysis domain of BmArgRS. Likewise, the His524Ala and Lys528Ala mutants of BmLamin-C exhibited no interactions with DA, which implied that Lamin tail domain is the DA-binding site (Figure 3).

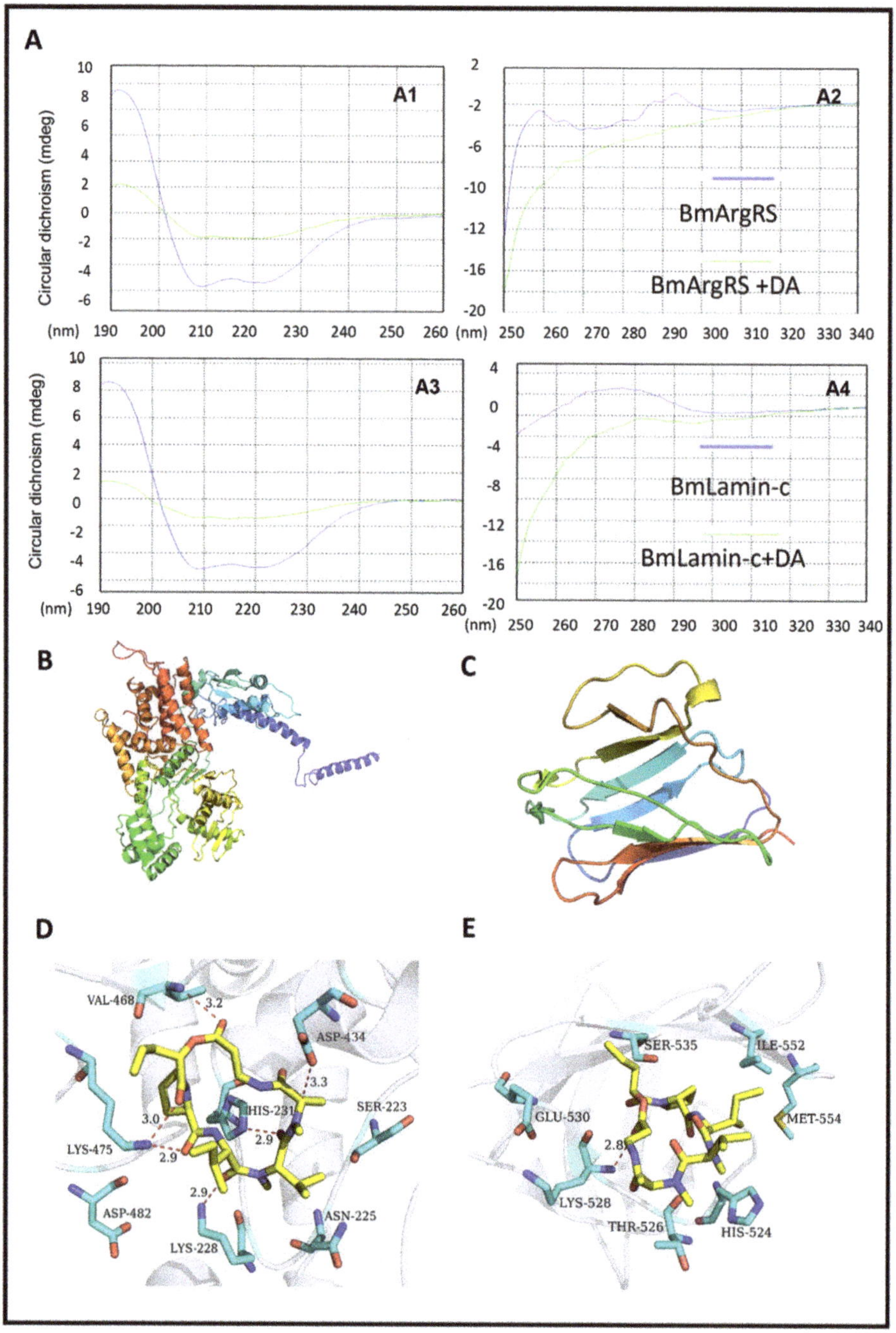

Figure 2. Structural evidences of interaction between DA with BmArgRS and BmLamin-C. (**A**) Profiles of circular dichroism tests indicating the effects of DA on proteins secondary structures. **A1**, **A2**, 190–260 nm and 250–340 nm ultraviolet region of BmArgRS interact with DA respectively. **A3**, **A4**, 190–260 nm and 250–340 nm ultraviolet region of BmLamin-C interact with DA respectively. (**B**,**C**) Homologous modeling of BmArgRS and BmLamin-C respectively. (**D**,**E**) Binding pose of DA with BmArgRS and BmLamin-C respectively.

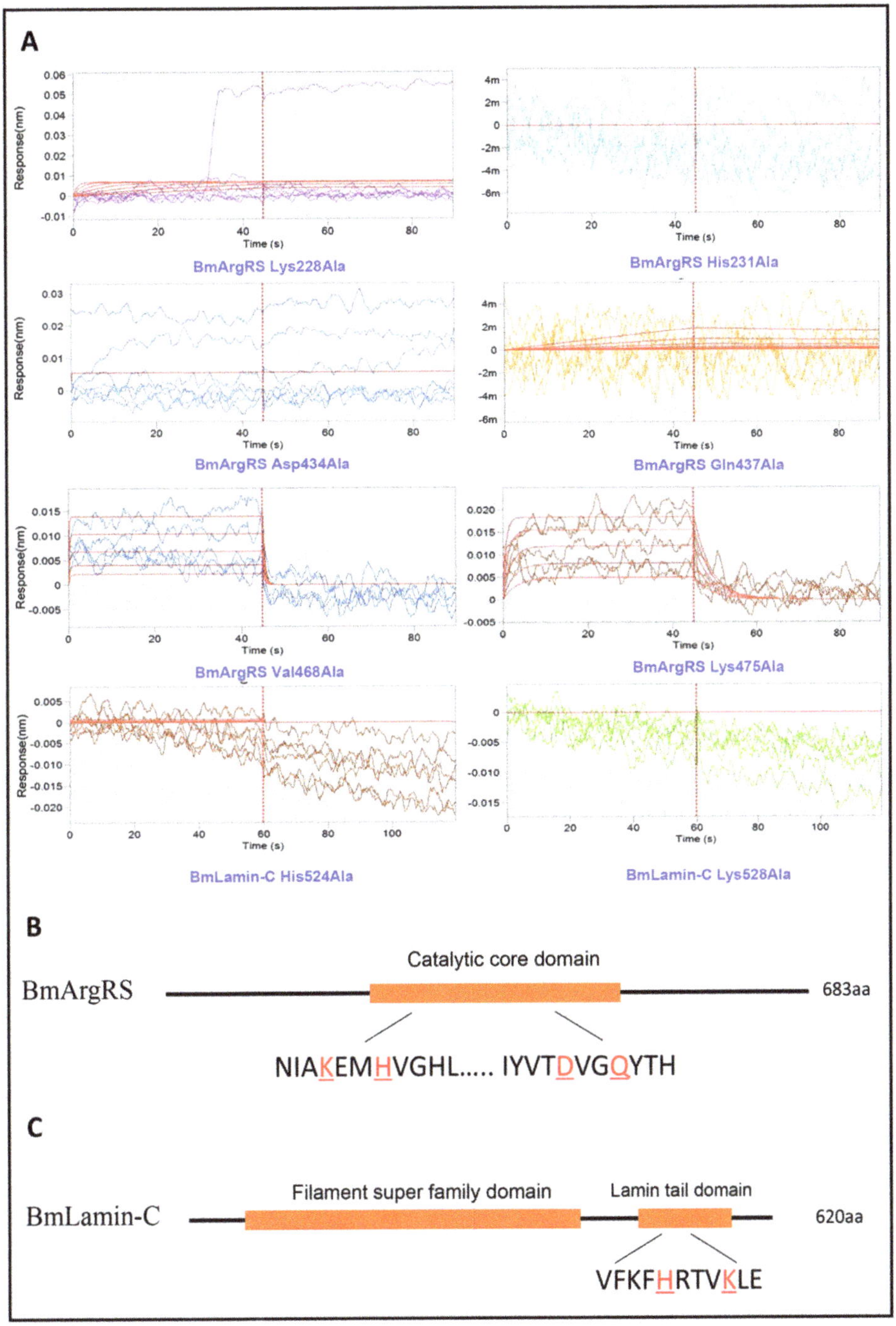

Figure 3. Key amino acid sites for interaction of DA with BmArgRS and BmLamin-C by BLI tests. (**A**) The interactions of DA with the mutants of BmArgRS and BmLamin-C. (**B**,**C**) Sketch of the domains of BmArgRS and BmLamin-C and key amino acid sites for DA binding.

2.3. Gene Expression Levels of Three Proteins in Bm12 Cells

We investigated DA dosage- and time-depend affecting expression three genes in Bm12 cells. The results indicated that there were no obvious relations between genes expression levels of three proteins in DA dosage- and time-depend manner. Totally, these genes had up-regulation of <2 folds, only BmArgRS was up-regulated by 3-fold in relative high dosage 200 μg/mL at 6 h post-treatment (Figure 4A). It is suggested that DA only leads to mild changes in gene expression levels of the three proteins.

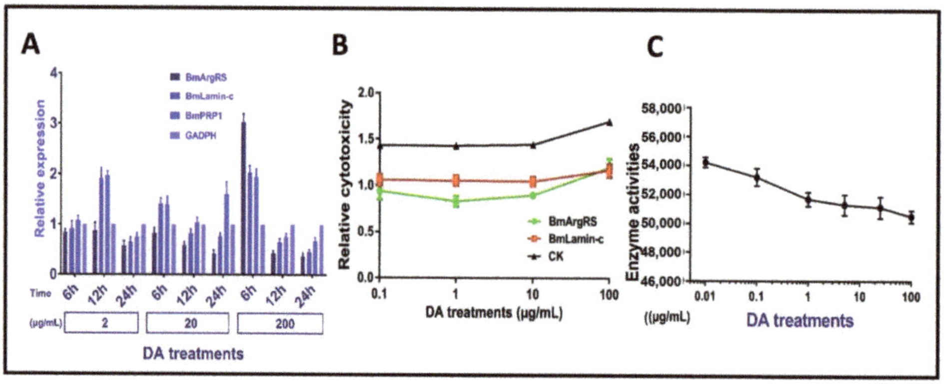

Figure 4. Effects of DA on BmArgRS and BmLamin-C of Bm12 cell. (**A**) Analysis of gene expression under DA stress by qPCR test. (**B**) Cytotoxicity of DA against Bm12 cells by RNAi treatments. (**C**) Enzyme activity of BmArgRS inhibited by DA.

2.4. Changes of DA Cytotoxicity and BmArgRS Enzyme Activity in Bm12 Cells

The results indicated that the toxicities of DA against Bm12 cells were decreased by more than 50% after the genes of *BmArgRS* and *BmLamin-C* were knocked down (Figure 4B). In addition, the enzyme activity of BmArgRS was decreased under DA exposure, because a negative correlation between enzyme activity and DA dosage was found (Figure 4C). This might explain that DA binds to enzyme active center of BmArgRS so as to inhibit its catalytic function.

3. Discussion

For research of small molecular drugs, it is of great importance to elucidate the target protein in special cells or tissues. In this study, we conducted the experiments of BLI, CETSA, qPCR, RNAi, and enzyme activity, as well as modeling and docking analysis. As results, we carefully validated that BmArgRS and BmLamin-C are the DA-binding proteins and elucidated their interaction modes. Obviously, it is significant for further developments of DA-like drugs and researches of target proteins. However, BmPRP1 was not DA-binding protein. In fact, similar to other RNA helicases, BmPRP1 was an important component of constitution of stress granules (SGs) under stimuli [16], while SGs, composed of mRNA and ribosomal subunit, expression initial factor and RNA-binding proteins, appear in cellular stress conditions such as hypoxia, oxidative stress, and virus infection so as to stall translation and expression for energy saving [17]. Interestingly, in our previous study, we found a DA-binding protein (BmTudor-sn) was also component of SGs [8]. In addition, there is a report showed that destruxin can induce oxidative stress in insect [18]. Therefore, it is more likely that DA injures cells in sorts of unknown mechanism to trigger mRNA translation and protein synthesis of related SGs components such as BmPRP1. It probably leads to a false-positivity of BmPRP1 in DARTS experiments.

Aminoacyl tRNA synthetases play an important role in protein synthesis and are usually considered as medicine targets [19–21]; among them, ArgRS is involved in the formation of arginyl-tRNA^{Arg} complex in peptide chain extension [22]. Sequence analysis indicates that BmArgRS contains a catalytic core domain of arginyl-tRNA synthetases in the region of 216–481. Interestingly, in this study, we proved that DA binds to a pocket of BmArgRS in the conserved active catalysis sites. It might be speculated that DA suppresses the synthesis of some proteins containing arginine, especially the arginine rich basic proteins (histone), subsequently causes and leads to cells chaos in insects. Our research results give some clues to development of ArgRS inhibitors. Although DA interacts with BmArgRS at lower level as 10^{-5} M, more other chemicals with higher bioactivity can be found on the basis of the quantitative structure-activity relationship (QSAR) of molecules and BmArgRS.

Lamins-C has many functions which usually acts as intermediate filament proteins providing stability and strength to cells, as supporting (scaffolding) components of the nuclear envelope regulating the movement of molecules into and out of the nucleus, and as a role in regulating the activity (expression) of certain genes [12]. Previously, researchers found out that DA showed no affinity to nucleus, but was abundant in cytosol [23]. As above indicated, nonpolar DA might access into nucleus at inner membrane to bind BmLamin-C but does not result in mechanical stress. In cytoplasm, lamins mainly function as response to eliminate heat shock and oxidative stress [7]. Interestingly, DA induced heat shock proteins upregulation and oxidative stress in cells. It is suggested that DA binds to BmLamin-C leading to maintain unsuitable environment in cells which constant to previous study that DA acts as immunosuppressor [2]. Intriguingly, C-terminal lamin tail domain is highly conserved and contains immunoglobulin fold. However, researches of Lamin-C were insufficient in *B. mori*, so it is hard to in-depth study in function with DA and make an assumption. But it provides new evidences and insight to further study owing to several nuclear related candidate proteins we have.

Reviewed in previous research on molecular mechanism of DA, the widely accepted hypothesis is that DA acts as immunosuppressor to inhibit innate immune system when *M. anisopliae* infected host. However, traditional molecular mechanism of DA target sites such as hemocyte and hemolymph are obscure. Here, we can speculate that DA stresses and leads to cell in uncomfortable environment and the meantime DA binds to those stress induced proteins to repress host defense as an immunosuppressor. Because we previously found that DA bond to heat shock protein [10], stress granule protein BmTudor-sn [8] and immunophilin peptidyl-prolylcis-transisomerase (BmPPI) [9], and interacted with BmArgRS to inhibit protein synthesis and bond to stress support protein BmLamin-C as well in this study.

In conclusion, we investigated the interaction between DA and three candidate proteins, and found that BmArgRS and BmLamin-C are DA-binding proteins but not BmPRP1. In addition, structurally, DA interacts with BmArgRS at Lys228, His231, Gln437 and Lys475 in catalysis active domain and with BmLamin-C at Lys528 and His524 in lamin tail domain. The above findings would offer new insight and evidence to DA target protein discovery.

4. Materials and Methods

4.1. Cell Culture and Destruxin A

The *Bombyx mori* Bm12 cell line was donated by our colleague Cao Yang (College of Animal Science, South China Agricultural University) and cultured in Grace's culture medium (Hyclone, Pittsburgh, MA, USA) and 10% fetal bovine serum (Gibco, Waltham, MA, USA). Cells were cultured at 27 °C and maintained at over a period of 2–4 days.

Destruxin A (DA) was isolated and purified from the *Metarhizium anisopliae* var. *anisopliae* strain MaQ10 in our laboratory [24]. Stock solution is 10,000 μg/mL in dimethyl sulfoxide (DMSO, Sigma-Aldrich, Darmstadt, Germany).

4.2. Bio-Layer Interferometry (BLI)

All proteins were prepared by expression in *E. coli*, and were tagged with His-tag and purified by nickel affinity chromatography. Protein accession number of BmArgRS, BmLamin-C, and BmPRP1 are XP_004931696.1, XP_004930078.1, and XP_004926349.1, respectively.

BLI analysis was performed on a ForteBio OctetQK System (K2, Pall Fortebio Corp, Menlo Park, CA, USA) [25]. Generally, the protein samples were coupled with a biosensor for immobilization. Dilutions of DA were used for treatment. PBST buffer (0.05% Tween20, 5% DMSO) was used for the running and dilution buffers. The working procedure was baseline for 60 s, association for 60 s, and dissociation for 60 s. Finally, the raw data were processed with Data Analysis Software (9.0, Pall ForteBio Corp, Menlo Park, CA, USA).

4.3. *Cellular Thermal Shift Assay (CETSA)*

The Bm12 cell line was used to conduct the CETSA experiments [26]. Firstly, Bm12 cells were treated with 100 μg/mL DA and divided into 8–10 aliquots. After heated at 37–58 °C at 3 min, cells were lysed by a freeze-thawcycle. After centrifugated, the supernatants of the lysed cells were used for the western blot analysis.

4.4. *RNAi and Toxicity Assessment RNAi*

SiRNAs were prepared by synthesis in vitro. The sequence of BmLamin-C siRNA: 5′-GCUGAUACCCGUAAGACUUTT-3′ and 5′-AAGUCUUACGGGUAUCAGCTT-3′. The sequence of BmArgRS: 5′-GCGAUCAAGAAGGAAGCUATT-3′ and 5′-UAGCUUCCUUCUUGAUCGCTT-3′. SiRNA and FuGENE (Promega, Beijing, China) transfection reagent were each diluted in serum-free medium and then mixed. The mixture was added to Bm12 cells and DA treatments. Toxicity assessment was performed by LDH-Glo™ Cytotoxicity Assay (Promega, Beijing, China) and detected in Synergy™ H1 (BioTek, Winooski, VT, USA).

4.5. *Survey of Gene Expression*

Expression of target gene was measured by RT-qPCR. Primer of BmLamin-C: 5′-CTTCACCACGGCTCTGCTCAAC-3′ and 5′- TGCGGCAATTCTCTTCACCTTCG-3′. Primer of BmArgRS: 5′-GAGGTTAGAAGAGCGAACCACCAG-3′ and 5′-CGCCGCTGAAGATTCGGTCTC-3′. Primer of BmPRP1: 5′-GGTGCTGTGATGGCGGAGTTC-3′ and 5′-GCATGGCAGTGATGGAGAGGATC-3′. The qPCR reactive program was subjected to 39 cycles at 95 °C for 10 s, 60 °C for 10 s, 72 °C for 30 s, then 95 °C for 10 s, and 65–95 °C for 5 s. The experiment was repeated three times. The silkworm GAPDH (glyceraldehyde-3-phosphate dehydrogenase) gene was taken as the reference gene. The qPCR data were analyzed by using the $2^{-\Delta\Delta Ct}$ method. The means and DMRT (Duncan multiple range test) were evaluated by employing SPSS software (IBM, Armonk, NY, USA).

4.6. *Homology Modeling and Molecular Docking*

The target sequence of BmArgRS and BmLamin-C were acquired from Uniprot, with the Uniprot ID H9JHD3 and H9J2B5. Template crystal structures of RARS and LAMC were identified through BLAST and downloaded from RCSB Protein Data Bank (PDB ID were 4R3Z1 and 6GHD2). Homology modeling and docking were conducted in MOE v2014.09014 (Chemical Computing Group, Montreal, Canada).

4.7. *Circular Dichroism Spectrum*

Circular dichroism (CD) experiments were conducted by Chirascan Plus V100 (Leatherhead, Surrey, United Kingdom) provided by Applied Photophysics Ltd. Analysis processing in 1.0 nm band width. Measurement range include 190~260 nm (far-UV region scan) and 250–340 nm (near-UV region scan). The test was repeated three times. All raw scanning data were processed in Pro-Data Viewer (Applied Photophysics, Leatherhead, Surrey, United Kingdom) with subtract baseline and smoothing analysis.

Author Contributions: Conceived the experiments and revised the manuscript, Q.H.; Performed the experiments, analyzed the data, and wrote the paper, J.W.; Analyzed the data, Q.W. and F.Y. All authors have read and agreed to the published version of the manuscript.

Funding: This research is supported by National Natural Science Foundation of China (U1901205).

Conflicts of Interest: The authors declare no conflict of interest.

References

1. Pedras, M.S.C.; Zaharia, L.I.; Ward, D.E. The destruxins: Synthesis, biosynthesis, biotransformation, and biological activity. *Phytochemistry* **2002**, *59*, 579–596. [CrossRef]
2. Liu, B.; Tzeng, Y. Development and applications of destruxins: A review. *Biotechnol. Adv.* **2012**, *30*, 1242–1254. [CrossRef] [PubMed]
3. Wang, B.; Kang, Q.; Lu, Y.; Bai, L.; Wang, C. Unveiling the biosynthetic puzzle of destruxins in Metarhizium species. *Proc. Nat. Acad. Sci. USA* **2012**, *109*, 1287–1292. [CrossRef] [PubMed]
4. Fan, J.Q.; Chen, X.R.; Hu, Q.-B. Effects of Destruxin A on Hemocytes Morphology of Bombyx mori. *J. Integr. Agric.* **2013**, *12*, 1042–1048. [CrossRef]
5. Chen, X.; Hu, Q.; Yu, X.; Ren, S. Effects of destruxins on free calcium and hydrogen ions in insect hemocytes. *Insect Sci.* **2014**, *21*, 31–38. [CrossRef] [PubMed]
6. Hu, W.; He, G.; Wang, J.; Hu, Q. The Effects of Destruxin A on Relish and Rel Gene Regulation to the Suspected Immune-Related Genes of Silkworm. *Molecules* **2016**, *22*, 41. [CrossRef]
7. Zuela, N.; Bar, D.Z.; Gruenbaum, Y. Lamins in development, tissue maintenance and stress. *EMBO Rep.* **2012**, *13*, 1070–1078. [CrossRef]
8. Wang, J.; Hu, W.; Hu, Q. BmTudor-sn Is a Binding Protein of Destruxin A in Silkworm Bm12 Cells. *Toxins* **2019**, *11*, 67. [CrossRef]
9. Wang, J.; Wen, Q.; Hu, Q. Effects of Destruxin A on Silkworm's Immunophilins. *Toxins* **2019**, *11*, 349. [CrossRef]
10. Zhang, H.; Hu, W.; Xiao, M.; Ou, S.; Hu, Q. Destruxin A induces and binds HSPs in Bombyx mori Bm12 cells. *J. Agric. Food Chem.* **2017**, *65*, 9849–9853. [CrossRef]
11. Lomenick, B.; Hao, R.; Jonai, N.; Chin, R.M.; Aghajan, M.; Warburton, S.; Wang, J.; Wu, R.P.; Gomez, F.; Loo, J.A. Target identification using drug affinity responsive target stability (DARTS). *Proc. Natl. Acad. Sci. USA* **2009**, *106*, 21984–21989. [CrossRef] [PubMed]
12. Al-Saaidi, R.; Peter, B. Do lamin A and lamin C have unique roles? *Chromosoma* **2015**, *124*, 1–12. [CrossRef] [PubMed]
13. Bence, A.K.; Crooks, P.A. The mechanism of L-canavanine cytotoxicity: Arginyl tRNA synthetase as a novel target for anticancer drug discovery. *J. Enzym. Inhib. Med. Chem.* **2003**, *18*, 383. [CrossRef] [PubMed]
14. Sloan, K.E.; Bohnsack, M.T. Unravelling the Mechanisms of RNA Helicase Regulation. *Trends Biochem. Sci.* **2018**, *43*, 237–250. [CrossRef] [PubMed]
15. Jankowsky, E. RNA helicases at work: Binding and rearranging. *Trends Biochem. Sci.* **2011**, *36*, 19–29. [CrossRef] [PubMed]
16. Xu, F. RNA Helicases and Stress Granules. *Chin. J. Biochem. Mol. Biol.* **2014**, *30*, 630–635.
17. Ivanov, P.; Kedersha, N.; Anderson, P. Stress Granules and Processing Bodies in Translational Control. *Cold Spring Harb. Perspect. Biol.* **2018**, *11*, a032813. [CrossRef]
18. Sree, K.S.; Padmaja, V. Destruxin from Metarhizium anisopliae induces oxidative stress effecting larval mortality of the polyphagous pest Spodoptera litura. *J. Appl. Entomol.* **2010**, *132*, 68–78. [CrossRef]
19. Chhibber-Goel, J.; Joshi, S.; Sharma, A. Aminoacyl tRNA synthetases as potential drug targets of the Panthera pathogen Babesia. *Parasit Vectors* **2019**, *12*, 482. [CrossRef]
20. Kim, E.Y.; Lee, J.G.; Lee, J.M.; Kim, A.; Yoo, H.C.; Kim, K.; Lee, M.; Lee, C.; P., N.; Han, G.; et al. Therapeutic effects of the novel Leucyl-tRNA synthetase inhibitor BC-LI-0186 in non-small cell lung cancer. *Ther. Adv. Med Oncol.* **2019**, *11*. [CrossRef]
21. Buckner, F.S.; Ranade, R.M.; Gillespie, J.R.; Shibata, S.; Hulverson, M.A.; Zhang, Z.; Huang, W.; Choi, R.; Ochida, A.; Akao, Y.; et al. Optimization of Methionyl tRNA-Synthetase Inhibitors for Treatment of Cryptosporidium Infection. *Antimicrob. Agents Chemother.* **2019**, *63*. [CrossRef]

22. Won, L.S.; Byeong Hoon, C.; Gyu, P.S.; Sunghoon, K. Aminoacyl-tRNA synthetase complexes: Beyond translation. *J. Cell Sci.* **2004**, *117*, 3725–3734.
23. Vey, A.; Dumas, C. Mechanism of action of insecticidal mycotoxins of the group of destruxins. *Toxicon* **1996**, *34*, 1096. [CrossRef]
24. Hu, Q.B.; Ren, S.X.; Wu, J.H.; Chang, J.M.; Musa, P.D. Investigation of destruxin A and B from 80 Metarhizium strains in China, and the optimization of cultural conditions for the strain MaQ10. *Toxicon* **2006**, *48*, 491–498. [CrossRef] [PubMed]
25. Abdiche, Y.; Dan, M.; Pinkerton, A.; Pons, J. Determining kinetics and affinities of protein interactions using a parallel real-time label-free biosensor, the Octet. *Anal. Biochem.* **2008**, *377*, 209–217. [CrossRef] [PubMed]
26. Martinez Molina, D.; Jafari, R.; Ignatushchenko, M.; Seki, T.; Larsson, E.A.; Dan, C.; Sreekumar, L.; Cao, Y.; Nordlund, P. Monitoring drug target engagement in cells and tissues using the cellular thermal shift assay. *Science* **2013**, *341*, 84–87. [CrossRef] [PubMed]

toxins

Review

Recent Advances on Macrocyclic Trichothecenes, Their Bioactivities and Biosynthetic Pathway

Muzi Zhu, Youfei Cen, Wei Ye, Saini Li and Weimin Zhang *

Guangdong Provincial Key Laboratory of Microbial Culture Collection and Application, State Key Laboratory of Applied Microbiology Southern China, Guangdong Institute of Microbiology, Guangdong Academy of Sciences, Guangzhou 510070, China; zhumz@gdim.cn (M.Z.); cenyoufei@163.com (Y.C.); yewei@gdim.cn (W.Y.); lisn@gdim.cn (S.L.)

* Correspondence: wmzhang@gdim.cn; Tel.: +86-20-8768-8309

Received: 23 May 2020; Accepted: 19 June 2020; Published: 23 June 2020

Abstract: Macrocyclic trichothecenes are an important group of trichothecenes bearing a large ring. Despite the fact that many of trichothecenes are of concern in agriculture, food contamination, health care and building protection, the macrocyclic ones are becoming the research hotspot because of their diversity in structure and biologic activity. Several researchers have declared that macrocyclic trichothecenes have great potential to be developed as antitumor agents, due to the plenty of their compounds and bioactivities. In this review we summarize the newly discovered macrocyclic trichothecenes and their bioactivities over the last decade, as well as identifications of genes *tri17* and *tri18* involved in the trichothecene biosynthesis and putative biosynthetic pathway. According to the search results in database and phylogenetic trees generated in the review, the species of the genera *Podostroma* and *Monosporascus* would probably be great sources for producing macrocyclic trichothecenes. Moreover, we propose that the macrocyclic trichothecene roridin E could be formed via acylation or esterification of the long side chain linked with C-4 to the hydroxyl group at C-15, and vice versa. More assays and evidences are needed to support this hypothesis, which would promote the verification of the proposed pathway.

Keywords: macrocyclic trichothecenes; bioactivities; putative biosynthetic pathway; macrocycle formation

Key Contribution: A new supposed biosynthetic pathway of macrocyclic trichothecene was proposed.

1. Introduction

Trichothecenes are a family of sesquiterpenoid mycotoxins produced by multiple genera of fungi, including plant and insect pathogens, and they are of great concern because they are toxic to animals and humans and frequently detected in cereal crops, especially in wheat, barley, maize and oats [1–4]. In the European Union, 57% of the collected food samples have been contaminated with deoxynivalenol (DON) [5], and a high proportion of UK oats were believed to contain high concentrations of the trichothecenes T-2 and HT-2 according to a survey of commercial crops [6]. These toxins consist of over 200 structurally distinct molecules, all of which are characterized by a three-ring molecule known as 12,13-epoxytrichothec-9-ene (EPT; Figure 1) [7,8]. One obvious structural variation can divide trichothecenes into two groups: the simple trichothecenes and the macrocyclic ones (also called Type D trichothecenes, Figure 1) [9,10]. The macrocyclic trichothecenes possess an additional ring at C-4 and C-15 of EPT, formed by esterification of the hydroxyls at relevant positions with a 12- or 14-carbon chain. On the contrary, the simple trichothecenes in the other group do not have a macrolide ring.

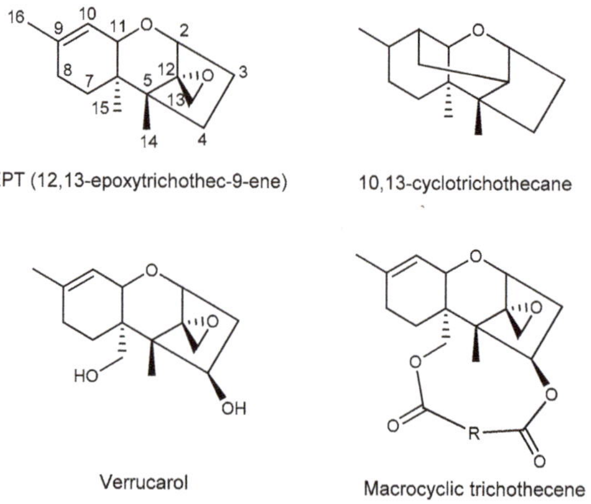

Figure 1. The tricyclic skeleton of trichothecene and macrocyclic trichothecene structure.

The biochemistry, bioactivity and biosynthesis of simple trichothecenes have been studied extensively [11,12]. In *Fusarium*, the biosynthetic pathway of the representative trichothecenes, e.g., DON, nivalenol and T-2 toxin, have been fully elucidated [11–13]. All trichothecenes share the same starting unit, initiated by cyclization of the primary metabolite farnesyl diphosphate to form trichodiene, which was catalyzed by the terpene cyclase trichodiene synthase (Tri5). Subsequently, trichodiene undergoes a series of oxygenations (Tri1, Tri4, Tri11 or Tri13), acylations (Tri3, Tri7, Tri16 or Tri101) and sometimes other modifications to create the simple trichothecene analogs [10,12]. Most genes responsible for these catalytic processes have been identified individually, and they are often located next to one another in the trichothecene biosynthetic gene (*TRI*) cluster [14–17]. However, the same gene homologs from different genera sometimes have diverse functions [10,18]. For instance, in *Myrothecium* sp. and *Trichoderma* sp., the *tri4*-encoded cytochrome P450 monooxygenase catalyzes oxygenation of trichodiene at three carbons (C-2, C-11, and C-13), but Tri4 of *Fusarium* catalyzes four carbons of trichodiene (combined with C-3) [19–21]. Proctor et al. declared that the ability of Tri4 to catalyze three oxygenations is more ancestral than the ability to catalyze four reactions [10]. Likewise, Tri8 exhibits two mutually exclusive deacetylation at C-3 or C-15 among different *Fusarium* species [22–24]. The numbers and arrangement of *TRI* genes per cluster also vary in different fungi [10,18,25]. The *TRI* cluster of *Fusarium sporotrichioides* contains 12 genes related to trichothecene biosynthesis, but the cluster of *Trichoderma arundinaceum* just contains 5 genes [10]. The other biosynthetic genes of *T. arundinaceum*, e.g., *tri5* initiating biosynthesis of trichothecene, are located in other loci [18]. In *Myrothecium* and *Stachybotrys* species, the *TRI* genes at other loci were paralogs of genes in the main cluster [10].

The genetic bases for most simple trichothecenes have been elucidated by functional analyses of *TRI* genes; however, the genetic bases for macrocyclic trichothecenes, namely Type D trichothecenes, are not completely elucidated, especially about the formation of the macrocycle, which is composed of polyketide- and isoprenoid-derived moieties [9,26,27]. Genes *tri17* and *tri18* were presumed to be involved in macrocycle formation [7,26]. The objective of this review is to summarize the latest developments on macrocyclic trichothecenes, including newly discovered compounds, bioactivities, hypothetic functions of *tri17* and *tri18*, and putative biosynthetic pathway. This review provides a new insight into the biosynthetic mechanism of macrocycle in macrocyclic trichothecene.

2. Macrocyclic Trichothecenes and the Producing Strains

Trichothecenes can be isolated from many fungal genera, such as *Fusarium*, *Isaria*, *Microcyclospora*, *Myrothecium*, *Peltaster*, *Spicellum*, *Stachybotrys*, *Trichoderma*, *Trichothecium*, *Cephalosporium*, *Cylindrocarpon*,

Memnoniella, *Phomopsis*, *Verticimonosporium* etc. [7,10,28]. Macrocyclic trichothecenes are produced by the genera *Myrothecium* [29–31], *Podostroma* [32], *Stachybotrys* [33], *Calcarisporium* [34], *Cercophora* [35], *Cylindrocarpon* [36], *Dendrodochium* [37], *Phomopsis* [38], and *Verticinimonosporium* [39]. It is worth noting that *Baccharis*, belonging to the *Asteraceae* family, is the only plant genus that can produce trichothecenes [40]. The macrocyclic trichothecenes can be further classified as verrucarins (mainly C27 compounds), or roridins and satratoxins (mainly C29 compounds) according to the carbon number of side chain [28,41,42]. The side chain with 12- or 14-carbon atoms was esterified to the tricyclic skeleton via hydroxyl groups at C-4 and C-15 of EPT [10].

New macrocyclic trichothecenes are constantly being discovered. Here, the novel macrocyclic trichothecenes isolated over the past decade are reviewed. There were 23 compounds related to macrocyclic trichothecene newly discovered between 2010 and 2019, and most of them were isolated from *Myrothecium* (Table 1; Figure 2). Only three compounds were isolated from *Podostroma*, and one from *Stachybotrys* (Figure 3). Four compounds belong to verrucarin-like trichothecenes (**1**, **2**, **11**, **18**), and the others with a side chain of 14-carbon atoms could be recognized as roridins or satratoxins. It was reported that roridin may be the precursor of the respective verrucarin, because the C_2-side chain at C-6′ of roridin might be cleaved by oxidation to form verrucarin [41,43]. Compounds **1–11** and **23** have a standard tricyclic core, namely EPT; however, compounds **12–20** lack the epoxide at C-12, C-13. Verrucarin Y (**1**) and verrucarin Z (**2**) were isolated from *M. roridum* M10 by Muhammad et al. [42]. Verrucarin Y (**1**) shares the same structure with epiroridin acid (**3**) [29], except that the latter possesses an additional C_2-side chain at C-6′, implying that epiroridin acid (**3**) may be the homologue of verrucarin Y (**1**) [41]. Verrucarin Z (**2**) has an epoxide ring at C-2′, C-3′ instead of the olefinic bond of verrucarin Y (**1**) at the same place, and the number of epoxide rings always has a significant impact on their biological activities [42]. Several macrocyclic trichothecenes with additional rings have also been isolated from *Myrothecium* (compounds **5–18**), such as mytoxin, satratoxin, vertisporin, roritoxin, and myrothecine, the names of which generally indicated the genus that this kind of toxins were firstly isolated from [41]. The second ring is closed by the connecting between C-6′ and C-12′ of the side chain. A third ring exists in some compounds, which is formed via an ester linkage between C-12′ and C-14′ (**9**, **10**, **15**) [30,44]. Roritoxin E (**10**) [30], 6′,12′-epoxymyrotoxin A (**11**) [45], and 2′,3′-epoxymyrothecine A (**18**) [46] have the epoxide ring at C-2′, C-3′; furthermore, 6′,12′-epoxymyrotoxin A (**11**) has an additional epoxide ring at C-6′, C-12′. Due to the absence of the epoxide at C-12, C-13, compounds **12–20** belong to 10,13-cyclotrichothecane derivatives [44,47]. Generally, 10,13-cyclotrichothecane macrolides have been proved to be less cytotoxic than the trichothecenes with the epoxide at C-12, C-13 [46–48]. Roridin F (**21**) and satratoxin I (**22**) discovered from *Podostroma cornu-damae*, a deadly poisonous mushroom, are not complete macrolides, because the macrocyclic ester bridge between C-4 and C-15 are not closed; however, they might be transformed into roridin E and satratoxin H, respectively, through a one-step esterification [32]. Chartarene D (**23**) is the only macrocyclic trichothecene isolated from *Stachybotrys* during the past decade [33]. This could be because the *Stachybotrys* fungi are not great source of trichothecenes, and most of them have been discovered before [28]. Search in the database Web of Science about macrocyclic trichothecenes reported during the last twenty years, implies that there is a possibility that more novel macrocyclic trichothecenes will be isolated from *Myrothecium* and *Podostroma*, especially the latter.

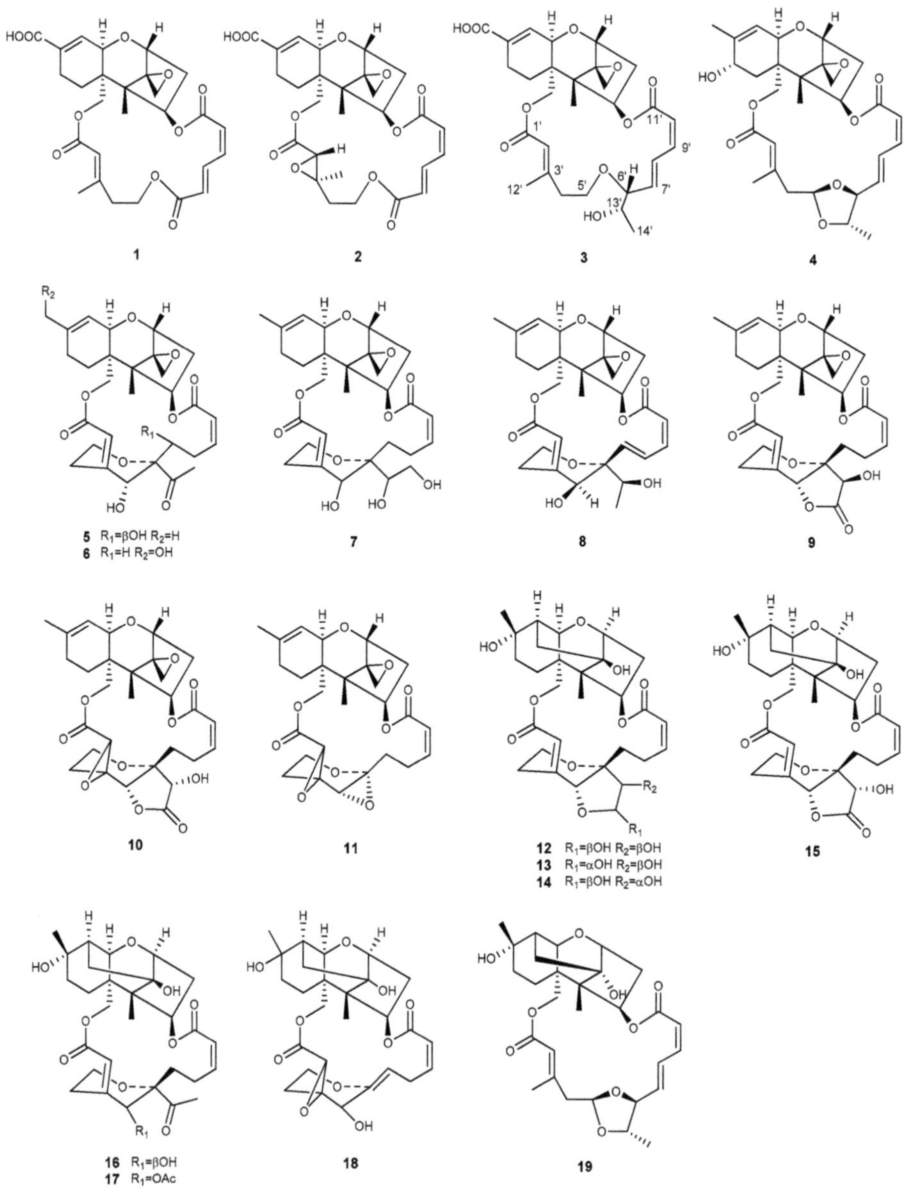

Figure 2. Structures of compounds **1–19** isolated from *Myrothecium*.

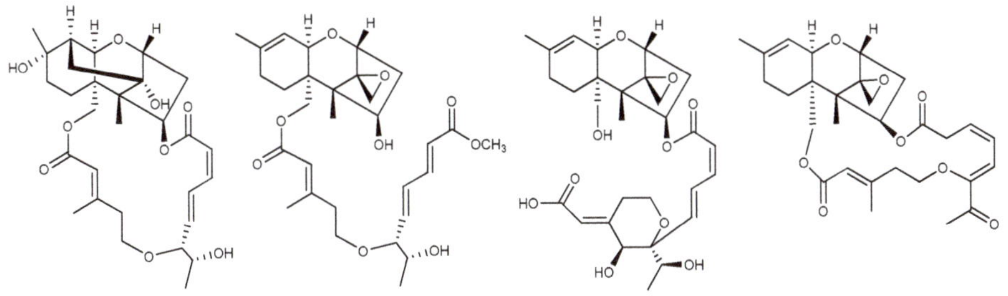

Figure 3. Structures of compounds isolated from *Podostroma* (**20–22**) or *Stachybotrys* (**23**).

Table 1. Macrocyclic trichothecenes newly discovered over the last decade.

Genera	No.	Compound	Ref.
Myrothecium	**1**	verrucarin Y	[42]
	2	verrucarin Z	[42]
	3	epiroridin acid	[29]
	4	8a-hydroxyroridin H	[49]
	5	7′-hydroxymytoxin B	[45]
	6	16-hydroxymytoxin B	[44]
	7	13′,14′-hydroxymytoxin B	[46]
	8	12′-episatratoxin H	[50]
	9	14′-dehydrovertisporin	[44]
	10	roritoxin E	[30]
	11	6′,12′-epoxymyrotoxin A	[45]
	12	dihydromyrothecine C, 1a	[47]
	13	dihydromyrothecine C, 1b	[47]
	14	myrothecine D	[44]
	15	myrothecine E	[44]
	16	myrothecine F	[44]
	17	myrothecine G	[44]
	18	2′,3′-epoxymyrothecine A	[46]
	19	myrothecin A	[49]
Podostroma	**20**	miophytocen D	[32]
	21	roridin F	[32]
	22	satratoxin I	[32]
Stachybotrys	**23**	chartarene D	[33]

3. Biological Activities of Macrocyclic Trichothecenes

Macrocyclic trichothecenes have been shown to possess diverse biological activities, such as antibiotic [51], antifungal [41], antimalarial [52], antiviral [53], and anticancer activities [54,55]. In this review, the biological activities of macrocyclic trichothecenes against cancer cell lines were collected and compared (Table 2). The cytotoxicities against the identical cancer cell line varied notably between different compounds, which could explain the structure-activity relationship of macrocyclic trichothecenes.

Table 2. Cytotoxicity of macrocyclic trichothecenes against diverse human cancer cell lines in vitro.

	Cytotoxicity (IC_{50})										
Compound	**HepG-2** [a]	**MCF-7**	**SF-268**	**K562**	**SW1116**	**KB**	**NCI-H187**	**A549**	**SMMC-7721**	**SGC-7901**	**Ref.**
3	0.380 ± 0.03 μM	0.170 ± 0.01 μM	0.751 ± 0.03 μM				0.360 ± 0.05 μM [b]				[29]
5						2.81 nM	5.99 nM				[45]
6				2.87 μM	0.18 μM						[44]
7	49 ± 3.35 nM	63 ± 2.38 nM						53 ± 3.36 nM	46 ± 2.88 nM		[46]
8	2.27 μM					1.42 μM					[50]
9				56 nM	200 nM						[44]
10									18.89 μM	0.46 μM	[30]
11						0.63 nM	0.79 nM				[45]
12						44.48 μM					[47]
14				8.2 μM	0.57 μM						[44]
15				15.98 μM	11.61 μM						[44]
16				0.97 μM	10.62 μM						[44]
17				1.53 μM	4.25 μM						[44]
18	32.03 ± 2.94 μM	18.13 ± 3.89 μM						36.45 ± 2.79 μM	30.33 ± 9.71 μM		[46]

[a] These cancer cell lines represent human hepatoma cell line (HepG-2), human breast adenocarcinoma cell line (MCF-7), human glioma cell line (SF-268), chronic myeloid leukemia cell line (K562), colorectal carcinoma cell line (SW1116), human nasopharyngeal carcinoma cell line (KB), human small cell lung cancer cell line (NCI-H187), human lung adenocarcinoma cell line (A549), human hepatocellular carcinoma cell line (SMMC-7721), and gastric carcinoma cell line (SGC-7901), respectively. [b] This datum was the cytotoxicity of compound **3** against NCI-H460 (human non-small cell lung cancer cell line).

Firstly, the existences of a double bond at C-9, C-10 and an epoxide at C-12, C-13 are the most important structural features, which contributes to the significant differences in biological activity (Table 2) [1,45,46,56]. The compounds lacking this epoxide and a double bond at C-9, such as compounds **12–20**, are not likely to show cytotoxicity with a nanomolar level. Secondly, an increase of the additional epoxide groups on the macrolide ring remarkably promote toxicity [1,57]. The 6′,12′-epoxymyrotoxin A (**11**), bearing an epoxide ring at C-6′, C-12′, showed quite strong cytotoxicity towards the KB and NCI-H187 cancer cell lines [45]. The substituent groups of other sites also affect the bioactivity. The carboxylation at C-16 could significantly reduce the cytotoxicity of epiroridin acid (**3**) compared to epiroridin [29]. The 12′-O-acetyl group in myrothecine G (**17**) enhanced bioactivity [44]. However, the hydroxylation of C-12′ decreased roridin E toxicity more than 1000-fold [58]. On the contrary, it has been reported that roridin H 8α-hydroxylation increased cytotoxicities towards MCF-7, Hela cells KB3.1, and skin cancer cells A431, but the acetylation of this hydroxy group or no oxidation at C-8 decreased activity towards all the mentioned cell lines [41]. Compounds **6**, **9**, **14–17** were evaluated for their in vitro cytotoxicities against K562 and SW1116, and the relatively large differences in IC_{50} values suggested that the slight changes of the substituent group have obvious effects on the biological selectivity of macrocyclic trichothecenes against cancer cell lines [44]. There have been some studies suggesting that the breakage of the macrocyclic ring could dramatically decrease the cytotoxicity [45,54], and it was supported by the fact that roridin F (**21**) and satratoxin I (**22**) without macrocyclic ring were almost inactive against cancer cell lines (data not included in Table 2) [32]. All these data indicated that even small alterations in the molecular structure can lead to a substantial change in biological activity or selectivity against cancer cell lines [41,59]. It should be noted that considerable research have pointed out that the macrocyclic trichothecenes have more potential than the other types of trichothecenes to become antitumor agents [41,60]. Therefore, more attention should be paid to exploration of the structure-activity relationships in the future.

There are some macrocyclic trichothecenes displaying other biological activities, such as antifungal and antimalarial activities. Verrucarin Z (**2**) showed a similar activity against *Mucor miehei* at a concentration of 50 μg/disk when compared with the positive drug nystatin [42]. The 8a-hydroxyroridin H (**4**) and myrothecin A (**19**) exhibited bioactivities against plant pathogenic fungi *Rhizoctonia solani* and *Fusarium oxysporum* [49]. Manami et al. suggested that the C-12-epoxide of trichothecene was essential for the antifungal activity against *Cochliobolus miyabeanus* [61]. Besides the cytotoxicity against the KB and NCI-H187 cell lines, 7′-hydroxymytoxin B (**5**) and 6′,12′-epoxymyrotoxin A (**11**) exhibited strong antimalarial activity against *Plasmodium falciparum* with 86.1% (1.84 nM) and 98.85% (2 nM) parasite inhibition, respectively [45].

4. Biosynthetic Pathway

Despite considerable published research on macrocyclic trichothecene, the biosynthetic pathway of Type D trichothecene remains obscure, especially on how the macrocycle is formed and linked to EPT. To date it has been well known that this mechanism is associated with genes *tri17* and *tri18*, but how they function is still being studied (Figure 4). According to previously reported BLAST analyses and function prediction [10,62], *tri17* is regarded as a polyketide synthase gene, and *tri18* as an acyltransferase gene. Based on the existence of *tri17* and *tri*18 in the *Stachybotrys TRI* cluster, Semeiks et al. speculated that the polyketide portion catalyzed by Tri17 protein participate in the biosynthesis of macrocyclic trichothecene in *Stachybotrys* [26]. Through gene deletion and complementation analyses, gene *tri17* in *Trichoderma arundinaceum* IBT 40,837 (Ta37) was confirmed to be essential for synthesis of the polyketide side chain of harzianum A (Figure 4). Furthermore, the complementation of *M. roridum tri17* into Ta37 could recover harzianum A production, demonstrating that *tri17* from different species played a similar role in biosynthesis of the polyketide-derived substituents of macrocyclic trichothecene [10]. Polyketide synthase is generally a delicate and complicate enzyme, containing several functionally diverse domains, including acyl carrier protein (ACP), acyl transferase (AT), ketosynthase (KS), ketoreductase (KR), dehydratase (DH), and enoylreductase (ER), all of which conjointly and sequentially function to generate a long branched-chain polyketide [63,64]. The polyketide synthases for other polyketide-derived compounds, such as tylosin [65], erythromycin A [63], and nanchangmycin [66], have been studied for many years. However, as a newly identified polyketide synthase gene, *tri17* has not been investigated thoroughly, and the functions of different domains have not been determined yet.

On the other hand, the only identification work for *tri18* was presented by Laura et al. in 2019 [62]. They proposed that the conversion of the intermediate trichodermol to harzianum A in Ta37 needed two acyltransferases, Tri3 and Tri18. Tri3 catalyzes 4-O-acetylation of trichodermol to give trichodermin, then Tri18 catalyzes the replacement of the resulting C-4 acetyl group with octa-2,4,6-trienedioyl (Figure 4). With deletion of gene *tri18* in Ta37, *tri18* mutants did not produce detectable levels of harzianum A, but the mutant genes increased trichodermol production, indicating that Tri18 accounts for the esterification of octa-2,4,6-trienedioyl to the C-4 of trichothecene. Moreover, Tri18 was presumed to be capable of transforming trichodermol to harzianum A directly, but the catalytic activity was quite low. This hypothesis requires more functional identification experiments in vitro to provide evidences.

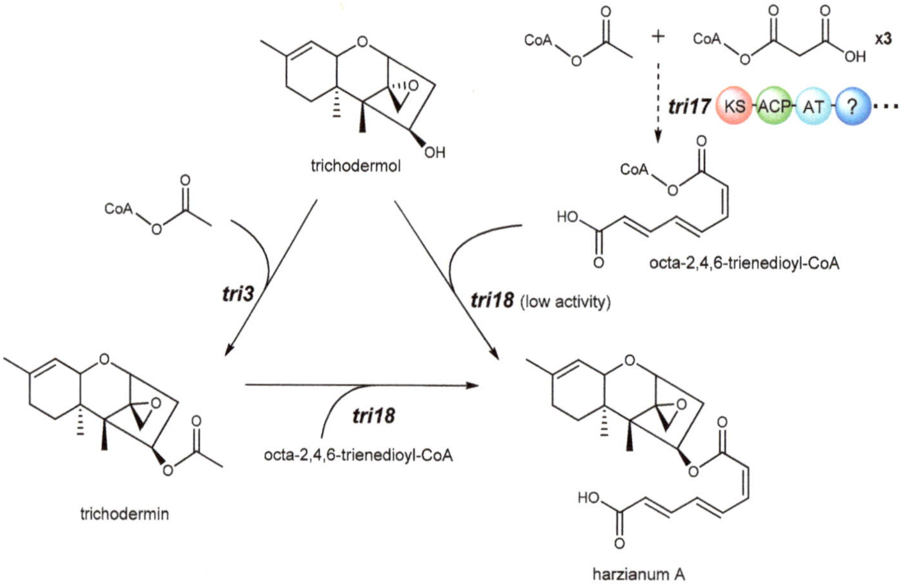

Figure 4. Biosynthetic pathway of harzianum A from trichodermol in *Trichoderma arundinaceum*. Genes are indicated in black italics.

To obtain insight into the distinction of gene homologs and the evolutionary relationship of the macrocyclic trichothecene-producing species, phylogenetic trees for *tri17* and *tri18* were generated in the present review (Figure 5). Some of these gene homologs came from the trichothecene-producing strain genomes, and some from the resulting sequences with high similarity according to NCBI BLAST algorithms (Table S1). There were still some species without any reports on their genome information, such as *Podostroma*, *Calcarisporium*, *Cercophora*, *Cylindrocarpon*, *Dendrodochium*, *Verticinimonosporium*, and *Baccharis*, therefore their genes were not included in phylogenetic trees. In the trees inferred from homologs of *tri17* and *tri18* genes, relationships among these species were generally consistent (Figure 5). Firstly, *Myrothecium*, *Monosporascus* and *Stachybotrys* formed a well-supported clade in both trees. *Monosporascus* is also one plant pathogen affecting muskmelon and watermelon, and there are just a few studies indicating that natural products of *Monosporascus* species included octocrylene, squalene, several hexaketide and pentaketide compounds [67,68]. Since *Myrothecium* and *Stachybotrys* are the predominant fungi producing macrocyclic trichothecenes, it is a reasonable hypothesis that *Monosporascus* could produce macrocyclic trichothecenes as well. Secondly, *Trichoderma* and *Trichothecium*, respectively, forms an independent clade, and *Trichoderma* is more close to the *Myrothecium-Stachybotrys* clade than *Trichothecium*. In fact, the representative trichothecene derived from *Trichoderma*, harzianum A, has a longer side chain at C-4 than the representative trichothecene of *Trichothecium*, trichothecin (octatrienoyl group vs. butenoyl group, Figure 5) [10]. Although *Trichoderma* and *Trichothecium* have *tri17* and *tri18* genes, there is no report to date showing that macrocyclic trichothecenes could be isolated from them. Since Tri17 may be responsible for formation of the octatrienoyl substituent or other polyketide-derived substituents, and Tri18 catalyzes acetylation of the consequent substituents to EPT, there is still a puzzle how the long chain polyketides of macrocyclic trichothecene were converted to a closed ring. Either the unique gene *tri18* from *Myrothecium* or *Stachybotrys* also participates in the process, or there is still an unknown gene contributing to closure. In addition, it should be noted that we did not find any homologs similar to *tri18* in the root species in *tri17* gene tree, *Phomopsis longicolla*, which was the only species of the genus with genome information in NCBI.

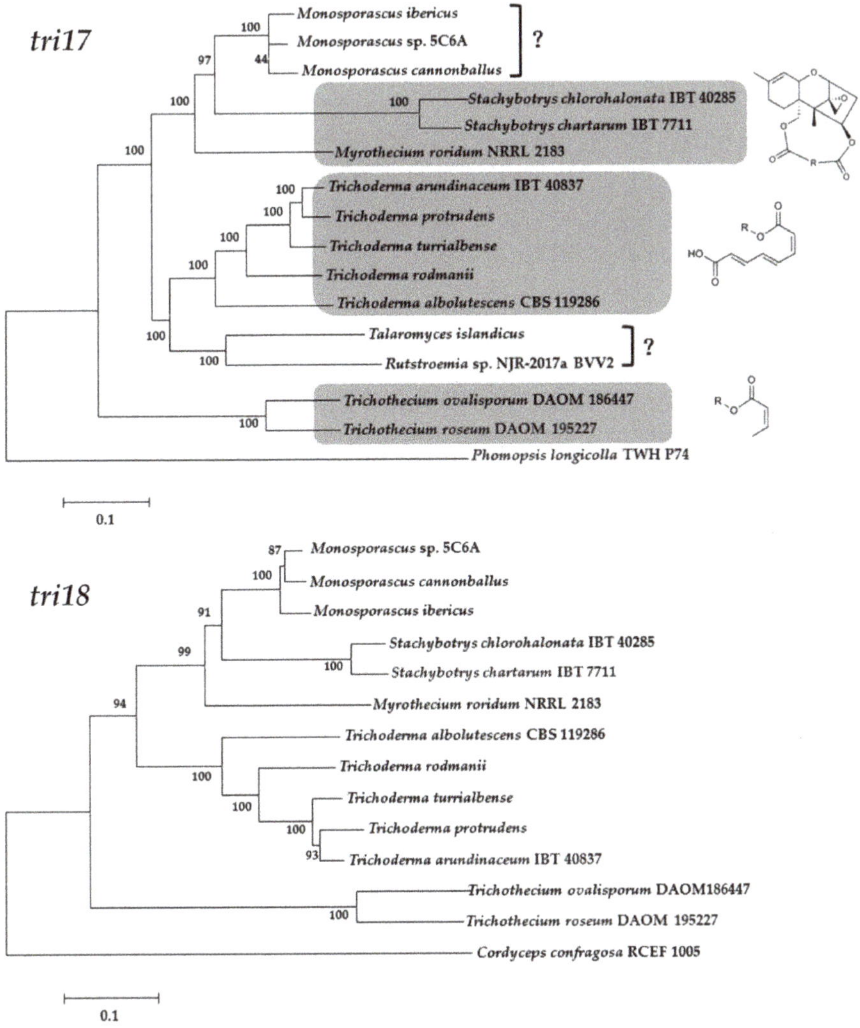

Figure 5. Maximum likelihood trees inferred from sequences of *tri17* (**top**) and *tri18* (**bottom**) and related homologs according to NCBI BLAST algorithms. Numbers near branch nodes are bootstrap values based on 1000 pseudoreplicates.

Although not all genes involved in the biosynthesis of macrocyclic trichothecene have been identified in detail, there are still a few studies proposing several possible biosynthetic pathways of macrocyclic trichothecenes [26,69–71]. The most commonly predicted biosynthetic pathway is shown as blue arrows in Figure 6. As initial compound of macrocyclic trichothecene, trichodermol can react with polyketide chains through esterification at two different sites: C-15 (left) or C-4 (right). A hydroxyl group at C-15 is a prerequisite for C-15 acetylation and subsequent esterification [10,72]. After oxidized, the 15-OH in trichodermol can be esterified with a 5-hydroxy-3-methylpent-2-enoic acid to form verrol, while the hydroxyl group at C-4 can be substituted by 6,7-dihydroxy-2,4-octadienoate to form trichoverrols [28]. If both the two hydroxyl groups are esterified consecutively, it will convert to trichoverrins. Subsequently, catalyzed by an unidentified protein, a dehydration between the two chains occurs to give the roridin E which constructs a macrocycle. Roridin E can be transformed to diverse derivatives by a series of slight modifications. As mentioned above, verrucarin J can be generated if the C_2-side chain at C-6′ of roridin E is oxygenated [41,43]. Similarly, after being continuously oxygenated at C-12′, C-6′ and C-12′ can be linked to form **8** with a pyran ring [50]. The hypothesis could explain the generation of the most macrocyclic trichothecenes; however, the isolations of several compounds, some of which were recently discovered, required the hypothesis to be modified. Roridin F (**21**) reported in 2019 [32] and roridin L-2 [33,73] seem to be formed by cutting off the connection at C-4 or C-15 of roridin E. For roridin L-2, it also needs to undergo a cyclization of the hydroxyl group at C-1′ and C-12′. Nevertheless, there is a possibility that **21** could be generated by attaching a free 6,7-dihydroxy-2,4-octadienoate to the hydroxyl group at C-5′ of verrol. Then, **21** could be sequentially converted to roridin E through acylation or esterification. Similar processes may happen to roridin L-2 and satratoxin I (**22**) [32]. Compound **22** could be created through hydrolyzing at C-15 of **8**, or attaching a free 5-hydroxy-3-methylpent-2-enoic acid to the end of octadienoate fused to trichoverrols. Until now, there is no obvious evidence showing how **21**, **22** or roridin L-2 is formed, and whether the conversion between roridin E and **21** or roridin L-2, between **8** and **22** is reversible. The puzzle may be explained by identifying the specific undiscovered gene accounting for construction of the macrocycle, or knocking out gene *tri18* in *Myrothecium*, *Podostroma*, and *Stachybotrys*, all of which are able to produce macrocyclic trichothecenes. Since gene *tri18* in Ta37 accounted for esterification of octa-2,4,6-trienedioyl, deletion of it in macrocyclic trichothecene-producing strains may cut off the formation of macrocycle, resulting in an accumulation of verrol, or roridin F (**21**) and their derivatives. If final products do contain **21** and its derivatives, it suggests that **21** could be generated from verrol, meaning that there is a second putative pathway to form macrocyclic trichothecenes. In addition, isolated from *Myrothecium* [73] and *Podostroma* [32], trichoverritone was generated by esterifying a free 5-hydroxy-3-methylpent-2-enoic acid to the hydroxyl group at C-15 of roridin L-2. It remains unclear whether the side chains of trichoverritone could be cyclized; if it did, the consequent novel compound would possess a 20-membered ring.

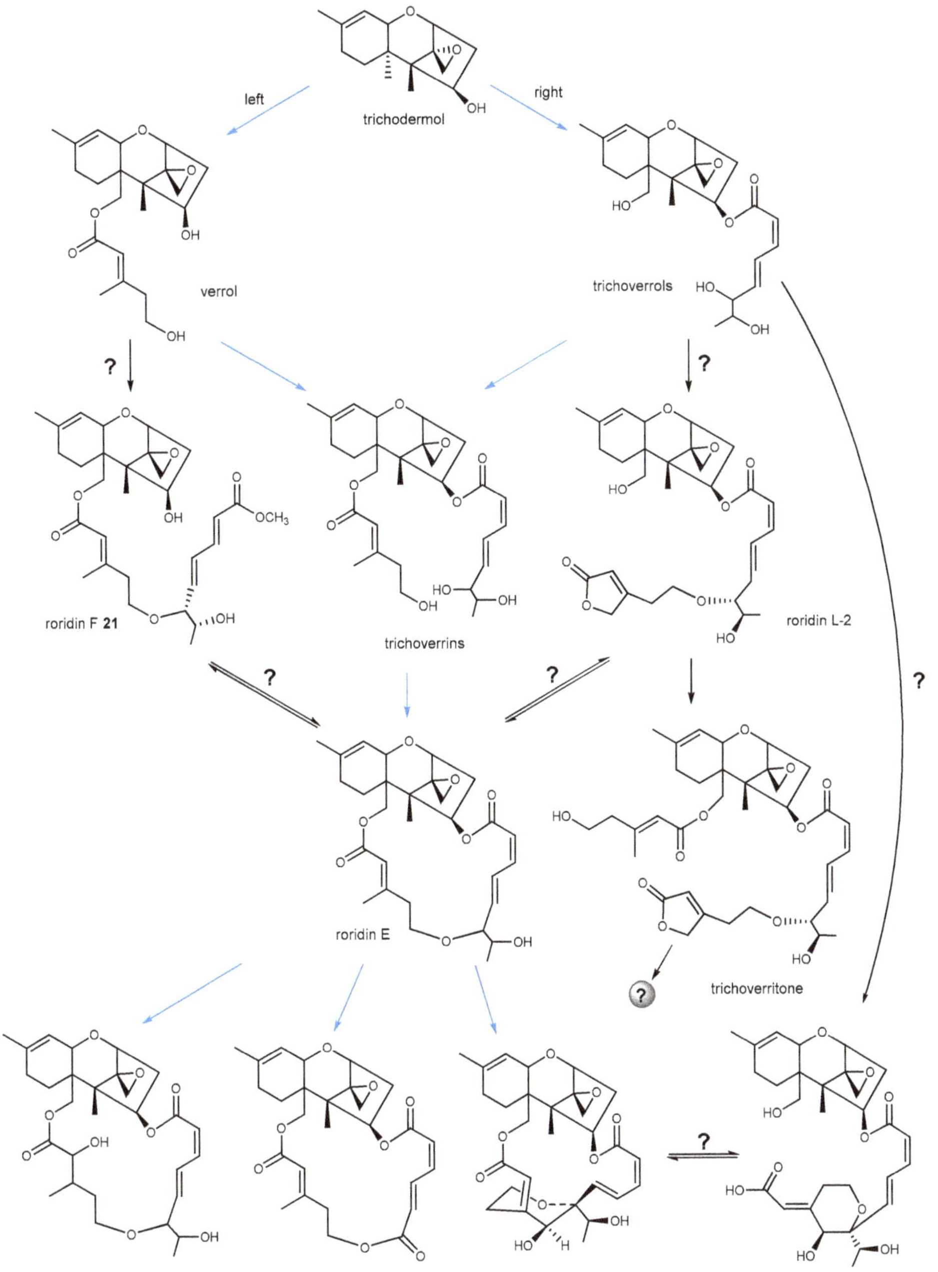

Figure 6. Plausible biogenetic pathway of macrocyclic trichothecenes. Blue arrows indicate the most predicted pathway; interrogation marks indicate that the process between two compounds still remains uncovered; gray ball represents a predicted unknown compound with a very large ring.

5. Conclusions and Outlook

Trichothecenes have been studied for more than 40 years. Initially, trichothecenes were well known and studied as the important contamination sources of grains [2,74], building materials [75,76], and air-handling systems [7]. However, because of a large number of identification of new macrocyclic trichothecenes and their diverse bioactivities, they have drawn much attention from chemists and pharmacists as research hotspots [41,77,78]. We have summarized the macrocyclic trichothecenes reported during the last ten years and their biological activities. Although there are many species capable of macrocyclic trichothecene production, the newly discovered compounds were isolated from *Myrothecium*, *Podostroma* and *Stachybotrys*. Meanwhile, summary review in bioactivity studies revealed that the small changes between structurally similar compounds isolated from different species can result in a considerable alteration on bioactivity and/or selectivity against cancer cell lines [41,59], which again confirmed the great potential of macrocyclic trichothecenes as antitumor drugs. We also overviewed the recent advances in the identification of genes involved in the formation of macrocycle and plausible biosynthetic pathways. Knowledge obtained from functional analyses of *tri17* and *tri18* genes in *Trichoderma* has contributed significantly to insights into the evolutionary history of macrocyclic trichothecene biosynthesis. In terms of phylogenetic trees generated in the review and the presence of the highly similar genes *tri17* and *tri18* in *Monosporascus*, it was suggested that these species would probably be a source of macrocyclic trichothecenes. Furthermore, based on several newly isolated intermediates, we propose that there is a second biosynthetic pathway of macrocyclic trichothecene. An identification assay of the genes responsible for constructing the macrocycle in macrocyclic trichothecene-producing strains (maybe *tri18* or other unidentified gene), will be critical to more precisely clarify the biosynthesis mechanism of potential anticancer compounds.

Supplementary Materials: The following are available online at http://www.mdpi.com/2072-6651/12/6/417/s1, Table S1: Information on fungal strains and genome sequences examined in the current study.

Author Contributions: Conceptualization, M.Z. and W.Z.; software and figure preparation, Y.C.; data collection, S.L.; writing—original draft preparation, M.Z.; writing—review and editing, W.Y. and W.Z. All authors have read and agreed to the published version of the manuscript.

Funding: This research was funded by the National Natural Science Foundation of China (grant 31800063), the National Natural Science Foundation of Guangdong Province (2019A1515011702, 2019A1515011829), GDAS' Project of Science and Technology Development (2020GDASYL-20200104012), Guangdong Provincial Special Fund for Marine Economic Development Project (Yue Natural Resources Contract No. [2020]042).

Conflicts of Interest: The authors declare no conflicts of interest.

References

1. Wu, Q.H.; Dohnal, V.; Kuca, K.; Yuan, Z.H. Trichothecenes: Structure-toxic activity relationships. *Curr. Drug Metab.* **2013**, *14*, 641–660. [CrossRef] [PubMed]
2. McMullen, M.; Jones, R.; Gallenberg, D. Scab of wheat and barley: A re-emerging disease of devastating impact. *Plant Dis.* **1997**, *81*, 1340–1348. [CrossRef] [PubMed]
3. Eriksen, G.S.; Pettersson, H. Toxicological evaluation of trichothecenes in animal feed. *Anim. Feed Sci. Technol.* **2004**, *114*, 205–239. [CrossRef]
4. Pascari, X.; Maul, R.; Kemmlein, S.; Marin, S.; Sanchis, V. The fate of several trichothecenes and zearalenone during roasting and enzymatic treatment of cereal flour applied in cereal-based infant food production. *Food Control* **2020**, *114*. [CrossRef]
5. Habrowska-Gorczynska, D.E.; Kowalska, K.; Urbanek, K.A.; Dominska, K.; Sakowicz, A.; Piastowska-Ciesielska, A.W. Deoxynivalenol modulates the viability, ROS production and apoptosis in prostate cancer cells. *Toxins* **2019**, *11*, 265. [CrossRef]
6. Opoku, N.; Back, M.A.; Edwards, S.G. Susceptibility of cereal species to *Fusarium langsethiae* under identical field conditions. *Eur. J. Plant Pathol.* **2018**, *150*, 869–879. [CrossRef]
7. McCormick, S.P.; Stanley, A.M.; Stover, N.A.; Alexander, N.J. Trichothecenes: From simple to complex mycotoxins. *Toxins* **2011**, *3*, 802–814. [CrossRef]
8. Grove, J.F. The trichothecenes and their biosynthesis. *Cheminform* **2007**, *38*, 63–130. [CrossRef]
9. Tamm, C.; Breitenstein, W. *The Biosynthesis of Mycotoxins: A Study of Secondary Metabolism*; Academic Press: New York, NY, USA, 1980; pp. 69–104.

10. Proctor, R.H.; McCormick, S.P.; Kim, H.S.; Cardoza, R.E.; Stanley, A.M.; Lindo, L.; Kelly, A.; Brown, D.W.; Lee, T.; Vaughan, M.M.; et al. Evolution of structural diversity of trichothecenes, a family of toxins produced by plant pathogenic and entomopathogenic fungi. *PLoS Path.* **2018**, *14*, e1006946. [CrossRef]
11. Kimura, M.; Tokai, T.; Takahashi-Ando, N.; Ohsato, S.; Fujimura, M. Molecular and genetic studies of *Fusarium* trichothecene biosynthesis: Pathways, genes, and evolution. *Biosci. Biotechnol. Biochem.* **2007**, *71*, 2105–2123. [CrossRef]
12. Alexander, N.J.; Proctor, R.H.; McCormick, S.P. Genes, gene clusters, and biosynthesis of trichothecenes and fumonisins in *Fusarium*. *Toxin Rev.* **2009**, *28*, 198–215. [CrossRef]
13. Brown, D.W.; Dyer, R.B.; McCormick, S.P.; Kendra, D.F.; Plattner, R.D. Functional demarcation of the Fusarium core trichothecene gene cluster. *Fungal Genet. Biol.* **2004**, *41*, 454–462. [CrossRef] [PubMed]
14. Garvey, G.S.; McCormick, S.P.; Alexander, N.J.; Rayment, I. Structural and functional characterization of *TRI3* trichothecene 15-O-acetyltransferase from *Fusarium sporotrichioides*. *Protein Sci.* **2009**, *18*, 747–761. [CrossRef] [PubMed]
15. Hohn, T.M.; Krishna, R.; Proctor, R.H. Characterization of a transcriptional activator controlling trichothecene toxin biosynthesis. *Fungal Genet. Biol.* **1999**, *26*, 224–235. [CrossRef] [PubMed]
16. Malmierca, M.G.; Cardoza, R.E.; Alexander, N.J.; McCormick, S.P.; Collado, I.G.; Hermosa, R.; Monte, E.; Gutierrez, S. Relevance of trichothecenes in fungal physiology: Disruption of *tri5* in *Trichoderma arundinaceum*. *Fungal Genet. Biol.* **2013**, *53*, 22–33. [CrossRef] [PubMed]
17. Garvey, G.S.; McCormick, S.P.; Rayment, I. Structural and functional characterization of the TRI101 trichothecene 3-O-acetyltransferase from *Fusarium sporotrichioides* and *Fusarium graminearum*—Kinetic insights to combating fusarium head blight. *J. Biol. Chem.* **2008**, *283*, 1660–1669. [CrossRef] [PubMed]
18. Cardoza, R.E.; Malmierca, M.G.; Hermosa, M.R.; Alexander, N.J.; McCormick, S.P.; Proctor, R.H.; Tijerino, A.M.; Rumbero, A.; Monte, E.; Gutierrez, S. Identification of loci and functional characterization of trichothecene biosynthesis genes in filamentous fungi of the genus *Trichoderma*. *Appl. Environ. Microbiol.* **2011**, *77*, 4867–4877. [CrossRef]
19. McCormick, S.P.; Alexander, N.J.; Proctor, R.H. *Fusarium Tri4* encodes a multifunctional oxygenase required for trichothecene biosynthesis. *Can. J. Microbiol.* **2006**, *52*, 636–642. [CrossRef]
20. McCormick, S.P.; Alexander, N.J. *Myrothecium roridum Tri4* encodes a multifunctional oxygenase required for three oxygenation steps. *Can. J. Microbiol.* **2007**, *53*, 572–579. [CrossRef]
21. Tokai, T.; Koshino, H.; Takahashi-Ando, N.; Sato, M.; Fujimura, M.; Kimura, M. *Fusarium Tri4* encodes a key multifunctional cytochrome P450 monooxygenase for four consecutive oxygenation steps in trichothecene biosynthesis. *Biochem. Biophys. Res. Commun.* **2007**, *353*, 412–417. [CrossRef]
22. Lee, T.; Han, Y.K.; Kim, K.H.; Yun, S.H.; Lee, Y.W. *Tri13* and *Tri7* determine deoxynivalenol- and nivalenol-producing chemotypes of *Gibberella zeae*. *Appl. Environ. Microbiol.* **2002**, *68*, 2148–2154. [CrossRef] [PubMed]
23. Brown, D.W.; McCormick, S.P.; Alexander, N.J.; Proctor, R.H.; Desjardins, A.E. Inactivation of a cytochrome P450 is a determinant of trichothecene diversity in *Fusarium* species. *Fungal Genet. Biol.* **2002**, *36*, 224–233. [CrossRef]
24. Alexander, N.J.; McCormick, S.P.; Waalwijk, C.; van der Lee, T.; Proctor, R.H. The genetic basis for 3-ADON and 15-ADON trichothecene chemotypes in *Fusarium*. *Fungal Genet. Biol.* **2011**, *48*, 485–495. [CrossRef]
25. Villafana, R.T.; Ramdass, A.C.; Rampersad, S.N. Selection of *Fusarium* trichothecene toxin genes for molecular detection depends on *TRI* gene cluster organization and gene function. *Toxins* **2019**, *11*, 36. [CrossRef] [PubMed]
26. Semeiks, J.; Borek, D.; Otwinowski, Z.; Grishin, N.V. Comparative genome sequencing reveals chemotype-specific gene clusters in the toxigenic black mold *Stachybotrys*. *BMC Genom.* **2014**, *15*. [CrossRef] [PubMed]
27. Corley, D.G.; Millerwideman, M.; Durley, R.C. Isolation and Structure of Harzianum A: A New Trichothecene from *Trichoderma harzianum*. *J. Nat. Prod.* **1994**, *57*, 422–425. [CrossRef]
28. Wang, A.R.; Xu, Y.B.; Gao, Y.X.; Huang, Q.; Luo, X.; An, H.M.; Dong, J.Y. Chemical and bioactive diversities of the genera *Stachybotrys* and *Memnoniella* secondary metabolites. *Phytochem. Rev.* **2015**, *14*, 623–655. [CrossRef]

29. Liu, H.X.; Liu, W.Z.; Chen, Y.C.; Sun, Z.H.; Tan, Y.Z.; Li, H.H.; Zhang, W.M. Cytotoxic trichothecene macrolides from the endophyte fungus *Myrothecium roridum*. *J. Asian Nat. Prod. Res.* **2016**, *18*, 684–689. [CrossRef]
30. Shen, L.; Wang, J.A.S.; Shen, H.J.; Song, Y.C.; Tan, R.X. A new cytotoxic trichothecene macrolide from the endophyte *Myrothecium roridum*. *Planta Med.* **2010**, *76*, 1004–1006. [CrossRef]
31. Zhao, L.; Liu, L.; Wang, N.; Wang, S.J.; Hu, J.C.; Gao, J.M. Potent Toxic Macrocyclic Trichothecenes from the Marine-Derived Fungus *Myrothecium verrucaria* Hmp-F73. *Nat. Prod. Commun.* **2011**, *6*, 1915–1916. [CrossRef]
32. Lee, S.R.; Seok, S.; Ryoo, R.; Choi, S.U.; Kim, K.H. Macrocyclic trichothecene mycotoxins from a deadly poisonous mushroom, *Podostroma cornu-damae*. *J. Nat. Prod.* **2019**, *82*, 122–128. [CrossRef] [PubMed]
33. Li, Y.; Liu, D.; Cheng, Z.B.; Proksch, P.; Lin, W.H. Cytotoxic trichothecene-type sesquiterpenes from the sponge-derived fungus *Stachybotrys chartarum* with tyrosine kinase inhibition. *RSC Adv.* **2017**, *7*, 7259–7267. [CrossRef]
34. Yu, N.J.; Guo, S.X.; Lu, H.Y. Cytotoxic macrocyclic trichothecenes from the mycelia of *Calcarisporium arbuscula* Preuss. *J. Asian Nat. Prod. Res.* **2002**, *4*, 179–183. [CrossRef] [PubMed]
35. Whyte, A.C.; Gloer, J.B.; Scott, J.A.; Malloch, D. Cercophorins A–C: Novel antifungal and cytotoxic metabolites from the coprophilous fungus *Cercophora areolata*. *J. Nat. Prod.* **1996**, *59*, 765–769. [CrossRef] [PubMed]
36. Matsumoto, M.; Minato, H.; Tori, K.; Ueyama, M. Structures of Isororidin E, Epoxyisororidin E, and Epoxy H and Diepoxyroridin H, New Metabolites Isolated from *Cylindrocarpon* Species Determined by C-13 and H-1 NMR Spectroscopy. Revision of C-2′:C-3′ Double-Bond Configuration of Roridin Group. *Tetrahedron Lett.* **1977**, *18*, 4093–4096. [CrossRef]
37. Panozish, K.P.; Borovkov, A.V. Roridin a from *Dendrodochium toxicum*. *Khimiya Prir. Soedin.* **1974**, *10*, 404–405.
38. Samples, D.; Hill, D.W.; Bridges, C.H.; Camp, B.J. Isolation of a mycotoxin (roridin A) from *Phomopsis* spp. *Vet. Hum. Toxicol.* **1984**, *26*, 21–23.
39. Minato, H.; Katayama, T.; Tori, K. Vertisporin, a New Antibiotic from *Verticimonosporium diffractum*. *Tetrahedron Lett.* **1975**, *16*, 2579–2582. [CrossRef]
40. Kupchan, S.M.; Jarvis, B.B.; Dailey, R.J., Jr.; Bright, W.; Bryan, R.F.; Shizuri, Y. Baccharin, a novel potent antileukemic trichothecene triepoxide from *Baccharis megapotamica*. *J. Am. Chem. Soc.* **1976**, *98*, 7092–7093. [CrossRef]
41. De Carvalho, M.P.; Weich, H.; Abraham, W.R. Macrocyclic trichothecenes as antifungal and anticancer compounds. *Curr. Med. Chem.* **2016**, *23*, 23–35. [CrossRef]
42. Mondol, M.A.; Surovy, M.Z.; Islam, M.T.; Schuffler, A.; Laatsch, H. Macrocyclic trichothecenes from *Myrothecium roridum* strain M10 with motility inhibitory and zoosporicidal activities against *Phytophthora nicotianae*. *J. Agric. Food Chem.* **2015**, *63*, 8777–8786. [CrossRef] [PubMed]
43. Jarvis, B.B.; Stahly, G.P.; Pavanasasivam, G.; Midiwo, J.O.; Geoghegan, R.F. Isolation and characterization of the trichoverroids and new roridins and verrucarins. *J. Org. Chem.* **1981**, *47*, 1117–1124. [CrossRef]
44. Shen, L.; Ai, C.Z.; Song, Y.C.; Wang, F.W.; Jiao, R.H.; Zhang, A.H.; Man, H.Z.; Tan, R.X. Cytotoxic trichothecene macrolides produced by the endophytic *Myrothecium roridum*. *J. Nat. Prod.* **2019**, *82*, 1503–1509. [CrossRef] [PubMed]
45. Lakornwong, W.; Kanokmedhakul, K.; Soytong, K.; Unartngam, A.; Tontapha, S.; Amornkitbamrung, V.; Kanokmedhakul, S. Types A and D trichothecene mycotoxins from the fungus *Myrothecium roridum*. *Planta Med.* **2019**, *85*, 774–780. [CrossRef]
46. Lin, T.; Wang, G.H.; Zhou, Y.Q.; Zeng, D.Q.; Liu, X.X.; Ding, R.; Jiang, X.; Zhu, D.; Shan, W.J.; Chen, H.F. Structure elucidation and biological activity of two new trichothecenes from an endophyte, *Myrothecium roridum*. *J. Agric. Food Chem.* **2014**, *62*, 5993–6000. [CrossRef]
47. Shen, L.; Zhu, L.; Tan, Q.W.; Wan, D.; Xie, J.; Peng, J.N. New cytotoxic trichothecene macrolide epimers from endophytic *Myrothecium roridum* IFB-E012. *J. Antibiot.* **2016**, *69*, 652–655. [CrossRef]
48. Shen, L.; Jiao, R.H.; Ye, Y.H.; Wang, X.T.; Xu, C.; Song, Y.C.; Zhu, H.L.; Tan, R.X. Absolute configuration of new cytotoxic and other bioactive trichothecene macrolides. *Chemistry* **2006**, *12*, 5596–5602. [CrossRef]
49. Zhang, S.Y.; Li, Z.L.; Guan, L.P.; Wu, X.; Pan, H.Q.; Bai, J.; Hua, H.M. Structure determination of two new trichothecenes from a halotolerant fungus *Myrothecium* sp. GS-17 by NMR spectroscopy. *Magn. Reson. Chem.* **2012**, *50*, 632–636. [CrossRef]

50. Piao, M.Z.; Shen, L.; Wang, F.W. A new trichothecene from *Myrothecium roridum* QDFE005, a symbiotic fungus isolated from *Mactra chinensis*. *J. Asian Nat. Prod. Res.* **2013**, *15*, 1284–1289. [CrossRef] [PubMed]
51. Matsumoto, M.; Minato, H.; Uotani, N.; Matsumoto, K.; Kondo, E. New antibiotics from *Cylindrocarpon* sp. *J. Antibiot.* **1977**, *30*, 681–682. [CrossRef] [PubMed]
52. Zhang, H.J.; Tamez, P.A.; Aydogmus, Z.; Tan, G.T.; Saikawa, Y.; Hashimoto, K.; Nakata, M.; Hung, N.V.; Xuan le, T.; Cuong, N.M.; et al. Antimalarial agents from plants. III. Trichothecenes from *Ficus fistulosa* and *Rhaphidophora decursiva*. *Planta Med.* **2002**, *68*, 1088–1091. [CrossRef] [PubMed]
53. Garcia, C.C.; Rosso, M.L.; Bertoni, M.D.; Maier, M.S.; Damonte, E.B. Evaluation of the antiviral activity against Junin virus of macrocyclic trichothecenes produced by the hypocrealean epibiont of *Baccharis coridifolia*. *Planta Med.* **2002**, *68*, 209–212. [CrossRef] [PubMed]
54. Amagata, T.; Rath, C.; Rigot, J.F.; Tarlov, N.; Tenney, K.; Valeriote, F.A.; Crews, P. Structures and cytotoxic properties of trichoverroids and their macrolide analogues produced by saltwater culture of *Myrothecium verrucaria*. *J. Med. Chem.* **2003**, *46*, 4342–4350. [CrossRef] [PubMed]
55. Jayasooriya, R.G.P.T.; Moon, D.O.; Park, S.R.; Choi, Y.H.; Asami, Y.; Kim, M.O.; Jang, J.H.; Kim, B.Y.; Ahn, J.S.; Kim, G.Y. Combined treatment with verrucarin A and tumor necrosis factor-alpha sensitizes apoptosis by overexpression of nuclear factor-kappaB-mediated Fas. *Environ. Toxicol. Pharmacol.* **2013**, *36*, 303–310. [CrossRef]
56. Brase, S.; Encinas, A.; Keck, J.; Nising, C.F. Chemistry and Biology of Mycotoxins and Related Fungal Metabolites. *Chem. Rev.* **2009**, *109*, 3903–3990. [CrossRef]
57. Steinmetz, W.E.; Rodarte, C.B.; Lin, A. 3D QSAR study of the toxicity of trichothecene mycotoxins. *Eur. J. Med. Chem.* **2009**, *44*, 4485–4489. [CrossRef]
58. Oda, T.; Xu, J.; Ukai, K.; Nakazawa, T.; Namikoshi, M. 12′-Hydroxyl group remarkably reduces Roridin E cytotoxicity. *Mycoscience* **2010**, *51*, 317–320. [CrossRef]
59. Wu, Q.H.; Wang, X.; Nepovimova, E.; Miron, A.; Liu, Q.Y.; Wang, Y.; Su, D.X.; Yang, H.L.; Li, L.; Kuca, K. Trichothecenes: Immunomodulatory effects, mechanisms, and anti-cancer potential. *Arch. Toxicol.* **2017**, *91*, 3737–3785. [CrossRef]
60. Smitka, T.A.; Bunge, R.H.; Bloem, R.J.; French, J.C. Two new trichothecenes, PD 113,325 and PD 113,326. *J. Antibiot.* **1984**, *37*, 823–828. [CrossRef]
61. Matsumoto, M.; Nishiyama, M.; Maeda, H.; Tonouchi, A.; Konno, K.; Hashimoto, M. Structure-activity relationships of trichothecenes against COLO201 cells and *Cochliobolus miyabeanus*: The role of 12-epoxide and macrocyclic moieties. *Bioorg. Med. Chem. Lett.* **2019**, *29*, 982–985. [CrossRef]
62. Lindo, L.; McCormick, S.P.; Cardoza, R.E.; Busman, M.; Alexander, N.J.; Proctor, R.H.; Gutierrez, S. Requirement of two acyltransferases for 4-O-acylation during biosynthesis of harzianum A, an antifungal trichothecene produced by *Trichoderma arundinaceum*. *J. Agric. Food Chem.* **2019**, *67*, 723–734. [CrossRef] [PubMed]
63. Weissman, K.J. Genetic engineering of modular PKSs: From combinatorial biosynthesis to synthetic biology. *Nat. Prod. Rep.* **2016**, *33*, 203–230. [CrossRef] [PubMed]
64. Xie, X.Q.; Garg, A.; Khosla, C.; Cane, D.E. Mechanism and stereochemistry of polyketide chain elongation and methyl group epimerization in polyether biosynthesis. *J. Am. Chem. Soc.* **2017**, *139*, 3283–3292. [CrossRef] [PubMed]
65. Valenzano, C.R.; Lawson, R.J.; Chen, A.Y.; Khosla, C.; Cane, D.E. The biochemical basis for stereochemical control in polyketide biosynthesis. *J. Am. Chem. Soc.* **2009**, *131*, 18501–18511. [CrossRef]
66. Liu, T.G.; Lin, X.; Zhou, X.F.; Deng, Z.X.; Cane, D.E. Mechanism of thioesterase-catalyzed chain release in the biosynthesis of the polyether antibiotic nanchangmycin. *Chem. Biol.* **2008**, *15*, 449–458. [CrossRef]
67. Al-Rawahi, A.Y.; Al-Mahmooli, I.H.; Al-Sadi, A.M.; Al-Sabahi, J.N.; Velazhahan, R. Toxin production by melon root rot fungus, *Monosporascus cannonballus*. *Australas. Plant Path.* **2018**, *47*, 543–546. [CrossRef]
68. Wheeler, M.H.; Bruton, B.D.; Puckhaber, L.S.; Zhang, J.X.; Stipanovic, R.D. Identification of 1,8-dihydroxynaphthalene melanin in *Monosporascus cannonballus* and the analysis of hexaketide and pentaketide compounds produced by wild-type and pigmented isolates of the fungus. *J. Agric. Food Chem.* **2004**, *52*, 4113–4120. [CrossRef]
69. Trapp, S.C.; Hohn, T.M.; McCormick, S.; Jarvis, B.B. Characterization of the gene cluster for biosynthesis of macrocyclic trichothecenes in *Myrothecium roridum*. *Mol. Gen. Genet.* **1998**, *257*, 421–432. [CrossRef]

70. Degenkolb, T.; Dieckmann, R.; Nielsen, K.F.; Grafenhan, T.; Theis, C.; Zafari, D.; Chaverri, P.; Ismaiel, A.; Bruckner, H.; von Dohren, H.; et al. The *Trichoderma brevicompactum* clade: A separate lineage with new species, new peptaibiotics, and mycotoxins. *Mycol. Prog.* **2008**, *7*, 177–219. [CrossRef]
71. Liu, L.; Tang, M.X.; Sang, X.N.; Chen, S.F.; Lu, X.J.; Wang, Y.B.; Si, Y.Y.; Wang, H.F.; Chen, G.; Pei, Y.H. Three new tetralol analogs from soil-derived fungus *Myrothecium verrucaria* with anti-inflammatory activity. *J. Asian Nat. Prod. Res.* **2018**, *21*, 33–42. [CrossRef]
72. Tokai, T.; Takahashi-Ando, N.; Izawa, M.; Kamakura, T.; Yoshida, M.; Fujimura, M.; Kimura, M. 4-O-acetylation and 3-O-acetylation of trichothecenes by trichothecene 15-O-acetyltransferase encoded by *Fusarium Tri3*. *Biosci. Biotechnol. Biochem.* **2008**, *72*, 2485–2489. [CrossRef] [PubMed]
73. Jarvis, B.B.; Vrudhula, V.M.; Pavanasasivam, G. Trichoverritone and 16-hydroxyroridin L-2, new trichothecenes from *Myrothecium roridum*. *Tetrahedron Lett.* **1983**, *24*, 3539–3542. [CrossRef]
74. Desjardins, A.E. *Fusarium Mycotoxins: Chemistry, Genetics and Biology*; APS Press: St. Paul, MN, USA, 2006; pp. 1–260.
75. Pestka, J.J.; Forsell, J.H. Inhibition of Human-Lymphocyte Transformation by the Macrocyclic Trichothecenes Roridin A and Verrucarin A. *Toxicol. Lett.* **1988**, *41*, 215–222. [CrossRef]
76. Dosen, I.; Andersen, B.; Phippen, C.B.W.; Clausen, G.; Nielsen, K.F. *Stachybotrys* mycotoxins: From culture extracts to dust samples. *Anal. Bioanal. Chem.* **2016**, *408*, 5513–5526. [CrossRef]
77. Jarvis, B.B.; Mazzola, E.P. Macrocyclic and Other Novel Trichothecenes—Their Structure, Synthesis, and Biological Significance. *Acc. Chem. Res.* **1982**, *15*, 388–395. [CrossRef]
78. Sy-Cordero, A.A.; Graf, T.N.; Wani, M.C.; Kroll, D.J.; Pearce, C.J.; Oberlies, N.H. Dereplication of macrocyclic trichothecenes from extracts of filamentous fungi through UV and NMR profiles. *J. Antibiot.* **2010**, *63*, 539–544. [CrossRef]

MDPI
St. Alban-Anlage 66
4052 Basel
Switzerland
Tel. +41 61 683 77 34
Fax +41 61 302 89 18
www.mdpi.com

Toxins Editorial Office
E-mail: toxins@mdpi.com
www.mdpi.com/journal/toxins

www.ingramcontent.com/pod-product-compliance
Lightning Source LLC
LaVergne TN
LVHW070629100526
838202LV00012B/760